Mentalization

Utilizing Reflection to Heal from
Borderline Personality Disorder

ROBERT P. DROZEK

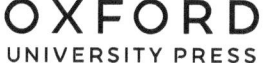

OXFORD
UNIVERSITY PRESS

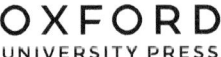

OXFORD
UNIVERSITY PRESS

Great Clarendon Street, Oxford, OX2 6DP,
United Kingdom

Oxford University Press is a department of the University of Oxford.
It furthers the University's objective of excellence in research, scholarship,
and education by publishing worldwide. Oxford is a registered trade mark of
Oxford University Press in the UK and in certain other countries.

Published in the United States of America by Oxford University Press
198 Madison Avenue, New York, NY 10016, United States of America.

British Library Cataloguing in Publication Data
Data available

Library of Congress Control Number: 2025935485

ISBN 978–0–19–891685–7

DOI: 10.1093/oso/9780198916857.001.0001

Printed and bound by
CPI Group (UK) Ltd, Croydon, CR0 4YY

Oxford University Press makes no representation, express or implied, that the
drug dosages in this book are correct. Readers must therefore always check
the product information and clinical procedures with the most up-to-date
published product information and data sheets provided by the manufacturers
and the most recent codes of conduct and safety regulations. The authors and
the publishers do not accept responsibility or legal liability for any errors in the
text or for the misuse or misapplication of material in this work. Except where
otherwise stated, drug dosages and recommendations are for the non-pregnant
adult who is not breast-feeding

The manufacturer's authorized representative in the EU for product safety is
Oxford University Press España S.A., Parque Empresarial San Fernando de Henares,
Avenida de Castilla, 2 – 28830 Madrid (www.oup.es/en or product.safety@oup.com).
OUP España S.A. also acts as importer into Spain of products made by the manufacturer.

MIX
Paper | Supporting
responsible forestry
FSC
www.fsc.org   FSC® C013604

Advance Praise for *Mentalization: Utilizing reflection to heal from borderline personality disorder*

"Robert Drozek brings his exceptional expertise as a mentalization-based treatment (MBT) practitioner and trainer to bear in this invaluable handbook for those impacted by the persistent and distressing relational challenges of borderline personality disorder (BPD). This volume offers both individuals facing these difficulties and their loved ones a compassionate and accessible framework for understanding and managing the emotional challenges they encounter. It is a remarkable and insightful work, with the potential to bring real, achievable solutions to millions. This is a major contribution to the mental health literature and an essential resource for anyone affected by these issues."

—PETER FONAGY, CBE, FMedSci, FBA, FAcSS, PhD,
co-developer of MBT and co-author of *Mentalization-Based Treatment for Personality Disorders: A Practical Guide*
Head of the Division of Psychology and Language Sciences,
University College London
National Clinical Advisor on Children's Mental Health,
National Health Service, England

"*Mentalization: Utilizing Reflection to Heal from Borderline Personality Disorder* is a practical, compassionate, and easy-to-use guide, packed full of powerful tools and strategies. This workbook will help you to better understand yourself, deal more effectively with difficult thoughts and feelings, effectively tackle your problems and challenges, improve your relationships, and build a better life."

—RUSS HARRIS, MBBS, acceptance and commitment therapy (ACT) trainer
and author of *The Happiness Trap*

"*Mentalization: Utilizing Reflection to Heal from Borderline Personality Disorder* is a clear, down-to earth self-help manual for people who suffer from shame and stigma. The book offers concrete, practical ways to develop a more accepting and open-minded attitude toward yourself and others, and to build the skills of emotional intelligence. Drozek writes in a conversational tone with a self-deprecating sense of humor, more like a trusted friend than an authority figure. A valuable resource for the many people with borderline personality disorder, their families, friends, and clinicians."

—JUDITH L. HERMAN, MD, author of *Trauma and Recovery*
Senior Lecturer, Department of Psychiatry, Harvard Medical School

"*Mentalization: Utilizing Reflection to Heal from Borderline Personality Disorder* is an essential aid for people struggling with BPD, and for clinicians dedicated to treating the disorder. The text is well-organized to help you understand and treat your difficulties in mentalization, complete with worksheets, exercises to assess your own style of mentalizing, and practical strategies to address the emotional dysregulation that causes so much pain in BPD. The book is a gem and an indispensable guide for patients and clinicians!"

—MICHAEL R. HOLLANDER, PhD, dialectical behavior therapy (DBT) trainer
and author of *Helping Teens Who Cut*
Co-founder and Endowed Director (retired),
3East DBT Continuum, McLean Hospital
Assistant Professor Emeritus of Psychology (part-time),
Department of Psychiatry, Harvard Medical School

We all use mentalizing, even though most of us have no idea what it is. Human beings are socially organized, form complex relationships with each other, and manage incredibly well at forming friendships, social groups, communities dedicated to tasks, and so on. We create things together that we could not create alone. Humans are naturally gregarious, working cooperatively and creatively in groups and collectives.

Intelligence of humans is higher when the group members have greater social sensitivity—that is, when we read and understand each other well. This is the success of humanity as a social species. To support our survival, natural selection has provided us with the tools necessary to interact and manage the hugely complex landscape of our social world. Understanding the thoughts, intentions, and mental states of our fellow humans is the key to the creation of human societies; it accounts for our attainment of dominance over other species on our planet. We constantly infer thoughts, feelings, and beliefs in the minds of other people, and we spend much of our mental lives engaging in the task of processing social information.

Dear reader, if you have gotten this far, it is likely that you are concerned about how you manage your relationships in a world of ever-increasing complexity. Yet it is only recently that there has been interest in how this social complexity works. How do you do it? And what can you do about it if it does not work satisfactorily for you?

Mentalizing is now known to be one of the main mental processes that enables you to navigate this complex social world. It underpins effective and satisfying personal and social relationships. "What an awkward and harsh and ungainly sounding word," you might think, "for what is essentially a soft and sensitive mental process used by all humans in their everyday lives." It refers to your ability to reflect on your own mind, the minds of others, and those minds in interaction.

If mentalizing is working well, you know who you are and how you feel when you get up in the morning. You are the same person who got up yesterday. You create in your mind an experience of yourself as you go out into the world. You identify how you feel, give it context and meaning, and are aware of what you think. You create a narrative of yourself over time with memories, linking everything together into a coherent story about yourself and other people.

When you meet someone, you naturally read their mind in the immediate moment. If you know them well, you understand their current mind in terms of your prior knowledge of their personal experience. You thus easily assess what they think and feel at any time. You don't even have to think about it. This is what friendships are. You understand someone, and they see you as understanding them in line with how they see themself.

The same applies the other way around: Your friends understand you, you see them as understanding you, and they recognize this—a somewhat complicated interaction, but in fact you do it all quite naturally. When it goes well, you no longer feel alone in the world. You are with someone. This is the key to experiencing a sense of belonging in the world; it builds relationships and protects you from painful feelings of loneliness and isolation.

Friendships generate mental resilience, helping you to bounce back from stressors and setbacks. Mentalizing does all of this for you.

Learning how to mentalize, then, is an important developmental and on-going life task. When it goes wrong, it causes no end of problems in your relationships, until eventually you experience persistent mental distress. So stabilizing mentalizing and using it more effectively in life becomes a necessity.

Now it so happens that there is a treatment which aims to improve mentalizing. Mentalization-based treatment (MBT) is an evidence-based intervention for borderline personality disorder (BPD), antisocial personality disorder, complex posttraumatic stress disorder, and a range of other mental health problems. MBT has been subjected to robust research right from its inception, and it is now recommended as a treatment for BPD in official national guidelines in many countries around the world.

To gain the most from treatment, you need to understand how a treatment might help you change, and how you can maximize any benefits. MBT focuses on improving your capacity to mentalize, on the basis that effective mentalizing increases your resilience to life stressors and enables you to progress over time. The first step in learning how to mentalize better is having access to accurate and up-to-date information. The second step is knowing how to practice it. So if you are offered MBT for your problems, have a look at this book before you start. But mentalizing is a general life skill, making this book one for all of us.

Mentalizing goes hand in hand with attachment. The two processes develop together from childhood to adulthood, determining how you relate to other people. When you are distressed, you look to others for help. This is a biological drive with which you are born, and a psychological drive that becomes wired-in over time. You seek proximity to someone who can help you, and you do so right from the start of life. Survival is at stake at this early point. In infancy, attachment processes propel you to connect to others: You cry, you reach out, you become agitated to attract attention.

You begin to learn who is helpful and who is not. Gradually you realize that other individuals have minds of their own, and they are not simply there to meet your needs. You also learn about your own mind, and about who you are through them. Amazingly, you learn about yourself and your feelings through others' minds. So it helps if people around you are consistent, reliable, and mirroring you accurately over time. You go to them for support and soothing. This is a secure attachment, and it is in this context that you learn how to trust other people, so that you can take in information from them. You trust that what they tell you—the knowledge that they pass on—is reliable and useful to you. In other words, it is *for* you, as a unique individual. As you will learn in this book, MBT refers to this experience as *epistemic trust* (see Chapters 4 and 15), which is enabled by mentalizing: "If I feel that I am understood, I will be disposed to learn from the person who understood me, who I feel is a trustworthy potential collaborator. This will include learning about myself, but also learning about others and the world in which I live."

Developing this kind of trust is quite a task, requiring you to have stable and effective mentalizing. First, you need to possess a coherent sense of yourself: You know yourself well enough to recognize that the other person is seeing your state of mind accurately. Second, you need a way of "taking in" the image of yourself that the other person is reflecting back to you. And finally, you need to judge the similarity or difference between your own self-perception and how the other person is describing you. (Of course this process also requires that the other individual has mentalized you well enough to have a fairly accurate understanding of you.)

But what if this mentalization-fueled process goes wrong, and when you look to others for help, there is a serious mismatch between how you experience yourself and how others see you? For example, you feel frightened and tense, and yet the other person tells you that you are horrible, you are being a nuisance, and you should stop creating such a fuss. You feel misunderstood, becoming confused about yourself and your experience. You are unsupported and fail to calm. This is the experience of trauma.

When this happens over time, your ability to know what you are feeling becomes muddled and uncertain. You are no longer able to learn about yourself and how to negotiate the world from other people. You naturally become wary and distrustful. Your mentalizing is unstable, and you feel alone in the world, which is a uniquely painful state. But you still need to feel safe. So naturally you try to get more help and support, resorting to more desperate strategies. You increase your demands from others, and if others continue to be unresponsive, you might give up and retreat. You close down. Then you are unable to use your social network to help you; the social network does not seem to *know* how to help you. This is a disrupted, disorganized attachment process. When you withdraw and close down your mind, your anxiety decreases, but this is only temporary. Loneliness and fear return, setting off your attempts to get help again. In effect, you are constantly trying to help yourself through others, but it is not working. Mentalizing is compromised.

So if you think of yourself as someone who is anxious in social situations, who worries constantly about relationships, and who feels uncertain about how you feel and how others feel about you, then improving your mentalizing is just the thing for you. But who can you trust to give you helpful information about how to do it better? This is where this book comes in.

Many people start looking things up on the web, which is a double-edged sword. On the one hand, you can learn a huge amount from the information provided, but on the other, it is difficult to know if the material is going to be accurate and useful to you. You can soon become bogged down in a tangle of information and misinformation, trapped in incomprehensible jargon, and discombobulated by overly complex descriptions of mental health disorders and their treatments.

You need someone to guide you through the maze. You need someone to attach to, someone you can trust. Bob Drozek takes on this task in this book, gently coaxing you to have confidence in reflecting on yourself, and providing ideas for practicing your mind-reading abilities on yourself and even with others. The mind is a dangerous place, and you should not have to go there alone. It plays tricks, uses imagination to fill in gaps when there is nothing there, and turns the lights out so you cannot see anything. All of this can lead to panic, unless you can conjure up someone in your mind to metaphorically hold your hand.

Use this book to learn how to conjure up your very own "Bob." Bob accompanies you by giving informed and kindly guidance about how to build a mentalizing toolbox for yourself. He gives you confidence to visit places in your mind you might otherwise avoid. There is no one more qualified to do this than Bob Drozek, a consummate clinician and great communicator. He transforms complex ideas into ordinary language in a way that maintains their meaning, while still making them useful in everyday life. Bob is a specialist with his feet on the ground, in the real world. A clinical social worker and psychotherapist at McLean Hospital, he spends most of his time providing individual and group MBT to patients with BPD and other personality disorders.

At the same time, he knows his mentalizing and MBT. He teaches and supervises MBT at Harvard Medical School, and he leads MBT trainings for the Anna Freud Centre (the epicenter of MBT in London), working hand in hand with MBT experts around the world. As clinical director of the MBT Clinic at McLean Hospital, he has contributed his original thinking and clinical interventions to the burgeoning field of mentalizing knowledge and clinical study. He has published numerous papers and book chapters about MBT (Drozek, 2018), is the lead developer (along with myself and Brandon Unruh) of MBT for narcissism (Drozek & Unruh, 2020; Drozek et al., 2023), and has also advanced MBT as an intervention to address the problem of law enforcement violence (Drozek et al., 2021). In addition, Bob created the domain-based theory of mentalization, a clear-cut pathway to simplify the teaching and practice of MBT (Drozek & Henry, 2021; Drozek et al., 2023). This is the conception of mentalizing on which this book is based.

This book is for anyone who wants to understand their mind better, take control of it, and deploy it effectively in their daily life to develop more satisfying relationships. For those of you who are starting MBT, this book provides all the information and support you need in order to hit the ground running. It is a companion to treatment, setting a practical mentalizing framework for use at home, at work, and during treatment itself. But even if you are not receiving MBT, you will benefit significantly from this carefully crafted book. Learn your own mentalizing at home, and practice it in your daily life. See how you go!

Each chapter builds on previous learning, allowing you to deepen your understanding of mentalization and strengthen your capacities step by step. You can even work out how to seamlessly mentalize with people you meet, and even with your friends. There is a trick here, though. Make sure that you carefully monitor the results of your mentalizing, rather than working out if you did it well or badly. The proof of the pudding is in the eating. How your social world responds to you is the best informant of your mentalizing capacities. You are not necessarily the best judge of yourself. You may be overly critical of yourself, as you could feel unsure if you have ever really been any good at anything. Contrariwise, you could over-estimate your capacities: You might not abide personal errors and feel unforgiving about others' weaknesses. So look to other people's responses to measure your mentalizing in complex social interactions, and even in personal relationships.

Once you have tried out all of the mentalizing tasks and toolkits in this book, you may find yourself wondering: "Is change really possible for me? And is it even worth it?" Learning mentalizing and integrating it into our daily life is hard work, and progress is not guaranteed. The good news is that even *trying* to mentalize creates the possibility of change. Go out into the world, and start practicing mentalizing with others, even if you don't feel too confident about it. Take an interest in their minds, and they will take an interest in yours. You will be amazed at how their responses to you begin to shift.

Whenever another person mentalizes you, you move out of social isolation. This experience frees you up, reactivating your capacity to learn and allowing you to grow in the context of your relationships in the world. You become the agent of change. You gain a sense of responsibility and personal effectiveness: You can create things, and you can evolve your relationships. You are no longer at the mercy of forces outside of you that blow you off course by triggering excessive uncertainty, intolerance, and inflexibility. You start to connect with other people, creating joint responsibility. Over time, you feel like you *belong* in the world, rather than feeling like the world owns and controls you.

I assure you that you will get all this and more out of this book. This is no idle promise. There is plenty of scientific evidence showing that people with secure attachment and stable mentalizing function more effectively in the world, negotiating the normal stressors of everyday life more successfully. Life becomes a pleasure rather than a chore. The good news is that attachment processes and mentalizing abilities are changeable, even though you might feel like they are set in stone.

Let Bob take you through the mentalizing steps so that you learn to dance, fluidly joining all the steps into rhythmic mental movements. Your capacity for social learning and thinking about mental states will improve immeasurably, simply because you become able to "use" your environment in a different way. Look forward to change.

Anthony Bateman
London, 2025

Robert P. Drozek, LICSW, is the clinical director of the Mentalization-Based Treatment (MBT) Clinic at McLean Hospital in Belmont, Massachusetts. He also serves as a staff psychotherapist in the Gunderson Outpatient Program and the Division of Alcohol, Drugs, and Addiction at McLean. He is a trainer and supervisor in MBT through the Anna Freud Centre in London, and a teaching associate in the Department of Psychiatry at Harvard Medical School. Mr. Drozek is a co-founder and co-director of MBT Boston, an organization dedicated to providing training and supervision in mentalization-based treatment. His publications examine the interface between psychotherapy and ethics, with an emphasis on the role of ethics in the patient's therapeutic change. He is author of the book *Psychoanalysis as an Ethical Process* (2019), and lead author of *Mentalization-Based Treatment for Pathological Narcissism: A Handbook* (2023). He is in private practice in Belmont, Massachusetts.

More so than anything I have ever written, this book owes its greatest debt to my patients. When I was hired at the Gunderson Outpatient Program in 2018, my role was to lead a weekly introductory Mentalization-Based Treatment (MBT) group, where we would cover the core concepts and treatment strategies of MBT. For some context, Gunderson is McLean Hospital's intensive outpatient program for patients with borderline personality disorder (BPD) and other personality disorders, offering daily group therapy, twice weekly individual therapy, family therapy, vocational support, family support groups, and psychopharmacology tailored to patients with personality disorders.

Gunderson's patients tend to be discriminating consumers of mental health treatment: curious, intelligent, educated, and highly "therapized," having received some of the world's best treatment for BPD and yet continuing to struggle with severe functional challenges. So on my first day leading the Gunderson MBT group, I felt very excited, and very intimidated. As a dutiful MBT therapist, my plan was to present the official MBT introductory materials, distributed by the Anna Freud Centre in London. I learned right away that our patients *really*, *really* did not like them. Feeling patronized by the material, they wanted to learn the "behind the scenes" version of MBT—the stuff we use to teach the therapists, not just the patients.

So with the blessing of Anthony Bateman (the co-developer of MBT—see more in Chapter 5), and with the encouragement of Gunderson's leadership Joe Flores, George Smith, and Kathryn Broge, I began reworking MBT's introductory materials. Developing worksheets and handouts about the core theoretical concepts of MBT, I created a short workbook that offered patients a "crash course" in the main elements of the therapy. The workbook caught on. Gunderson patients reported feeling more stimulated and "seen" by this manner of framing MBT, and the Anna Freud Centre began distributing it to clinicians who attended their trainings in MBT. The current book is a significantly expanded version of that workbook, and it would not exist if not for the dogged self-advocacy of our Gunderson patients.

Elsewhere in my practice, I was providing individual MBT, as well as longer-term group MBT to patients with BPD and other personality disorders. These patients raised a different sort of concern. After I delivered a written MBT formulation to a patient, or when I helped someone to mentalize a difficult situation in their lives, the most common response I would receive is: "This all makes sense, but what do I actually DO to address the problem? I don't understand how 'mentalizing' is going to make me feel any better." These objections underscored the fact that, despite the wealth of research supporting MBT's efficacy, there were no written materials in the psychotherapy literature written FOR patients about how to actually apply MBT's principles in their everyday lives.

So I began to write down tailored "mentalizing prompts" for my patients, which were essentially *questions* they could ask themselves when they were starting to go down especially destructive lines of thought. Patients found such questions notably helpful, as they offered some level of direction and focus about how to work through their challenges. In this case, the "how" was simply *reflection on mental states*, targeted to the particular area of patients' lives where they were struggling. The more that I developed these prompts for my individual and group patients, I began to realize that this could be done at a broader scale as well—developing *general* mentalizing prompts to address the core emotional and interpersonal challenges of BPD. These prompts serve as the informal archetypes for the mentalizing practice points that fill this book. They are thus indebted to these group and individual patients, especially their deep wish to get better, and their perceptiveness about the "gaps" in the current state of MBT.

Outside of my clinical work, I am grateful to all of the colleagues who have supported me in my work with patients with BPD. Lois Choi-Kain, Amy Gagliardi, and John Gunderson: Thank you for giving me my first job in personality disorders treatment, and for creating a role for me where literally none had existed before. My colleagues and supervisors in the Gunderson Outpatient Program—Joe Flores, George Smith, Kathryn Broge, Julia Lustick, Elizabeth Murphy, Elsa Ronningstam, and Igor Weinberg—have taught me the foundational importance of *change* in the treatment of BPD. You are tireless champions of our ethical mandate to help patients recover and flourish, in order to live more fulfilling and meaningful lives.

In the world of MBT, I am grateful to all of our supervisees in our MBT Boston supervision groups. I look forward to our time together every two weeks, and I feel especially appreciative of your incisive questions and challenges to the model. You consistently inspire me to reapproach these principles from a fresh perspective, and to wrestle with them at a deeper level.

To my wonderful team in the MBT Clinic: Caleb Demers, Adam Henderson, Halsey Niles, Brandon Unruh, Hillary Woodworth, Mary Zanarini, our research assistants, and all of our incredible trainees—I have been so fortunate to present on the ideas in these pages throughout the writing process, finding myself consistently enriched by your perceptive and compelling feedback. I see this book as reflecting not simply my own mind, but the warm and vibrant community that we have built together in the MBT Clinic.

Brandon, you are my mentalizing partner in crime! You have always encouraged me to develop these constructs, and even to "road test" them in our introductory MBT groups. I cherish our friendship, and I admire your humility, wisdom, and gentle but steady leadership. I learn so much from you, about how to "pick your battles" when it really matters, and to be flexible when it doesn't. You embody the true spirit of MBT—not just in your technique, but in who you are as a person.

It continues to blow my mind that I have been able to learn this highly effective form of therapy from the developers of the modality itself, Anthony Bateman and Peter Fonagy. You have both served as responsive mentors to me, even when I was a young therapist with no publications to my name. This speaks to your generosity, and your lack of pretense as human beings. Peter, thank you for your kind endorsement of this book, and your support of this project since its inception. Anthony: This book really represents a "translation" of your brilliant, therapist-focused MBT techniques for patients to utilize in their everyday lives. In that respect, you are as much an author of this text as I am. Never territorial or precious, you have always welcomed "other minds" into MBT, encouraging other thinkers to elaborate, build upon, and rework your ground-breaking formulations. This book is no exception. Thank you for writing your thoughtful foreword, and for always encouraging my development as an author and trainer in MBT.

Martin Baum and all the staff at Oxford University Press, thank you for believing in this project from the outset and shepherding it across the finish line. David Klee, you have graced us all with another arresting cover, this time depicting the joy, complexity, and wonder of recovery from BPD.

Finally, I am so thankful for my incredible family: Rose, Margaret, Kipling, and our miniature schnauzer Elsa. You have been so understanding of how much time I have spent working on the book, and you have helped me to sort out so many knotty conceptual problems, whenever I was confused about how to explain or present things. Rose, you have graciously read so many of these pages, always with an eye toward making things accessible and clear to the reader who is new to these concepts. You are the love of my life, and the center of our family. None of this would be possible without you.

PUBLISHER'S ACKNOWLEDGMENTS

Chapters 1 and 2 contain selected narrative from

Drozek, R. P., & Unruh, B. T. (2022). Mentalization-based treatment for a physician with borderline personality disorder. *American Journal of Psychotherapy*, *75*(1), 51–54.

Reprinted with permission from the *American Journal of Psychotherapy*, Mentalization-Based Treatment for a Physician With Borderline Personality Disorder, Robert P. Drozek, L.I.C.S.W., and Brandon T. Unruh, M.D. (Copyright © 2022). American Psychiatric Association. All Rights Reserved.

Chapter 8 contains statements drawn and adapted from the Experiences in Close Relationships scale, utilized with permission from P. R. Shaver.

Chapter 8 contains statements drawn and adapted from the Relationship Style Questionnaire, utilized with permission from D. W. Griffin.

Chapter 9 contains selected narrative from

Drozek, R. P. (2015). The dialectics of dignity: Clinical applications: Reply to commentaries. *Psychoanalytic Dialogues*, *25*(4), 472–480. https://www.tandfonline.com/

Chapters 9 and 10 contain selected narrative from

Drozek, R. P., Unruh, B. T., & Bateman, A. W. (2023). *Mentalization-based treatment for pathological narcissism: A handbook.* Oxford University Press.

CONTENTS

TABLES

WORKSHEETS

The above worksheets can be accessed freely online by searching for this book's title on the Oxford Academic platform, at academic.oup.com.

CHAPTER REVIEWS

The above chapter reviews can be accessed freely online by searching for this book's title on the Oxford Academic platform, at academic.oup.com.

PART 1

Mentalization and Borderline Personality Disorder

What Is Making You Feel So Unstable?

Katherine was in her mid-20s when she presented to treatment to address her challenges with depression, suicidal thinking, and self-injurious behavior. Raised in the Midwest, Katherine moved to Boston to complete her residency in obstetrics and gynecology at a prestigious local hospital. As an only child, Katherine was cherished by her parents, but only conditionally so. She experienced her mother as highly intrusive and controlling, easily injured if Katherine ever displayed any emotions that seemed "negative" or critical toward her. Katherine's father was more reasonable, but he remained largely passive, never intervening when her mother would direct aggression toward Katherine.

Katherine thus learned to keep her head down and "be a good girl": excelling in school, joining athletic teams, participating in extracurricular activities, and above all, always appearing happy, hiding any emotions that would trigger her mother's discomfort. When she left home for college, the façade finally began to crack. She experienced periods of extreme emotional instability, often triggered by phone conversations with her mother, or by interpersonal interactions with her classmates where she felt rejected. Katherine would feel intense anger toward the other person, alternating quickly with feelings of self-hatred and self-loathing: *I am bad, disgusting, ugly, and worthless. No one wants to be with me, and that is never going to change.*

Katherine fantasized about suicide in these moments, even writing suicide letters to her family, which she would never send. By the time she had reached residency, she started cutting herself with razors. This felt like a well-deserved punishment, but it also gave her a momentary feeling of internal peace, "shutting off" her mind by creating an experience of physical rather than emotional pain. For reasons she could not explain, Katherine increasingly began to feel emotionally numb, separated from herself, even dead inside. She felt like she was leading two lives: the highly functional doctor, who cared for her patients and always had the right answers; and her "depressed" self, who was so incapacitated that she could only be the recipient of caretaking, not the provider of it.

UNDERSTANDING THE PROBLEM OF BORDERLINE PERSONALITY DISORDER

Borderline personality disorder, or "BPD" for short, is a serious mental health condition marked by challenges with *instability*—more specifically, instability in emotions, self-esteem, relationships, and behavior. BPD is more common than you might think. In the United States, the estimated prevalence of BPD is 1.6%, with a lifetime prevalence as high as 5.9% (Grant et al., 2008). This amounts to over five million people who struggle with the symptoms of BPD, and over **19 million people** who will experience these symptoms at some point in their lives. In treatment settings, these numbers shoot up even more: 12% of outpatients and 22% of inpatients have BPD (Ellison et al., 2018). BPD is associated with a range of significant psychosocial challenges: interpersonal instability (Javaras et al., 2017), work impairment (Juurlink et al., 2018), suicidal behavior (Grilo & Udo, 2021), and other

Mentalization. Robert P. Drozek, Oxford University Press. © Oxford University Press 2025.
DOI: 10.1093/oso/9780198916857.003.0001

distressing psychiatric conditions, such as depression, anxiety, addiction, eating disorders, and PTSD (Frías & Palma, 2015; Martinussen et al., 2017; Tomko et al., 2014).

If you have BPD, then you are probably all too familiar with these forms of instability. One barrier to accurately recognizing and understanding BPD is that the disorder can take so many different shapes, depending on the individual person struggling with these problems. Recent research suggests that there are several different presentations or "subtypes" of BPD, varying in interpersonal style, emotionality, and level of functionality (Hallquist & Pilkonis, 2012; Salzer et al., 2013; Smits et al., 2017). Like Katherine, the physician mentioned at the start of the chapter, you might be extremely functional and competent in the workplace, but on the inside, you experience intense feelings of emptiness and self-loathing, which you feel like you need to hide from the world around you. Or perhaps you have truly struggled to effectively manage your responsibilities at work or school: falling into interpersonal conflicts; over-sharing about your emotional troubles; finding it difficult to concentrate when you are feeling upset; or missing work or class due to your depression, emotional sensitivity, or inpatient hospitalizations.

You might be more directly *seeking* of connectedness in your relationships, for example by "jumping into" relationships or friendships quite quickly, having multiple sexual partners, engaging in frequent texting and DMs, and feeling insecure when other people are not responsive enough to you. Or you might be more withdrawn or avoidant in your relationships. On the inside, you desperately want to connect with others, but you feel overwhelmed by these feelings, and terrified that other people would reject you, if they knew what you are *really* like.

Other variations in BPD center on how people relate to feelings of anger and frustration. When you feel hurt or rejected by people, or if you feel like something wrong or unjust is happening, you could experience intense anger or even rage, feeling drawn to criticize, argue, or lash out at the offending party. That is the stereotype of BPD. However, you could share similarities with the more "quiet" subtype of BPD, where you are more likely to direct your anger toward yourself, especially when other people disappoint you. *This is a sign that there is something wrong with me. If I were different—if I were* better—*then people would be nicer to me, the way that they are with everyone else.*

As outlined in the official manual of psychiatric conditions, in order to carry the diagnosis of BPD, the individual needs to meet at least five out of nine diagnostic criteria (American Psychiatric Association, 2022, pp. 752–757). This means that, as BPD researchers Oladottir and colleagues (2022) point out, "There are 256 combinations that can result in the same BPD diagnosis and it is possible for two individuals with BPD to share only one criterion" (p. 1). This underscores the significant diversity in experiences of people with BPD. To understand the diagnosis further, let's review these criteria, and the various shapes they might take in your everyday life.

1. Frantic efforts to avoid real or imagined abandonment

This criterion really encompasses two related processes in BPD: internal fears of abandonment, and behavioral efforts to prevent those fears from being realized. Often people assume that "fears of abandonment" refer only to worries that other people will leave or break up with you. While that is definitely the case, these fears can also involve *emotional* abandonment— that is, concerns that others will judge you, criticize you, dislike you, reject you, become angry with you, withdraw from you, get bored with you, see you in a negative light, or value other people more than you.

You might feel like you genuinely *need* others' physical and emotional presence, or that other people must feel a certain way about you (e.g., loving you, desiring you, admiring you) in order for you to feel good about yourself. This gives rise to the aforementioned fears of abandonment. If you require another person in order to feel grounded in yourself, then of course you would worry about losing the person—it is tantamount to losing yourself. John Gunderson, the widely recognized "father" of the borderline diagnosis who founded many of our programs for BPD here at McLean Hospital, variously referred to this experience as "intolerance of aloneness" (Gunderson, 1996), as well as the problem of *interpersonal hypersensitivity*: "a paradoxical, seemingly contradictory combination of intense needs for closeness and attention with equally intense fears of rejection or abandonment" (Gunderson & Lyons-Ruth, 2008, p. 23).

These fears manifest themselves in a range of visible behaviors, which can be seen as your efforts to avoid abandonment: engaging in frequent communications (e.g., talking, calling, or texting extensively; posting on social media); quickly escalating the intensity and close-ness of relationships; pursuing sexual intimacy ("trading sex for love"); sacrificing your own needs and wishes so as not to alienate the other person; giving gifts, money, or services to others; utilizing criticism, control, and arguments when people are insufficiently responsive to you; discussing your difficulties and challenges, so that others provide you with care and attention; and pushing people away (e.g., breaking up with them, withdrawing from them, ghosting them) before they can reject or abandon you.

2. A pattern of unstable and intense interpersonal relationships characterized by alternating between extremes of idealization and devaluation

Here, "relationships" encompass dynamics with romantic or sexual partners, and also with family members, friends, and co-workers. These relationships can be marked by disruptions and instability: arguments; break-ups and estrangement; suspended communications; getting back together; other people distancing themselves from you due to these difficulties with instability; and in some cases, relationships only lasting for brief periods of time. Such relationships are "intense" in that they are often marked by powerful emotions: strong feelings of love, passion, and desire, as well as acute feelings of anxiety, panic, anger, or rage.

This is where the idealization and devaluation come in. If you have BPD, you likely have the tendency to idealize particular people—that is, to put them up on a pedestal, to make them into a "favorite person," and to extensively rely on certain individuals in order to meet your emotional needs. *I need this person in order to feel OK. If they were to leave me, I am not sure that I could function.* Sometimes you might actually believe that the person is quite amazing, in some respects "better" than other people in your life. *My new boyfriend is so much more caring and understanding than my exes. He would never treat me the way that they did.* At other times, you might cognitively "know" that the person has their flaws, but at an emotional level, you continue to relate to them as if they are the key to your stability and psychological well-being.

You may also have a pattern of *devaluing* other people—that is, seeing them as highly bad, problematic, or flawed, and focusing extensively on their defects when you are thinking about or interacting with them. If you are devaluing someone, you could genuinely see the person in a primarily negative light. *He is a narcissistic abuser, just like they talk about on TikTok. I was completely taken in by him, but now I can see that he was manipulating me the whole time.* Or you might intellectually recognize that the person has both positive and negative traits, but at an emotional level, you continue to *feel* victimized by them, and you find it challenging to consider the potentially valid aspects of their perspective ("I guess they could have a point, too . . .").

These tendencies toward idealization and devaluation are components of what is commonly referred to as *splitting* in psychology, which the psychoanalytic theorist Otto Kernberg (1975) defines as "the division of external objects into 'all good' ones and 'all bad' ones, with the concomitant possibility of . . . sudden and complete reversals of all feelings and conceptualizations about a particular person" (p. 29). Splitting can take several different shapes in BPD:

- Shifting between idealizing and devaluing the same individual, depending on how they are treating you (or how you are feeling about them) at the time
- Idealizing certain people and devaluing others. For example, you experience resentment and hatred toward your parents, but you feel connected and supported in your romantic relationship.
- Feeling highly "picky" about the people with whom you connect. You might find it challenging to find people who really excite you, but when you meet one of those people, you become emotionally invested quite quickly. With most other people, you feel bored, impatient, or irritated.
- "Flipping a switch" and devaluing specific people, groups, or situations. For example, you feel largely positive about your work relationships for an extended period of time. However, after a conflictual interaction at work, the whole environment feels stressful and unsafe, and you start noticing problematic issues you had overlooked before.

3. Identity disturbance: markedly and persistently unstable self-image or sense of self

People with BPD often struggle with identity disturbance—that is, instability in self-image, self-worth, and self-esteem (Richetin et al., 2017). You might feel like you lack a coherent sense of self, a state referred to as *identity diffusion*: You do not "know who you are," and your goals, values, and wishes feel like they are constantly changing (Kaufman & Meddaoui, 2021). Or your self-experience could be significantly influenced by the people around you. You may absorb other people's characteristics, a tendency known as "chameleoning" or the "chameleon effect" in BPD. In addition, others' views of you might determine how you feel about yourself. For example, you feel happy and good about yourself when others express their approval of you, but you descend into self-doubt and self-hatred when other people criticize or reject you. In addition, you might carry around a consistently *negative* view of yourself: feeling bad, worthless, and disgusting, like there is something inherently wrong with you. This can manifest itself in a pervasive sense of shame and embarrassment, which persists across different situations and relationships (Buchman-Wildbaum et al., 2021).

4. Impulsivity in at least two areas that are potentially self-damaging

People with BPD are increased risk for engaging in impulsive behavior, especially while under stress (Cackowski et al., 2014). When you experience intense emotions (e.g., hurt, anger, sadness, shame), you may be drawn to take actions that make you feel better in the moment but over time lead to negative consequences in your life. These actions could include:

- overspending
- promiscuity, or risky sexual behavior
- excessive use of alcohol, marijuana, or other substances

- addictive behaviors not connected to substances (e.g., involving gambling, exercise, technology, video games)
- maladaptive eating: binging, restricting, purging
- law-breaking behaviors: theft, violence, destruction of property
- thrill-seeking or "sensation-seeking" behaviors: reckless driving, extreme sports, going to exciting or dangerous places
- impulsive interpersonal approaches: making provocative comments, being dishonest, sharing too much about yourself, starting conflicts with people

Can you identify at least two forms of impulsivity in which you have engaged? These might include actions not on the above list.

5. Recurrent suicidal behavior, gestures, or threats, or self-mutilating behavior

Many individuals with BPD experience powerful impulses to harm their own bodies. *Suicidal behavior* includes thinking about, fantasizing about, researching, planning, threatening, or taking actions aimed at taking your own life. Research suggests that 30% of people with BPD attempt suicide (Grilo & Udo, 2021), and 6% of individuals with BPD die from suicide (Temes et al., 2019). In BPD, suicidal behavior can be triggered by a range of internal experiences, including feeling overwhelmed by intense emotions (e.g., sadness, anger, panic); feeling hurt, rejected, or abandoned by other people; or feeling hopeless about whether or not your circumstances will improve over time. In such moments, you might feel like you *have* to think about ending things—that is the only way you can get the pain to stop.

Self-mutilating behavior—also referred to as self-harm or non-suicidal self-injury—is the deliberate destruction of your own body, without the intention to die. 90% of patients with BPD have engaged in some form of self-injury (Goodman et al., 2017), which could include cutting, burning, scratching, head banging, or hitting oneself. The motives for engaging in these forms of self-harm are complex and multifaceted (Snir et al., 2015; Zanarini, Laudate, et al., 2013). From an internal perspective, you might hurt yourself in order to relieve anxiety, to punish yourself, to gain a sense of agency, to generate some positive emotion in yourself, or to decrease your emotional suffering—to shift the pain "from the inside to the outside."

You could feel numb or dead inside, and harming your body helps you feel connected to yourself again. If you are feeling overwhelmed and unstable, hurting yourself might temporarily regulate your emotions, "clearing your head" so that you are able to think again (see Hollander, 2017). For some people with BPD, self-injury can serve an interpersonal function as well: expressing anger or frustration at other people, creating distance between yourself and others, communicating your distress to people in your life, or "asking for help" (e.g., care, attention, support) from others. Research suggests that self-injurious behavior leads to significant reductions in distress for individuals with BPD, and that these processes are likely grounded in the neurobiology of BPD (Olié et al., 2018; Reitz et al., 2015).

Despite popular opinion, while many people with BPD struggle with suicidality and self-injury, many other patients never experience these problems. **Safety-related difficulties are not a requirement in order to carry the diagnosis of BPD.** So if you have never struggled with these challenges but you still identify with the other symptoms we have been discussing, I hope that you keep reading. In this book, we will be considering strategies to address the full spectrum of BPD symptoms: problems with safety, but also instability in emotions, self-esteem, and interpersonal relationships.

6. Affective instability due to a marked reactivity of mood

Emotional dysregulation and instability are defining features of BPD (D'Aurizio et al., 2023). *Affective instability* refers to a range of different processes (Koenigsberg, 2010), outlined below.

- You might easily and frequently "switch" from one emotion to another (e.g., from fear to anger, from contentment to sadness).
- These switches can happen quite suddenly, without your full awareness or control.
- You could experience your emotions at a high level of intensity: despair or hopelessness rather than mild sadness; anger or rage rather than just frustration; anxiety or panic rather than simply worry.
- Once you fall into an intense painful emotion, it may take longer for you to return to your emotional baseline. Whereas many people easily bounce back from a challenging emotion, you might find it challenging to simply "let it go." This can then make it difficult to reengage with your life, or to focus on the task or situation in front of you.
- You could also *show or express* your emotions in a more intense manner: raising your voice, crying, using dramatic language, or "wearing your heart on your sleeve" through your posture, facial expressions, or bodily movements. You might struggle to hide what you are feeling from other people, which can make you feel vulnerable, exposed, or socially awkward.

"Marked reactivity of mood" essentially means that you are exquisitely emotionally sensitive, such that how you feel at any given moment can be significantly impacted by the world around you: interpersonal interactions, how people treat you, what they say to you, or others' non-verbal communications (e.g., facial expression, eye contact, bodily posture and movements, voice tone and volume). Your emotions may also be strongly influenced by other people's emotional states, a tendency in BPD referred to as *emotional contagion* (Sosic-Vasic et al., 2019). When you have BPD, you might lack a firm membrane between yourself and others, such that you naturally "absorb" other people's feelings. The people around you seem anxious, and you feel worried. Your partner gets irritated, and you start to feel on edge and frustrated yourself.

In addition, you could be acutely impacted by events in your environment: You feel overwhelmed by chaotic situations, or you find it difficult to concentrate when surrounded by noise and external stimuli. Your moods also might be greatly affected by your own bodily experiences: lack of sleep, hunger, fatigue, menstrual cycles, physical pain, and so on.

7. Chronic feelings of emptiness

"Chronic feelings of emptiness" involve a sense of disconnection or separateness from yourself and other people (Miller et al., 2020). This can manifest in an experience of numbness, nothingness, or feeling "dead inside." At other times, emptiness shows itself in a lack of meaning, purpose, or fulfillment—a perpetual feeling of restlessness and dissatisfaction that has no clear focus or resolution. You might then try to cope with these feelings through impulsive behaviors, hurting yourself, or distracting yourself by filling up your life with productive activities (Miller et al., 2021).

8. Inappropriate, intense anger or difficulty controlling anger

People with BPD often experience powerful, intense feelings of anger, as well as related emotions along the anger spectrum: irritation, annoyance, impatience, resentment, frustration, and rage. You might feel like you have a short fuse, a quick temper, or that you can "go from 0 to 60" without much warning. Behaviorally, these feelings can escalate into

- criticizing other people
- trying to make others feel guilty
- saying hurtful things
- passive aggressive behaviors: sarcasm, sulking, giving the silent treatment, withdrawing in order to punish people
- getting into arguments
- yelling or raising your voice
- throwing or breaking things, slamming doors or cupboards
- physical violence and aggression

As mentioned earlier, if you have more of a "quiet" subtype of BPD, your anger likely shows itself in a less overt fashion in your life. You might "act in" instead of "acting out"—directing your aggression toward yourself rather than other people, in the form of shame, self-loathing, self-neglect, suicide, and self-injury. Or your anger could arise only in certain relationships (e.g., with parents, with romantic partners), but you tend to be more people-pleasing and self-negating in other relationships. At the same time, you might *feel* anger toward other people, but you avoid showing or expressing such feelings, instead engaging in more "private" expressions of anger: focusing extensively on other people's perceived wrongs or defects, ruminating about problematic things that others have done or said to you, fantasizing about ways to get back at them, or rehearsing what you might say the next time that you see the person.

Research links anger and aggression in BPD to challenges regulating emotions, as well as to a high sensitivity to feeling rejected by other people (Mancke et al., 2015; Scott et al., 2017). So when you feel hurt or abandoned by others, you might reflexively assume a more judgmental, antagonistic stance in relation to them. This can lead to significant instability in relationships (e.g., conflicts, estrangement, break-ups), ultimately pushing people away from you and making you feel more alone.

9. Transient, stress-related paranoid ideation or severe dissociative symptoms

People with BPD are significantly impacted by feelings of stress and anxiety (Shah & Zanarini, 2018). "Stress-related paranoid ideation" does not mean that you are delusional, or that you endorse bizarre beliefs, for example that people are spying on you or that aliens are about to invade the Earth. Rather, it means that when you are under stress, you are more likely to feel suspicious about other people's motives, feelings, and behaviors. For example, you might feel worried that people are judging you, that they do not care about you, that romantic partners are cheating on you, or that your loved ones are going to abandon you. At an intellectual level, you might "know" these things are unlikely, but at an emotional level, it *feels* like these things are true.

This is consistent with extensive research suggesting that people with BPD can struggle with trusting other people, in myriad ways:

- Feeling highly suspicious of others (Zanarini, Frankenburg, et al., 2013)
- Interpreting neutral or ambiguous facial expressions in a negative light (Mitchell et al., 2014)
- Focusing more attention on "negative" emotional words, rather than neutral ones (Kaiser et al., 2016)
- Assuming that others will harm, betray, abandon, and abuse you (Barazandeh et al., 2016)
- Engaging with other people in a less trusting, cooperative manner (King-Casas et al., 2008; Liebke et al., 2018)

But there is a limit to what the mind can take. This is where the "severe dissociative symptoms" come in. When you feel too anxious or overwhelmed, you might cope with this by shutting down—by disconnecting from yourself and the world around you (Al-Shamali et al., 2022; Scalabrini et al., 2017). Examples of BPD-related dissociation include:

- Feeling separate from your emotions and desires
- Disconnecting from your body and bodily sensations
- Feeling like you are seeing yourself from the outside, or as if you are in a dream
- Daydreaming, fantasizing, and "getting lost in your thoughts"
- Zoning out and "losing time." You know that you have been awake, but you do not recall what has been happening or what you have been doing.
- Memory problems. You cannot remember familiar objects and places; you forget information that you usually know, including how to do certain things.
- Identity or personality alterations: feeling like you are not yourself, or behaving in a manner that is not customary for you

---

Mentalizing Warm-up

Now that you understand the diagnostic criteria for BPD, return to Katherine's story at the start of the chapter, on page 3. What symptoms of BPD do you observe in Katherine's experience?

WRAPPING UP THE DIAGNOSTIC CRITERIA FOR BPD

With all of these diagnostic criteria under your belt, it's time to shift the focus onto *you*. Take a crack at completing Worksheets 1.1 and 1.2, which walk you through applying these ideas to your own life and challenges.

Worksheet 1.1
Diagnostic Criteria for Borderline Personality Disorder #1–4

Criterion #1: How have you worked to avoid abandonment, rejection, or criticism in your relationships? Describe at least three observable behaviors (e.g., frequent communications, pursuing sexual intimacy, self-sacrifice, criticizing or avoiding others when they disappoint you) you have utilized along these lines.

Criterion #2: "Relationships" encompass dynamics with romantic or sexual partners, and also with family members, friends, and co-workers. Share at least three examples where you have experienced intensity and instability in your relationships.

Idealization involves focusing extensively on someone's positive qualities, while minimizing their negative ones. *Devaluation* entails focusing on a person's flaws or deficiencies, while ignoring their potentially positive traits. Utilize the spaces below to describe times where you have idealized or devalued certain people or groups.

Idealizing People, AKA "All Good"	Devaluing People, AKA "All Bad"

[continued on next page]

Criterion #3: How have you encountered instability in your sense of self? This could include feeling confused about who you are, struggling with shame and self-hatred, or being highly influenced by the people around you.

Criterion #4: *Impulsiveness* refers to taking actions suddenly and without reflection, usually in a manner that results in negative consequences in your life. Circle any of the impulsive behaviors listed below with which you can identify.

Overspending

Excessive substance use

Thrill-seeking behaviors: reckless driving, extreme sports, going to exciting or dangerous places

Maladaptive eating: binging, purging, restricting

Promiscuity or risky sex

Law-breaking behaviors

Addictive behaviors not connected to substances: involving gambling, exercise, technology, video games

Impulsive interpersonal approaches: provocativeness, dishonesty, oversharing, starting arguments

Impulsive actions not listed here:

Worksheet 1.2
Diagnostic Criteria for Borderline Personality Disorder #5–9

Criterion #5: *Suicidal behavior* includes thinking about, fantasizing about, researching, planning, threatening, or taking actions aimed at taking your own life. Describe any examples of suicidal behavior with which you have struggled.

Self-injurious behavior is the deliberate destruction of your own body, without the intention to die. This can include cutting, burning, scratching, head banging, or hitting oneself. Sketch out any examples of self-injurious behavior you have experienced.

Criterion #6: Share about at least three examples of emotional instability you have experienced, where your emotions are significantly impacted by outside factors (e.g., interpersonal interactions, how people treat you, external situations, your physical states).

Criterion #7: *Chronic feelings of emptiness* involve a sense of disconnection or separateness from yourself and other people. This can manifest in experiences of numbness, nothingness, feeling dead inside, and a lack of meaning or purpose in life. Detail any experiences with emptiness you have encountered.

[continued on next page]

Criterion #8: Outline at least three ways in which you have struggled with anger issues, or difficulties controlling your frustration and anger in your interactions with others.

Criterion #9: *Stress-related paranoid ideation* means that, when you are under stress, you are more likely to feel suspicious about other people's motives, feelings, and behaviors. Provide any examples where you have experienced this sort of suspiciousness and mistrust.

See below for a list of dissociative symptoms that some people with BPD encounter. Circle any of the symptoms that resonate with you.

Feeling separate from your emotions and desires

Disconnecting from your body and bodily sensations

Feeling like you are seeing yourself from the outside, or as if you are in a dream

Daydreaming, fantasizing, and "getting lost in your thoughts"

Identity or personality alterations: feeling like you are not yourself, or behaving in a manner that is not customary for you

Memory problems (e.g., forgetting objects, places, past events and experiences, how to do things)

Zoning out and "losing time"

Dissociative symptoms not listed here:

THE GOOD NEWS: BORDERLINE PERSONALITY DISORDER GETS BETTER

Reviewing the diagnostic criteria for BPD can bring up a lot of different emotions for people, especially if you identify with them. You might experience a sense of relief or comfort knowing that other people struggle in similar ways that you do, or hope that this is a known problem with effective forms of treatment. You also could feel embarrassed or ashamed reading about these symptoms: They can sound a bit "crazy," and that might make you feel bad about yourself. This is not helped by the nasty social stigma associated with BPD, where individuals with BPD can be portrayed as manipulative, unempathetic, and untreatable (Ring & Lawn, 2019).

If you have been suffering from any of the symptoms we have been discussing, hopefully this book can bring some good news. Led by seminal research completed here at McLean Hospital (Zanarini et al., 2005), research suggests that BPD tends to improve over time (see Choi-Kain et al., 2020; Temes & Zanarini, 2018; Zanarini et al., 2010, 2012). In fact, one recent analysis found that 50–70% of people with BPD no longer meet criteria for the diagnosis over the long term, with significant improvements in depression and overall functionality in their lives (Álvarez-Tomás et al., 2019). We also have a range of highly effective therapies for BPD, which offer relief from many of its most painful symptoms (Cristea et al., 2017; Oud et al., 2018; Storebø et al., 2020; Witt et al., 2021). These scientific findings directly dispel the myth of BPD as some untreatable or hopeless condition. So if there are any take-aways from all of this research, let them be this:

You are not alone.

You will get better.

There is help.

This is what Katherine ended up learning, just when she was at her lowest point in her struggle with BPD. Let's return to Katherine's story, to see how things unfolded for her as she was getting started on her journey toward recovery.

RETURNING TO KATHERINE: LEARNING ABOUT BPD

Katherine was not a newcomer to the therapy game. She first started therapy in college, in order to address her worsening depression and emotional dysregulation. She had always liked therapy, especially the experience of having someone listen to her, support her, and validate her in the midst of her suffering. She saw herself as having simply "treatment-resistant depression," and her therapists largely agreed with that view. The problem was that, while she appreciated *being* in therapy, it never seemed to resolve the challenges that were causing her so much pain. She would try every antidepressant on the market, but she continued to hate herself, and her suicidal thinking and self-injury just got worse.

Katherine was referred to the Mentalization-Based Treatment (MBT) Clinic at McLean Hospital following a month-long inpatient admission, prompted by increased cutting and a plan to overdose on her psychiatric medications. In her initial appointments with her MBT therapist, the therapist introduced the potential relevance of the BPD diagnosis as a manner of understanding Katherine's difficulties with instability. Katherine *really, really* did not like the idea of having a personality disorder. As a physician, she knew all about the stigma connected with BPD. Her colleagues would snicker whenever they had to deal with patients with BPD, calling them "attention-seeking," "selfish," and "manipulative"—the exact opposite of how she saw herself. But when her new therapist reviewed the diagnostic criteria with her, she could not deny that many of these symptoms resonated with her: efforts to avoid abandonment and rejection; instability in self-esteem and identity; suicidality and self-injury; extreme sensitivity of mood; chronic feelings of emptiness; difficulties with anger; and challenges trusting people when she was under stress.

Katherine started to learn that BPD can present itself in a variety of different ways, depending on the particular person with the disorder. Even before the treatment had officially started, she started feeling a newfound sense of hope. She had long assumed that there was something intrinsically wrong with her—that she was defective in a way that meant she would never get better. But if her challenges were simply related to a common diagnosis that was highly responsive to treatment, this opened up the possibility that change could actually happen for her. It almost gave her shivers to think this way: *There might be a way out.*

Katherine was having the experience shared by many patients with BPD, when they first start receiving treatment that is evidence-based for their unique needs and vulnerabilities. This book is about the form of therapy that Katherine ended up receiving, which is one of the most effective forms of treatment for BPD: mentalization-based treatment, or "MBT." So let's transition to learning a bit about MBT—how MBT explains the problem of BPD, and how it can help.

Chapter Review 1.1
What Is Making You Feel So Unstable?

Key Facts about Borderline Personality Disorder

- Borderline personality disorder, or "BPD" for short, is a serious mental health condition marked by challenges with instability—more specifically, instability in emotions, self-esteem, relationships, and behavior.

- In the United States, the estimated prevalence of BPD is 1.6%, with a lifetime prevalence as high as 5.9%.

- In treatment settings, 12% of outpatients and 22% of inpatients have BPD.

- BPD is associated with a range of psychosocial challenges

  - Interpersonal instability

  - Work impairment

  - Suicidal and self-injurious behavior: 30% of people with BPD attempt suicide, 90% have engaged in some form of self-injury, and 6% die from suicide

  - Other psychiatric conditions, such as depression, anxiety, addiction, eating disorders, and PTSD

- Research suggests that people with BPD get better: 50–70% of people with BPD no longer meet criteria for the diagnosis over the long term, with significant improvements in depression and overall functionality.

- The treatment of choice for BPD is psychotherapy. There are a range of highly effective therapies for BPD, including mentalization-based treatment (MBT).

The Diagnostic Criteria for BPD from the DSM-5-TR

Individuals with BPD meet five out of the following nine criteria.

1. Frantic efforts to avoid real or imagined abandonment.

2. A pattern of unstable and intense interpersonal relationships characterized by alternating between extremes of idealization and devaluation.

3. Identity disturbance: markedly and persistently unstable self-image or sense of self.

4. Impulsivity in at least two areas that are potentially self-damaging.

5. Recurrent suicidal behavior, gestures, or threats, or self-mutilating behavior.

6. Affective instability due to a marked reactivity of mood.

7. Chronic feelings of emptiness.

8. Inappropriate, intense anger or difficulty controlling anger.

9. Transient, stress-related paranoid ideation or severe dissociative symptoms.

2

Borderline Personality Disorder as a Deficit in Mentalization

Mentalization, also referred to as "mentalizing," is defined as the ability to "read," access, and reflect on mental states in yourself as well as other people. "Mental states" are all the invisible stuff of the mind: thoughts, beliefs, emotions, desires, needs, attitudes, values, feelings about yourself, and personality traits. Mentalizing is thus a fundamentally imaginative capacity. You cannot literally see such things, but you imagine them, and you make presumptions and conjectures about them.

Mentalization-based treatment (MBT) utilizes this conception of mentalization to explain the challenges that you experience in borderline personality disorder (BPD). MBT observes that people with BPD can often mentalize quite well, in that you are often sensitively and empathically attuned to other people's thoughts and feelings. However, there are two key conditions under which your mentalizing can get disrupted:

- situations where you feel rejected, criticized, or abandoned; or
- whenever you are experiencing an intense emotion.

These experiences fall under the heading of *attachment insecurity*—that is, scenarios where your need to connect with other people gets stimulated or threatened. Studies show that BPD is associated with increased attachment anxiety (Smith & South, 2020), such that people with BPD can struggle with negative feelings about themselves, relying extensively on other people for a sense of self-worth and stability. (More on all of this in Chapter 8, "What is Your Attachment Style?")

Under those circumstances, your mentalizing can sometimes "go offline"—that is, you struggle to reflect on mental states in yourself and others in a careful, flexible, emotionally engaged manner. This theory has been supported by extensive research suggesting that people with BPD can experience significant problems reflecting on mental states in themselves and other people (Bora, 2021; Johnson et al., 2022; Németh et al., 2018).[1] These problems in mentalizing can take a range of shapes in BPD:

- Confusion about what you are feeling and wanting, or only noticing a narrower range of feelings in yourself
- Struggling to accurately "read," interpret, and understand what other people are thinking and feeling

---

[1] It is important to note that deficits in mentalizing are not unique to BPD. Science shows that these deficits are actually associated with a range of different psychiatric challenges, including anxiety (Sloover et al., 2022), depression (Rifkin-Zybutz et al., 2021), trauma and PTSD (Stevens & Jovanovic, 2019), eating disorders (Gagliardini et al., 2020), psychotic disorders (Lysaker et al., 2021), substance use disorders (Imperatori et al., 2020), and personality disorders other than just BPD (Bateman et al., 2023; Drozek & Unruh, 2020; Luyten et al., 2020; Newbury-Helps et al., 2017).

Mentalization. Robert P. Drozek, Oxford University Press. © Oxford University Press 2025.
DOI: 10.1093/oso/9780198916857.003.0002

- Reflexively assuming that others are judging you, disliking you, not caring about you, or wanting to reject or abandon you
- Uncertainty about "why" you are feeling the way you are feeling, especially when you are struggling
- Finding it challenging to understand and modify your own contributions to problematic dynamics in relationships
- Relying extensively on other individuals' minds in order to understand your own feelings and opinions
- Depending on other people (e.g., their physical presence, validation, and support) to feel safe, secure, and stable in yourself
- Encountering panic, rage, and hopelessness when you feel rejected or abandoned by others
- Failing to consistently "pause" and reflect when you feel rejected or mistreated by others
- Feeling compelled to engage in concrete behaviors (e.g., reassurance-seeking, angry outbursts, self-injury, suicidal actions) in order to manage feelings of overwhelming distress
- Falling into dissociation, or disconnection from your own emotions and desires. At times, you might be more "in your head," rather than "in your heart."
- Experiencing deficits in empathy toward others, especially when you are feeling frustrated or angry with them
- Perhaps most importantly, feeling CERTAIN that particular things are true. These experiences do not *feel* like mental states or perspectives—they feel like facts.
  - "I am bad, disgusting, and worthless."
  - "The only way for me to feel better is to hurt myself."
  - "I need this person to be with me in order to feel OK."
  - "This individual is problematic and unkind, and they have treated me horribly."

MBT suggests that, when you are struggling to mentalize in the above ways, you lose the presence of mind to see and do things in a different way, naturally sliding back into destructive patterns: interpersonal reactivity, arguments with other people, impulsive actions, and desires to hurt yourself. These maladaptive behaviors can be seen as an unfortunate but inevitable "side effect" of problems in mentalizing. On this theory, you are not fully choosing to take these actions. Rather, these actions just sort of *happen* to you, given that you have temporarily lost your ability to reflect on mental states.

Mentalizing Warm-up

Now that you have a clearer sense of the different problems in mentalizing, consider what you have learned about Katherine, the physician with BPD discussed in Chapter 1. Where do you observe deficits in mentalization in Katherine's history of depression and emotional instability?

You might know what you "should" think or do; you might even know "why" you are struggling. But this knowledge is unable to translate into a different outcome. Things can go fine 90% of the time in your life, but during the remaining 10% of time, the whole system can unravel. And unfortunately, that 10% of time ends up causing 100% of your difficulties. **In MBT's view, the problem is that you have already lost the ability to mentalize.** In that state, all of the skills and insights in the world will not make much difference. See Figure 2.1 for a visual rendering of this theory.

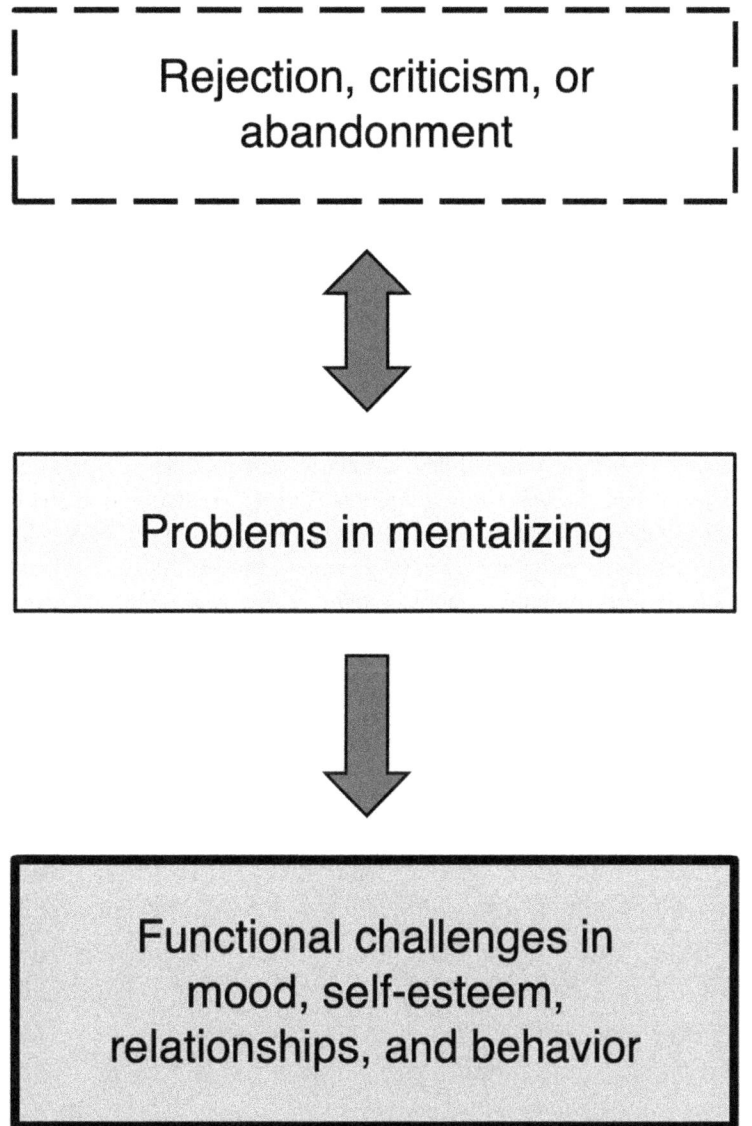

Figure 2.1 MBT's theory of borderline personality disorder (BPD). When encountering experiences of rejection, criticism, or abandonment, people with BPD struggle to mentalize in flexible, adaptive, and effective ways. This leads to the functional difficulties associated with BPD: instability in mood, self-esteem, relationships, and behavior.

To illustrate these ideas, let's return to Katherine, the patient discussed in Chapter 1. From the perspective of mentalizing, Katherine's challenges reflecting on mental states might include:

- Basing her sense of self-esteem and self-worth on academics, success, functionality, her mother's view of her, and always "appearing happy" to the world
- Difficulties with emotional instability triggered by experiences of rejection or criticism (e.g., by her mother, by classmates)
- Struggling to "pause" and reflect in those moments on her own mental states, and on the mental states of others
- Rigid, overly certain views of herself and other people, which then lead her to experience intense, volatile emotions surrounding the issue in question.
  - "My mother is aggressive, intrusive, and controlling."
  - "I am bad, disgusting, ugly, and worthless."
  - "I deserve to be punished."
  - "No one wants to be with me, and that is never going to change."
- Feeling like she can only alleviate her psychological distress by engaging in specific behaviors: fantasizing about suicide, writing suicide notes, cutting herself

According to MBT, these problems with reflectiveness served as the primary driver of Katherine's difficulties with emotional instability. Since she based her self-esteem on these external markers of success, she *had* to pursue success and achievement—without these things, she lacked a coherent sense of self. Similarly, since Katherine's self-stability rested on others' views of her, she was thrown into states of dysregulation and shame when she felt rejected or criticized by other people. Having lost her ability to reflect, Katherine felt overwhelmed by a sense of certainty about own badness and worthlessness. This badness did not feel like a belief or assumption—it was a *felt fact*. For Katherine, she *was* bad in these moments, and so she needed to act accordingly: by fantasizing about suicide, writing suicide notes, and cutting herself. In MBT's view, these experiences were not fully "chosen" by Katherine. Without the ability to mentalize, she was acting on reflex, lacking any meaningful sense of agency to regulate her emotions and behaviors.

Can you relate to any of these difficulties with reflectiveness? Try completing Worksheet 2.1, which examines the connection between your insecurities and problems with mentalization.

Worksheet 2.1
Identifying Your Attachment Insecurities
and Problems in Mentalizing

(1) MBT suggests that there exists an inverse connection between attachment insecurity and mentalizing abilities. List at least three areas where you tend to feel more insecure, about yourself or in your relationships.

(2) Now looking at those three areas, how have you struggled to mentalize when you are feeling insecure in those ways? Remember that mentalizing involves "holding on to your mind" when you are under stress, and deficits in mentalizing involve *losing* your ability to reflect in these moments.

(3) See below for a list of troubles in mentalizing that many individuals with BPD experience. Circle any difficulties with which you can identify—where you struggle to flexibly reflect on mental states in yourself and other people.

Confusion about what you are feeling and wanting, or only noticing a narrower range of feelings in yourself

Struggling to accurately "read," interpret, and understand what other people are thinking and feeling

Reflexively assuming that other people are seeing you negatively, or wanting to reject or abandon you

Uncertainty about "why" you are feeling the way you are feeling, especially when you are struggling

Finding it challenging to understand and shift your own contributions to problematic dynamics in relationships

Relying extensively on other people's minds in order to understand your own feelings and opinions

Depending on other people (e.g., their physical presence, validation, and support) to feel safe, secure, and stable in yourself

Experiencing deficits in empathy toward others, especially when you are frustrated or angry with them

[continued on next page]

Failing to consistently "pause" and reflect when you feel rejected or mistreated by others

Feeling CERTAIN that particular things are true (e.g., regarding yourself, other people, the future)

Falling into dissociation, or disconnection from your own emotions and desires

Encountering panic, rage, and hopelessness when you feel rejected or abandoned by others

Feeling compelled to engage in concrete behaviors (e.g., reassurance-seeking, angry outbursts, self-injury, suicidal actions) in order to manage overwhelming distress

Other problems in mentalizing not included here:

(4) What challenges in functionality have you encountered when you have struggled to mentalize in the above ways? These could involve instability in mood, self-esteem, relationships, or behaviors.

THE AIM OF MBT: LEARNING HOW TO REFLECT RATHER THAN REFLEX

Hopefully you are starting to consider the implications of this theory for your own experiences with instability. If we see BPD as involving deficits in mentalization, that means that your challenges with emotional dysregulation are not truly "your fault." In the moments of dysregulation, there is not enough of a "you" to have a fault! This also informs MBT's approach to addressing these difficulties. The aim of MBT is helping you to reflect on mental states, specifically in the areas where you tend to get "stuck" in your life and relationships. MBT focuses on the areas of your experience where you struggle with insecurities or instability, working with you to

- **START** reflecting on relevant mental states (e.g., in yourself, in other people) related to the problem areas;
- **RESUME** reflecting on mental states in those areas, when you have fallen out of a mentalizing stance; and
- **CONTINUE** reflecting on mental states, even when you are under emotional and interpersonal stress.

The research on MBT suggests that, when people with BPD are able to mentalize in these ways, they experience significant functional improvements in their lives, including decreased depression, anger issues, paranoia, hostility, self-injury, suicidality, medication usage, and inpatient hospitalizations, as well as notable advances in social, academic, and vocational functioning (Bateman & Fonagy, 1999, 2001, 2008, 2009; Bateman et al., 2016; Bateman, Constantinou, et al., 2021).

As you learn how to "hold on to your mind" in your key areas of insecurity, you gain an increased sense of internal freedom and autonomy. The world exerts less control over you, you are less dominated by your maladaptive tendencies, and you are more able to make choices that reflect your best self. For all of these reasons, MBT targets the "upstream" issue of problems in reflectiveness, working to bring mentalization back online whenever it has become disrupted. This then indirectly resolves the "downstream" problems of functional impairment, as illustrated in Figure 2.2.

In reviewing MBT's emphasis on mentalizing, it is also useful to consider the things that MBT does NOT seek in treatment. Some of these might surprise you.

- MBT does not work to change the content of your thoughts, for example by trying to get you to think more positively.
- MBT does not attempt to directly modify your behavior, nor does it teach behavioral skills.
- MBT does not try to offer you insight, whether about the past, the present, or unconscious dynamics.

All of these techniques (e.g., cognitive restructuring, behavioral activation, self-understanding) sound lovely on paper. As long as you are "in the zone" and feeling OK, they work just fine. But without mentalizing, it becomes nearly impossible to consistently and effectively implement these strategies. Accordingly, while many types of therapy try to change and evolve the content of patients' experience (e.g., through modifying thoughts or behavior, or by generating insight), MBT simply seeks to stimulate a *process* of reflectiveness about mental states. As you are able to do this in the areas where you struggle, you will naturally start to feel better, like yourself more, and engage more effectively in your life and relationships.

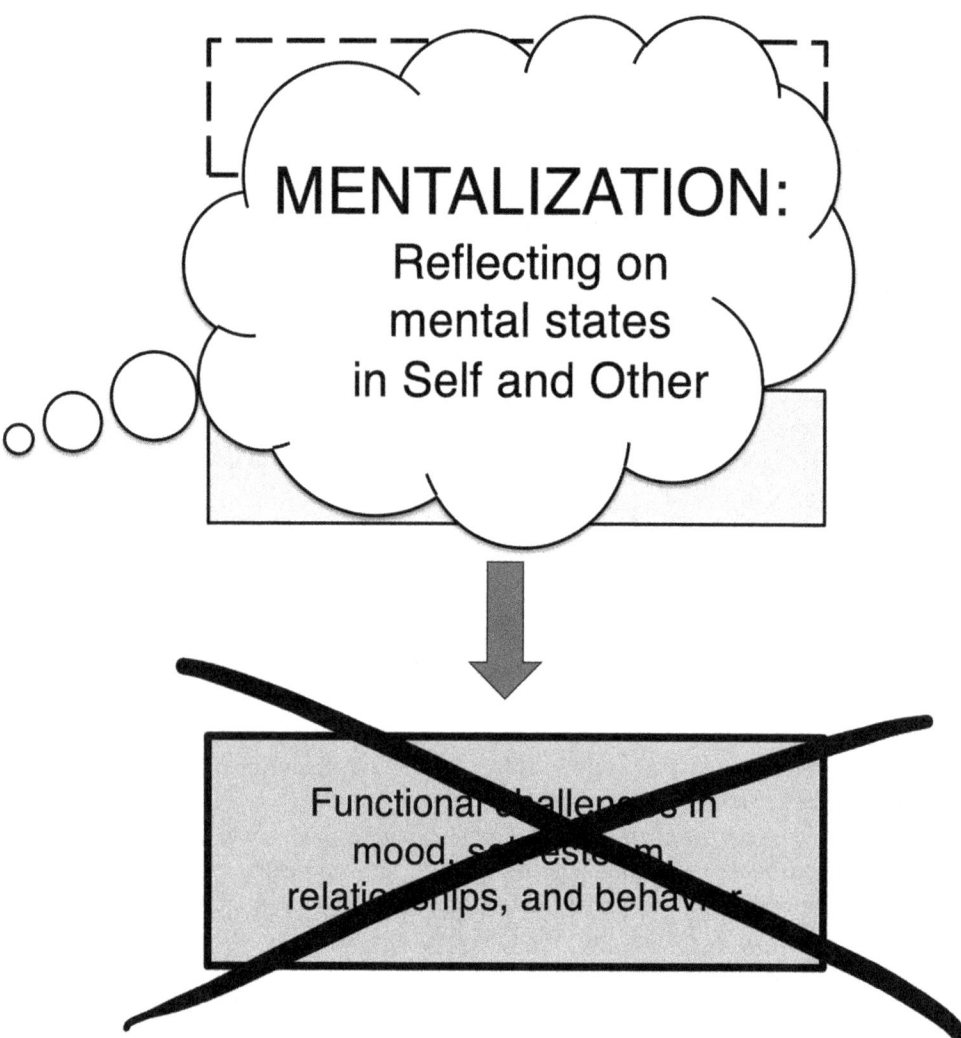

Figure 2.2 The aim of MBT as a therapy. MBT's primary focus is helping people to mentalize—to reflect on mental states in themselves and others. As individuals gain the ability to mentalize around their core areas of insecurity, they experience improvements in mood, self-esteem, relationships, and behavior.

"Wait," you might be thinking. "This all sounds too good to be true. Why would 'reflection' make my life any better? I already worry too much. If anything, I need to be thinking LESS about all of my insecurities!" I hear your point, and I can assure you that many patients starting MBT share similar concerns. However, mentalization is not the same thing as obsessing, ruminating, and worrying. In fact, such preoccupations are usually *anti*-mentalizing!

The purpose of this book is to show you how to mentalize, in a manner that does not just replicate the areas where you have struggled. In other words, we are going to help you to productively REFLECT about mental states, rather than engaging with them reflexively or reactively. As a trainer in MBT through the Anna Freud Centre in London, and as faculty at Harvard Medical School, I have the opportunity to train other clinicians in how to deliver MBT in an evidence-based manner, consistent with what the research shows about MBT's effectiveness. In my current position at McLean Hospital, I am privileged to work in some of the leading treatment programs in the world for patients with BPD, including the Gunderson Outpatient Program and the Mentalization-based Treatment Clinic. In those roles, I provide individual and group MBT to patients with a wide range of diagnoses, including BPD, mood disorders, anxiety disorders, addiction, and trauma and dissociative disorders. When patients are starting in our treatment programs, I regularly hear the same sorts of questions:

- "What really IS mentalizing? I am kind of confused about what it even means."
- "What would it look like to mentalize about this situation? How do I even do it?"
- "Are there any books that I can read about what MBT is, and how it works?"
- "Do you have any worksheets that you can give me about this, like they have in DBT?"

Unfortunately, despite the fact that MBT is one of leading therapies for BPD, there is not a single book about MBT written primarily for people struggling with the symptoms of BPD. Whereas dialectical behavior therapy (DBT) has Linehan's (2015a) landmark *DBT skills training handouts and worksheets*, there is no corollary in MBT. This means that MBT's wisdom resides primarily in the mind of a relatively small group of skilled clinicians, whom the majority of patients with BPD are unable to access.

This book aims to finally address this deficit: walking you through the core elements in MBT as a therapy, and outlining the therapeutic strategies that make MBT so effective. As the first book for non-clinicians about MBT, it will show you how to apply MBT's principles in your everyday life, so that—like the tens of thousands of patients whose lives have already been changed by MBT—you can get relief from the suffering of BPD. With the help of worksheets, mentalizing prompts, and case examples from actual treatments of patients with BPD, I will try to keep things clear, practical, and always accessible. The symptoms of BPD are painful enough—you should not have to be working so hard to discover techniques that can genuinely make a difference in your life.

More on all of this, and the structure of the book, in the upcoming chapters. For now, let's return to Katherine, one of the many patients we have treated here in the MBT Clinic at McLean. We can consider how things progressed for her, once she started applying the principles of MBT to address her difficulties.

CONTINUING WITH KATHERINE: HER EXPERIENCE IN MBT

Getting started in MBT, Katherine identified her primary goal as remaining out of the hospital, which she understood would involve decreasing her depression, suicidality, and self-injurious behavior. The therapist worked with Katherine to consider the ways in which she struggled with reflecting on mental states in herself and others, synthesizing these ideas in writing in the form of an *MBT formulation* of her difficulties (see Chapter 5). This formulation reviewed Katherine's triggers for emotional dysregulation (e.g., criticism by her mother, feeling ignored by colleagues, feeling insecure about her appearance); her strengths in mentalizing (e.g., a high capacity for empathy and self-reflection when not dysregulated); and her main challenges with mentalizing (e.g., rigid beliefs about her badness, tendencies toward intellectualization and abstraction, feeling compelled to engage in visible behaviors like cutting in order to regulate her internal states).

The earliest phase of the treatment focused on Katherine's episodes of what she then called "my depression." Katherine initially described her depression in largely physical terms (e.g., lack of motivation, decreased energy, desire to sleep, feelings of deadness and numbness), adamantly denying any psychological or relational dimensions to the mood state: "My depression is not 'about' anything—there's no content to it. Everything in my life is really fine, other than this feeling."

Recognizing this seemingly intractable area of Katherine's experience, the therapist diverted attention to a related domain where Katherine appeared more capable of reflection: her difficulties with self-hatred. Katherine was able to articulate her deep feelings of insecurity about her appearance. She saw herself as ugly and disgusting, leading to powerful feelings of hopelessness about ever being able to have a romantic relationship. When the therapist inquired if this meant Katherine *wanted* such a relationship, Katherine reluctantly admitted this, also expressing her shame for desiring something that would never be possible for her. As the therapeutic work progressed, Katherine revealed something she had never disclosed before—namely, that she actually *was* in an intimate relationship at the time, with a fellow resident in her program. When she first met this person, she had liked him and wanted to date him, but the resident was only interested in a "friends with benefits" arrangement. "It is really nice to be with him, to have just some sort of physical contact with someone. But every time he leaves, I just feel horrible about myself, like 'See, this is all you are good for, but no one will ever want to be with you because you are so disgusting and pathetic.'"

Recognizing a much broader array of mental states in Katherine's experience, the therapist invited her to reflect on the possible connection between these states and her experience of her "depression": "It sounds like, whenever he leaves, you end up feeling much worse about yourself. Do you see any connection between these feelings and how things play out with your depression?" Katherine recognized that she would often feel less depressed on the days she was planning to see this person, but her desires to hurt herself would intensify on the days *after* these sexual encounters, or whenever he would decline spending time with her.

After five months in treatment, Katherine decided to end the relationship with the fellow resident: "I think I would rather be alone than be in this thing that just makes me feel so ashamed." While Katherine felt confident about this decision, it also sent her into a period of intense loneliness and despair, during which she was overcome by desires to cut herself with razors—a behavior in which she had not engaged since starting treatment.

This led to a highly productive period of the treatment where Katherine began reflecting on what she experienced as the most compelling form of caretaking—where she felt paralyzed and incapacitated in her illness, and others took physical actions (e.g., holding her, offering explicit reassurance) to comfort her. As Katherine described it, "When I'm helping my patients, I'm not allowed to have any needs. They are the sick ones, not me. But it just builds up over time, and it reaches the point where *I* need caretaking, too. That's when I get depressed, and wanting to cut more."

The therapist observed, "You seem to be equating 'needs' with 'illness.' What leads to the connection there for you?"

Katherine explained further: "I don't WANT to need anything from anybody. It makes me feel pathetic, disgusting. I guess the only way I feel justified asking for attention is if I am really sick, like so sick that I am unable to move or function."

This recognition opened up a new and generative path in the treatment: helping Katherine to imagine ways in which she might *experience* her emotions and desires outside the context of designated psychiatric illness. When she was treating patients, Katherine started to give herself permission to engage with feelings formerly reserved for her depressive episodes, including sadness, loneliness, and a desire to be comforted by others. With friends, Katherine tried to share less about her psychiatric symptoms, instead engaging with them around topics like work, relationships, and common interests. Perhaps most strikingly, Katherine created a profile on a dating app. To her surprise, she was flooded with people wanting to go out with her. As she began to date again after many years, she noticed a lift in her mood, and a sense of satisfaction from moving toward her goal of pursuing a stable relationship with a long-term partner.

A pivotal moment in the treatment came when Katherine finally threw away the razors she had used for cutting, which she had been saving "just in case I needed them." By the end of her first year in MBT, Katherine had evinced notable functional improvements (e.g., improved attendance at work, no hospitalizations, no incidents of self-injury), as well as a subtle but notable shift in her experience of herself: "I can't really say that I like myself yet. That would be going too far. But I do feel a little less convinced that I am completely awful, and every once in a while, I actually feel OK. That gives me a bit more hope about my future—that I could have a life where I feel more connected to other people, and maybe even connected to myself as well."

Chapter Review 2.1
Borderline Personality Disorder as a Deficit in Mentalization

Mentalization

Mentalization is the ability to "read," access, and reflect on mental states in yourself and other people.

Mental states are the invisible stuff of the mind: thoughts, beliefs, emotions, desires, needs, attitudes, values, feelings about oneself, and personality traits.

Mentalization and BPD

- Science shows that people with BPD can experience significant problems reflecting on mental states in themselves and other people.

- Mentalization is significantly impacted by *attachment insecurity*, or experiences where your need to connect with other people gets stimulated or threatened.

- In BPD, there are two key conditions under which mentalizing gets disrupted:

  - Situations where you feel rejected, criticized, or abandoned; or

  - Whenever you are experiencing an intense emotion.

- Problems in mentalizing include:

  - Confusion about what you are feeling and wanting

  - Struggling to accurately "read" other people, or assuming that they are seeing you negatively

  - Relying on others to understand yourself, and to feel safe and secure

  - Failing to "pause" and reflect when you feel rejected or mistreated

  - Needing to engage in concrete behaviors to manage distress

  - Feeling CERTAIN that particular things are true (e.g., regarding yourself, other people, the future)

- These problems in mentalizing lead to the functional difficulties of BPD: instability in mood, self-esteem, relationships, and behavior.

[continued on next page]

Rejection, criticism, or abandonment

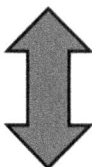

Problems in mentalizing

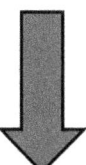

Functional challenges in mood, self-esteem, relationships, and behavior

Chapter Review 2.2
The Aim of MBT for Borderline Personality Disorder:
Learning How to Reflect Rather than Reflex

The Aims of Mentalization-Based Treatment

MBT's primary aim is helping you to mentalize—to reflect on mental states in yourself and others.

MBT focuses on the areas of your experience where you struggle with insecurities or instability, working with you to

- **START** reflecting on relevant mental states (e.g., in yourself, in other people) related to the problem areas;

- **RESUME** reflecting on mental states in those areas, when you have fallen out of a mentalizing stance; and

- **CONTINUE** reflecting on mental states, even when you are under emotional and interpersonal stress.

What MBT Does Not Do

MBT does **NOT** work to change the content of your thoughts, for example by trying to get you to think more positively.

MBT does **NOT** attempt to directly modify your behavior, nor does it teach behavioral skills.

MBT does **NOT** try to offer you insight, whether about the past, the present, or unconscious dynamics.

The Benefits of MBT

Multiple studies show that MBT leads to significant benefits for people with BPD, including

- Reductions in depression, anger issues, paranoia, hostility, self-injury, suicidality, medication usage, and inpatient hospitalizations; and

- Notable advances in social, academic, and vocational functioning.

As you gain the ability to mentalize around your core areas of attachment-related insecurities, you experience improvements in mood, self-esteem, relationships, and behavior.

[continued on next page]

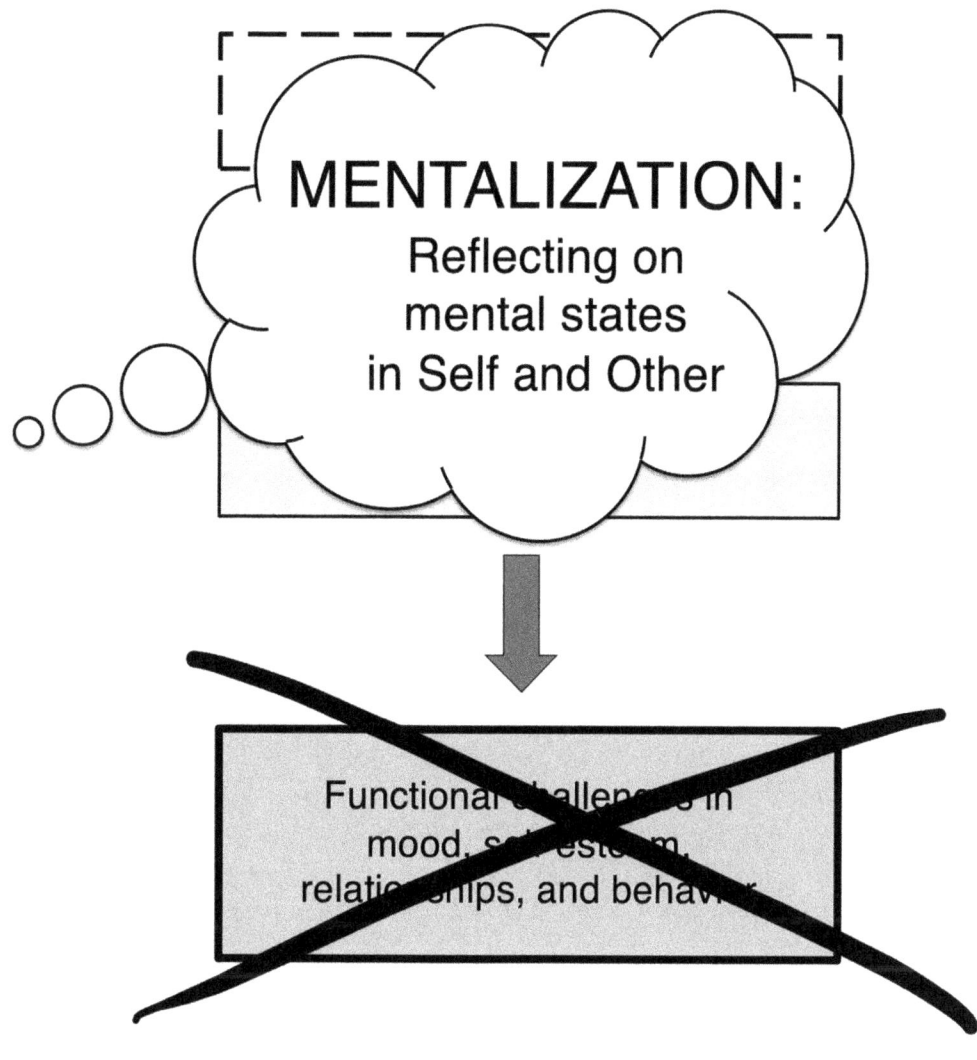

3

Mentalization: What Is It?

Looking inward, you notice a rumbling inside of you. You seem to be feeling something, but it is not immediately clear what that feeling is. It could be anxiety, but it also feels like anticipation and excitement. Perhaps a bit of both? At another time, when interacting with a colleague, you notice her looking away from you, grimacing with a pained expression on her face. Is she upset with you in some way, or is something else on her mind that has nothing to do with you? It is difficult to tell. In a different scenario, seemingly out of nowhere, you experience a sudden surge of joy, satisfaction, and comfort arising within you. Now the emotions are unmistakable, but it is not obvious what these feelings are *about*. Where are they coming from? What is going on—inside of you, or in your life—that is leading you to feel this way?

All of these experiences are examples of *mentalization*. Mentalization can variously focus on yourself as well as other people. You look at other people, and you consider a wide range of visible data—facial expressions, eye contact, verbal communications, tone and volume of voice, bodily posture and movements—in order to understand what they are going through. You go from the "outside" to the "inside."

You also do something analogous with yourself. You are able to look inward, to introspect and consider what *you* are going through: what you are feeling, wanting, and believing. Mentalization is thus a two-pronged capacity. At any given moment, it can be directed toward Self or Other, to a greater or lesser degree and with varying levels of intentionality. Sometimes you might mentalize quite deliberately, "slowing things down" in order to figure out what another person is experiencing. In other moments, you mentalize more reflexively and automatically, drawing conclusions about yourself and others without really pausing to consider what you are presuming.

In more experience-near ways, mentalization is variously described as:

- Attending to mental states
- Holding mind in mind
- Making things mental: to "mental" "-ize"
- Thinking about thinking
- Understanding misunderstanding
- Seeing others from the inside and yourself from the outside

In different ways and with different emphases, all of these definitions underscore the essence of mentalization: It involves forming some idea or image about psychological processes in yourself or other people.

A BRIEF HISTORY OF MENTALIZATION

The idea of mentalizing has a long and storied ancestry throughout the history of philosophy and psychology. Mentalization was foreshadowed in Plato's tripartite conception of the soul, where *logos* is able to reflect upon (and thus regulate) both spirits and appetites. With his famous dictum "I think, therefore I am," the 17th century philosopher René Descartes

Mentalization. Robert P. Drozek, Oxford University Press. © Oxford University Press 2025.
DOI: 10.1093/oso/9780198916857.003.0003

similarly prioritized reflective process as a foundational dimension of human experience. Contemporary analytic philosopher Daniel Dennett (1971) took a giant leap towards mentalization with his notion of "the intentional stance," understood as the tendency to explain and predict other people's behavior in terms of beliefs and desires.

Within cognitive psychology, researchers in the 1980s utilized the false belief experiment to show that children as young as 4–6 years of age already possess a robust "theory of mind," or "an ability to impute mental states to themselves and others" (Wimmer & Perner, 1983, p. 104). In research on autism, Simon Baron-Cohen (1990) suggested that children with autism suffer from "mind-blindedness," or a developmental delay in attributing mental states to other people.

This brings us firmly into the arena of what is now commonly referred to as "mentalization." While the term had been floating around within psychoanalysis since the 1950s, our current understanding of mentalization was first expounded in 1989 by Peter Fonagy, a Hungarian-born British psychoanalyst and clinical psychologist. Deeply committed to understanding and treating people with borderline personality disorder (BPD), Fonagy (1989) introduced the theory reviewed in Chapter 2—namely, that individuals with BPD struggle with intermittent deficits in the ability to flexibly reflect on mental states in themselves and other people. Synthesizing concepts from attachment theory, psychoanalysis, and developmental psychology, Fonagy and his colleagues (2002) proposed a comprehensive theory explaining how healthy mentalization develops in adaptive parent–child relationships, as well as how disruptions in these relationships can impair the ability to mentalize, leaving people vulnerable to instability in emotions, relationships, and sense of self.

More on all of this in Chapter 4. In the meantime, let's take a deeper dive into the various shapes that mentalizing takes in everyday life and relationships.

DOMAINS OF MENTALIZATION

When people are first starting to learn about mentalizing, they often feel confused about the different meanings of the single term. Mentalization clearly involves considering "what" you are feeling. Does it also entail trying to understand "why" you are feeling that way? And then there is the issue the *intensity* of the feeling: Does mentalizing also cover "how" you are relating to these feelings in yourself? The answer to all of these questions is an emphatic YES!

In order to help people understand the various meanings and usages of "mentalization," some colleagues and I have suggested that mentalizing tends to unfold across three different domains of experience. We refer to this as the domain-based theory of mentalization (Drozek & Henry, 2021; Drozek et al., 2023). Let's take a look at these three different domains. This will help you get better acquainted with the nuances involved in mentalizing, while also recognizing how you are already doing it, in ways that really make a difference in your life.

Content-mentalizing: Reflecting on "what" people are feeling

When you are mentalizing about content, you focus on "what" people are experiencing: thoughts, emotions, desires, and so on. With other people, you seek to "read," perceive, and understand what they are going through. With yourself, you try to identify and "put words on" what is happening inside of you.

I was going on a walk with my kids one day, trying to explain the differences between the three different types of mentalizing. (These poor children!) Since they are young, I came up with a metaphor to illustrate content-mentalizing. It was a beautiful, crisp autumn day in New England, and I noticed a bright orange leaf on the ground. I explained that content-mentalizing is like when you are just looking at the leaf itself. What does it look like? What is its shape, color, and texture? What are the edges of the leaf like? How does the blade attach to the stalk? Does the leaf seem fresh, new, and strong? Or is it more brittle and fragile, about to break apart into little pieces?

Analogously, when considering your own emotions, you try to regard the feeling in and of itself. What does this emotion feel like inside of you? What are its qualities: its intensity, pressure, or direction? Where do you feel the emotion in your body? Is the feeling more static, or can you notice any changes in the emotion across time—any shifts as you are observing it?

Common Mental States Involved in Mentalizing

- **Thought:** a verbal idea or opinion that a person has at any given moment. "Given all of the traffic, it is going to take so long to get home today." "I cannot believe that he said that to me. He is such a jerk!"

- **Belief:** a viewpoint about oneself, other people, or reality that one takes to be true. "I am too emotionally sensitive." "My husband is pulling away from me." "The two-party system is fundamentally flawed and ruining our country."

- **Emotion:** a feeling, sentiment, or mood, usually accompanied by some bodily experience. While thoughts and beliefs are "in your head," emotions are more "in your heart." Often emotions have a positive or negative valence to them, and they can often be described with one word: sadness, anxiety, anger, happiness, exhilaration.

- **Desire:** a wish or impulse that some event will happen, or that some other scenario will *not* happen. Desires are always focused on the future, or some hypothetical scenario that does not yet exist. "I want you to see me as a good person." "She is hoping to get a promotion at work." "I wish that I were more intelligent." "You don't seem to want to talk about this right now."

- **Self-state:** a feeling about oneself—who one is as a person, usually concerning one's own value and worth. Self-states are essentially a sub-category of emotions; they are emotions *about the self*. Examples include pride, insecurity, self-confidence, self-hatred, shame, and embarrassment. More abstractly, a person might consider issues of self-esteem and self-worth. "What is my sense of self-esteem like?" "He seems to have a pretty low opinion of himself."

- **Value:** an experience to which someone ascribes personal importance, worth, or meaning. Values can thus encompass ethical principles ("I always try to be honest"); standards for oneself or others ("I need to get straight A's in order to have value"); esteemed qualities or interpersonal approaches (e.g., kindness, intelligence, humility, authenticity); or domains of life that an individual takes to be meaningful (e.g., family, work, friendships).

Being able to recognize and identify mental states is foundational to issues of *identity and connectedness*. When you understand what is happening inside of you—what you believe, what you want, what you are feeling, what matters to you—you are able to remain grounded in your own experience. Content-mentalizing allows you to understand other people as well: who they are as people, what they are feeling, and what they care about in their lives. You "make sense" to yourself, and other people make sense to you as well. This provides you with a secure base from which you can safely and comfortably explore the world.

With these ideas in place, spend some time on Worksheet 3.1. This will help you to assess your own strengths in content-mentalizing, as well as the consequences of these capacities in your everyday life.

Worksheet 3.1
Recognizing Strengths in Mentalizing: Reflecting on Content

Mentalizing Yourself

(1) List mental states (e.g., thoughts, beliefs, emotions, desires, values, feelings about yourself) that you are easily able to recognize and describe in yourself.

(2) Recount a recent situation in which you were able to successfully identify a particular mental state in yourself. What (e.g., in the situation, in yourself) enabled you to effectively mentalize in this way?

(3) In this situation, what were the consequences of your adaptive mentalizing of yourself? For example, did it impact what you felt, how you behaved, or how you saw this situation?

Mentalizing Other People

(4) List mental states (e.g., thoughts, beliefs, emotions, desires, values, feelings about themselves) that you are easily able to "read" and recognize in other individuals.

[continued on next page]

(5) Describe a recent situation in which you were able to successfully understand a specific mental state in another person. What (e.g., in the situation, in yourself) allowed you to mentalize in this way?

(6) In this situation, what were the consequences of this adaptive mentalizing? For example, did it impact how you saw or related to the person?

[continued on next page]

Context-mentalizing: Reflecting on "why" people are feeling a certain way

You can also consider the connection between mental states and other elements "around" the experience: situations, behaviors, other psychological processes, and past history. This is the "why" of mentalizing: reflecting upon what has led to the feeling in question, and how that feeling ends up impacting other aspects of the situation. See Figure 3.1 for an illustration of these forms of mentalizing.

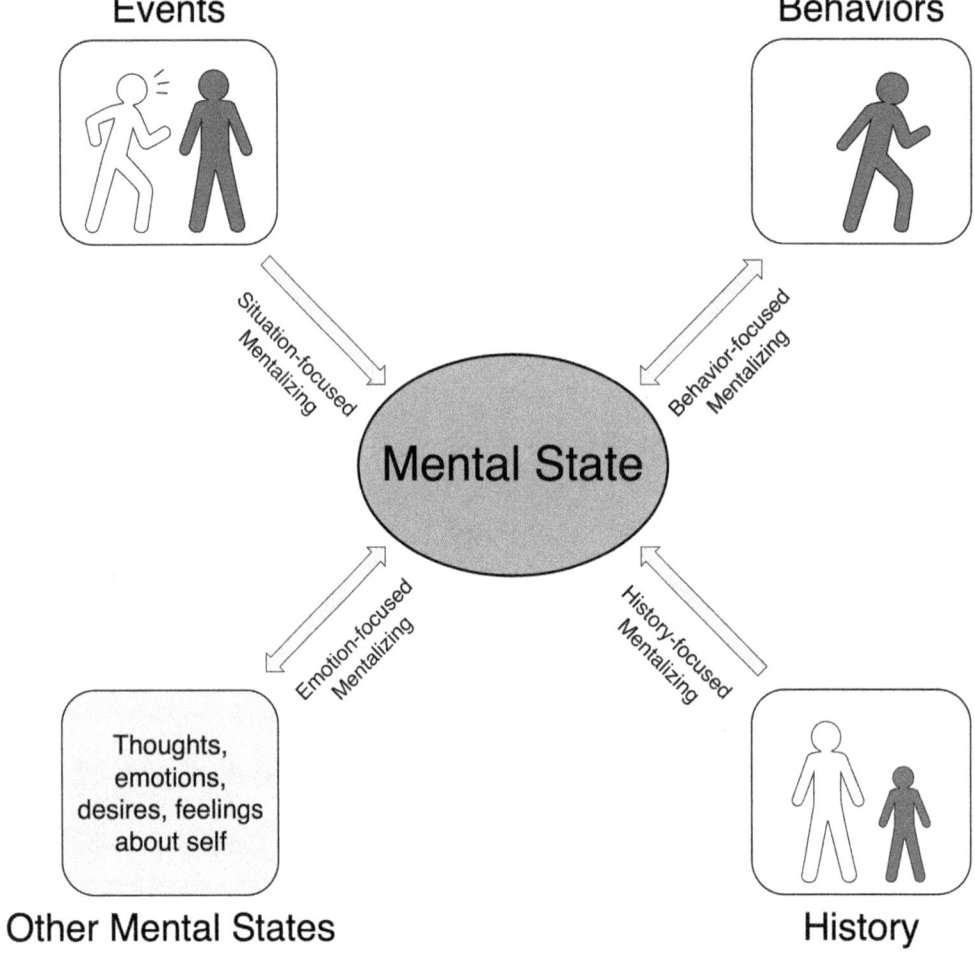

Figure 3.1 Types of context-mentalizing. Context-mentalizing involves considering the connection between mental states and other elements "around" the experience: situations, behaviors, other psychological processes, and past history.

Continuing with the metaphor of the leaf, you do not simply look at the leaf itself. You "expand your field of vision" to consider how the leaf is related to other parts of the environment. You notice that it is actually sitting on a pile of other leaves, which are supporting it and holding it up. Now you are also recognizing the leaf's backdrop: a tapestry of red, orange, brown, and even some green stretching out across the knotted earth. You think about the cool air surrounding the leaf. It is of course invisible, but you are now aware that the coldness is likely making the leaf itself cold. Zooming out even further, you can reflect upon how the leaf itself came to be sitting here in the first place: its origins as a tiny bud on the branch, its growth into a healthy green adult leaf, and its cell walls weakening as the tree prepared for the winter, leaving it vulnerable to the wind that finally whisked it away from its branch.

You can engage in analogous forms of reflection with context-mentalizing. To illustrate this, consider Mitchell, a 19-year-old college student with BPD who was experiencing increased anxiety about his grades and academic performance in his undergraduate courses. Mitchell had long struggled with perfectionism surrounding his schoolwork: holding himself to extremely strict standards, criticizing himself if he ever failed to meet them, and on several occasions while in high school, even hitting and scratching himself if he felt like he had done poorly on an assignment.

Now in college, as his feelings of anxiety were worsening, Mitchell was able to successfully reflect on the content of what he was feeling: "I am afraid that I am going to fail out of school. I'm doing fine so far, but I'm worried that is not going to continue: I'll get a bad grade on an assignment, and then I'll stop trying in the class. And if get a bad grade in a class, I'm terrified that I'll just stop trying at school in general. Like, what's the point of anything if my whole transcript has this black mark on it?"

Mitchell decided to stretch himself beyond simply *identifying* his feelings to considering the broader context of them.

Situation-focused mentalizing. *Situation-focused mentalizing* is reflecting on the connection between external events (e.g., interactions with others, visible circumstances, impersonal events) and feeling states in yourself or other people. Attempting to practice situation-focused mentalizing, Mitchell started to wonder, "What could be causing this sudden spike in my anxiety about failing out of school? I mean, I have always been anxious about my grades, but this is at a whole 'nother level." Mitchell realized that he had signed up for an advanced writing seminar this semester, with a professor who was notorious for being a very tough grader. As a biology major, Mitchell did not feel especially competent about his writing skills. Could that be contributing to his increased anxiety recently?

Behavior-focused mentalizing. *Behavior-focused mentalizing* is considering the link between feelings and actions: how a person's feelings impact their behavior, and also how their behavior influences how they feel. Along these lines, Mitchell examined the reciprocal relationship between his anxiety and his various actions and behaviors. Initially, he dealt with the anxiety by spending more time on all of his assignments, and by fastidiously working to make sure that "everything was perfect" before turning an assignment in. But as he felt increasingly overwhelmed by his coursework, he started to avoid even *looking* at his assignments until right before they were due. The more that he thought about them, the more anxious he felt. Reflecting on these issues, he was curious: How much of his anxiety was being caused by the schoolwork itself, versus his recent shift toward procrastination and avoidance?

Emotion-focused mentalizing. *Emotion-focused mentalizing* is contemplating the relationship between different emotions, desires, and self-states within yourself or other people. Mitchell then tried to tackle the question: "Other than just the anxiety, are there additional feelings in me that I have not been examining in all of this?" Mitchell was aware that college was not the only area of concern for him. He was quite socially isolated, and he felt highly insecure about his ability to build connections and friendships with other people. Privately obsessed with tabletop board games and roleplaying games, he had been hoping to start attending his school's Board Game Club, but now he was just focusing on his classes, the way that he always did. Mitchell wondered: Could his insecurities about socializing ever be impacting his academic anxieties? Even with all of the stress, it was a bit easier to think about school than relationships with other people—an area where he felt *completely* incompetent.

History-focused mentalizing. *History-focused mentalizing* is pondering the possible association between a person's feelings and their history and background. Mitchell asked himself: "Could anything from my past be playing into how stressed out I have been?" His parents were both successful engineers, and they always put a lot of pressure on him to do well in school. He would get grounded whenever he did *not* get straight A's. Over time, he started applying these same standards to himself: feeling good about himself whenever he did really well, and feeling worthless and ashamed whenever he made even little mistakes on tests and assignments. Mitchell thought to himself, "These used to be my parents' expectations, but now they have found their way into me. It's hard to escape when the attack is coming from the inside!"

All of these forms of reflection illustrate Mitchell not simply identifying "what" he was feeling, but considering "why" he was feeling that way. This is the heart of context-mentalizing. This type of mentalizing leads to a sense of agency and accountability in your life. When you are able to recognize what is impacting your emotions, they end up feeling less overwhelming to you, and you are able to take constructive steps to curb and modulate your feelings. Similarly, when you consider all of the different factors potentially impacting other people, those people seem more reasonable and understandable to you. You engage with others more effectively, in a manner consistent with their unique needs and personalities.

Let's try applying these ideas to your everyday experience, using Worksheet 3.2. How are you already context-mentalizing yourself and other people?

Worksheet 3.2
Recognizing Strengths in Mentalizing: Reflecting on Context

Situation-focused Mentalizing

(1) Describe a recent example where some external situation (e.g., event, interaction with another person) impacted how you were feeling.

(2) At the time, were you aware that the situation was affecting you? If so, what enabled you to understand this? If not, what interfered with that awareness?

(3) Detail a recent instance when you recognized how another person was being impacted by what was going on around them. What allowed you to be attuned to this?

Behavior-focused Mentalizing

(4) Share about some situation where your feelings significantly influenced how you behaved or engaged in that situation. What were those feelings, and what were those behaviors?

[continued on next page]

(5) Now relay another situation where your behaviors significantly impacted your feelings (e.g., emotions, desires, feelings about yourself). What were those behaviors, and what were those feelings?

(6) Describe a situation in which you noticed the connection between another person's feelings and behaviors. What enabled you to be attuned to this?

Emotion-focused Mentalizing

(7) Recount a recent experience when you were simultaneously aware of TWO feeling states in yourself (e.g., emotions, desires, feelings about yourself), which you saw as potentially related. What were those feelings, and what were your ideas about their connection to each other?

(8) Discuss a recent instance when you considered the potential presence of TWO feeling states in another person (e.g., emotions, desires, feelings about themself), which you saw as potentially linked. What were those feelings, and what were your ideas about their connection to each other?

Process-mentalizing: Reflecting on "how" people relate to mental states

So far we have explored two key domains of mentalizing: considering "what" you are feeling and examining "why" you are feeling that way. The final mentalizing domain concerns the process of "how" you relate to mental states in yourself and other people: psychologically versus concretely, flexibly versus rigidly, and authentically versus disconnectedly.

First, by definition, mentalizing focuses on the internal, psychological dimensions of everyday life. You do not just attend to objective aspects of reality when mentalizing: events, circumstances, behaviors, visible objects or characteristics. Rather, you prioritize considering *subjective* processes in Self and Other: thoughts, beliefs, emotions, motives, self-states, and so on.

Second, effective mentalizing always involves some level of flexibility. Part of focusing on mental states entails understanding the pervasive influence of *your* mental states on whatever you feel like you are "perceiving" about reality. You only have access to your perspective on any issue. This perspective is saturated with your personal biases, meanings, and personality, and so it likely says more about *you* than about the issue in question. Accordingly, you remain humble and tentative about what you can ever definitively "know" about yourself and other people. There are multiple valid ways to see the same topic, and thus, to borrow the oft-quoted adage, no one possesses "a monopoly on the Truth." This approach disallows any level of certainty, rigidity, or confidence about your own belief states.

Third, mentalizing means that you are authentically connected to mental states in yourself and other people. Within yourself, you are able to access and actually *feel* your emotions and desires, rather than simply "being aware" that they are happening in you. With others, you do not only "read" other people; you empathically resonate with (and care about) their feelings and needs. Their feelings move you and motivate you. Similarly, you feel genuinely interested in and curious about what is happening inside of yourself and other people. You are inquisitive, and you want to learn more.

Continuing with the metaphor of the leaf, you can imagine getting so close to the leaf that you are unable to see anything else: the other leaves, the ground below, or the tree above. The leaf is the only thing you see! (This is the rigidity and certainty.) Or you could focus so much on the outside visage of the leaf that you never consider its internal workings: the veins, the stomata, the mesophyll. (This is the concreteness and externalization.) Or you could back up so far away from the leaf that you can barely see it. You "know" the leaf is there, but it becomes just a vague shape in the distance you cannot really appreciate. (This is the disconnection.) In contrast, there is a stance you adopt where you can fully see the leaf, while also being able to take in all of the things around it. You are aware of the external features of the leaf (e.g., the now-orange skin, the stalk, the blade, the tip), but you also know that there is more to the leaf than meets the eye, just beneath the surface.

Analogously, at the level of process, mentalizing involves flexibility, connectedness, and a focus on psychological processes. These qualities play an essential role in stability and functionality in life. When you are aware of your initial perspectives *as* perspectives, they do not automatically control you as much. And when you are authentically connected to emotions in yourself and others, you are able to make choices that reflect your fullest self, and to engage with other people with authenticity, empathy, and emotional depth.

To illustrate, let's return to the college student Mitchell we discussed in the last section. Mitchell ended up starting on a course of individual mentalization-based treatment. At the outset of the therapy, Mitchell and his therapist prioritized exploring Mitchell's conviction that he was going to fail out of school. Mitchell came to gradually relate to this conviction as a psychological state, rather than an objective "fact" about reality. As he saw this experience as a changeable aspect of his own psychology, he became more able to question and interrogate it, and to see his academic capacities in new and different ways. Mitchell's avoidance and procrastination improved, and he felt less anxious and hopeless about his schoolwork.

Mitchell also began to talk about, and to become more connected to, his wish for deeper relationships with other people. He finally took the leap of trying out the Board Game Club, attending their weekly game nights in order to cultivate a greater sense of community. He laughed as he told his therapist: "I had thought I was the most socially inept person at this school, but now I'm hanging out with a bunch of people who are just as a socially awkward as I am! I am starting to feel like I might actually belong somewhere." While Mitchell continued to struggle with insecurities and fears of rejection, he expressed a growing confidence in himself, and an enjoyment of his everyday life—feelings that persisted even alongside the anxieties he was addressing in treatment.

Through engaging in therapy, Mitchell displayed notable progress in process-related mentalizing. Now try your hand at Worksheet 3.3, which invites you to consider your own strengths in these forms of mentalizing.

Worksheet 3.3
Recognizing Strengths in Mentalizing: Reflecting on Process

Flexibility and Humility

(1) Where have you shown flexibility and humility in your beliefs about yourself? Provide at least one example when you revised a viewpoint based on something that happened, or feedback that you received from someone else.

(2) Where have you shown flexibility and humility in your beliefs about other people? Provide at least one example when you revised your perspective based on something that happened, or feedback that you received from another person.

(3) Identify any conditions (e.g., situations, specific relationships, doing particular things or feeling certain emotions) that make it easier for you think in a more flexible, humble manner. What about those circumstances is helpful for you?

Focus on Psychological Process

(4) How do you tend to focus on internal processes (e.g., thoughts, beliefs, emotions, desires, values, feelings about yourself) in yourself, rather than just considering external factors in the environment (e.g., events, behaviors, visible objects or qualities)?

[continued on next page]

(5) How do you tend to focus on internal processes (e.g., thoughts, beliefs, emotions, desires, values, feelings about self) in other people, rather than just considering external factors in the environment (e.g., events, behaviors, visible objects or qualities)?

(6) List any conditions (e.g., situations, specific relationships, doing particular things, or feeling certain emotions) that make it easier for you to focus on mental states in yourself and other people. What about those circumstances is helpful for you?

Authentic Connectedness

(7) Describe your strengths in accessing and connecting to your emotions, desires, or feelings about yourself. Include at least three feelings that you are most easily able to access in an authentic way.

(8) Recount any conditions (e.g., situations, activities, interacting with particular people or types of people) that make it easier for you to authentically connect with your own emotions. What about those circumstances is helpful for you?

[continued on next page]

(9) Discuss your strengths in empathizing, caring about, and emotionally resonating with other people's feeling states. Include at least three feelings in others with which you are most easily able to empathize.

(10) Detail any conditions (e.g., situations, activities, interacting with particular people or types of people) that make it easier for you to empathize with others. What about those circumstances is helpful for you?

Chapter Review 3.1
Mentalization: What Is It?

Mentalization

Mentalization is the ability to "read," access, and reflect on mental states in yourself and other people.

Mentalization is variously described as:

- Attending to mental states

- Holding mind in mind

- Making things mental: to "mental" "-ize"

- Thinking about thinking

- Understanding misunderstanding

- Seeing others from the inside and yourself from the outside

---

Common Mental States Involved in Mentalizing

- *Thought:* a verbal idea or opinion that a person has at any given moment

- *Belief:* a viewpoint about oneself, other people, or reality that one takes to be true

- *Emotion:* a feeling, sentiment, or mood, usually carrying some positive or negative valence

- *Desire:* a wish or impulse that some event will happen, or that some other scenario will *not* happen

- *Self-state:* a feeling about oneself—who one is as a person, usually concerning one's own value and worth

- *Value:* an experience to which someone ascribes personal importance, worth, or meaning

---

Domains of Mentalization

Content-mentalizing: Reflecting on "what" you and other people are thinking and feeling

Context-mentalizing: Thinking about "why" you and other people are feeling some way

[continued on next page]

Context-mentalizing examines the relationship between mental states and other factors: events, behaviors, other mental states, and a person's history.

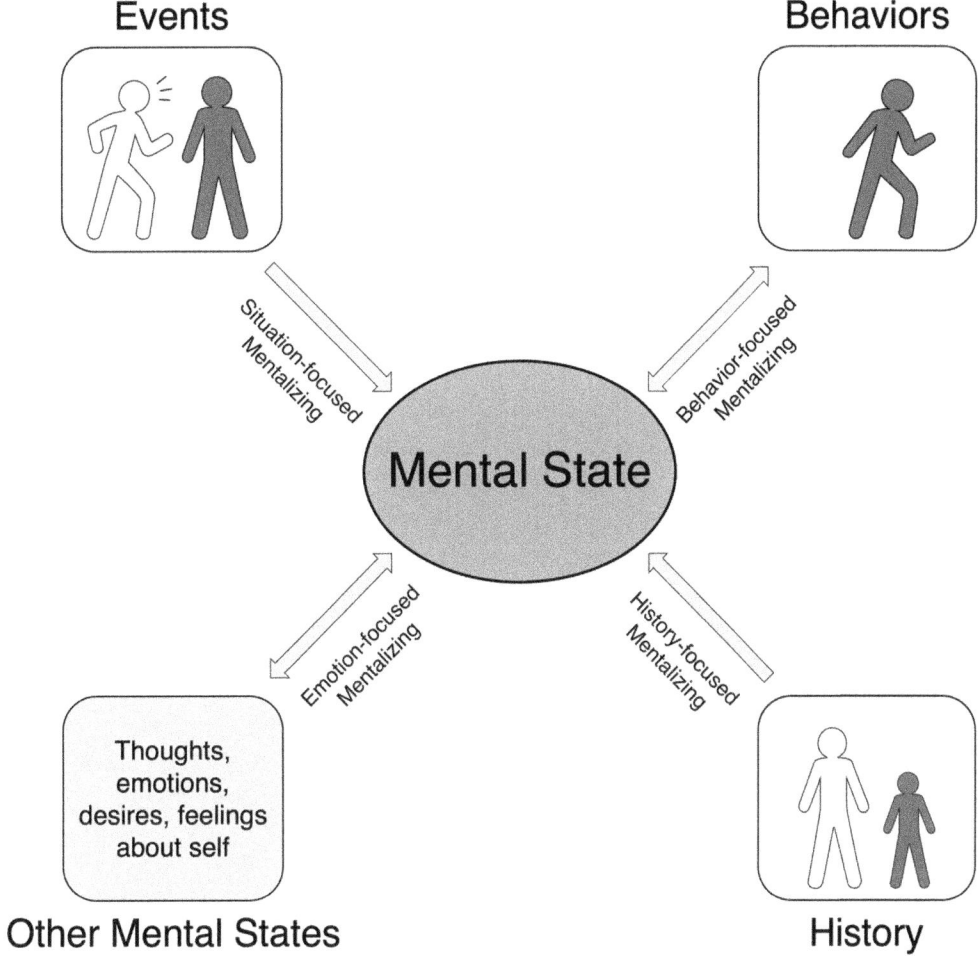

Process-mentalizing: Considering "how" you relate to mental states in yourself and other people

At the level of process, effective mentalizing involves:

- Flexibility, tentativeness, and humility
- Focus on psychological rather than strictly visible factors
- Authentic, engaged connection to your own emotions and desires
- Empathic resonance with others' feelings
- Genuine curiosity and interest in understanding mental states

4

How Does Borderline Personality
Disorder Develop?

There are multiple theories about how borderline personality disorder (BPD) develops. By and large, existing research suggests that a combination of genetic factors, neurobiology, and adverse child experiences likely interact to increase the probability that someone will develop BPD (Cattane et al., 2017). At the genetic level, BPD is highly hereditary: It is more common in people with a family history of BPD (Belsky et al., 2012), as well as among identical twins and full siblings (Skoglund et al., 2021). From the perspective of neurobiology, studies show that people with BPD often exhibit functional and structural abnormalities in frontolimbic brain regions, which are essential in regulating emotions and behavior (Krause-Utz et al., 2017). In addition, extensive research suggests that people with BPD are more likely to have suffered adverse childhood experiences, including physical, emotional, and sexual abuse, as well as physical and emotional neglect. In fact, compared to the general population, individuals with BPD are **14 times** more likely to have a history of childhood adversity, especially emotional abuse and neglect (Porter et al., 2020).

The prevailing theories of "what causes" BPD could be referred to as *trauma–vulnerability* models (Belsky et al., 2012; Crowell et al., 2009; Linehan, 2015b). Consistent with the aforementioned research on genetic/neurobiological differences in people with BPD, these theories suggest that children who end up developing BPD are often quite emotionally sensitive: experiencing more intense affective states, struggling to regulate their emotions and behaviors, and finding it difficult to "come back down" when experiencing heightened emotions. Marsha Linehan (1993), the developer of dialectical behavior therapy, refers to these traits as forms of *emotional vulnerability*. When these children encounter the abuse and neglect often associated with BPD, their existing vulnerabilities are intensified, placing them at increased risk for developing the disorder.

As Herman and colleagues (1989) suggest in their landmark study on childhood trauma in BPD, "It is possible that trauma is most pathogenic for children with vulnerable temperaments or for those most lacking protective factors, such as positive relationships with other caretakers or siblings" (p. 493). Along similar lines, in a long-term study that followed infants from the first year of life, Lyons-Ruth and colleagues (2013) found that both abuse and "maternal withdrawal" were independent contributors to BPD symptoms, leading them to conclude that exposure to abuse, the quality of the caregiver–child relationship, and genetic vulnerabilities are all key precursors to the development of BPD. On these views, no single factor is sufficient to explain how people acquire BPD. However, all of these factors—genes, neurobiology, and trauma—can mutually influence and reinforce each other throughout the course of development, resulting in the pervasive challenges with insecurity and instability that lie at the heart of BPD.

Mentalization-based treatment (MBT) offers its own version of the trauma–vulnerability model (Fonagy & Bateman, 2008; Fonagy et al., 2002), which we will review in this chapter. According to this theory, when parents fail to adequately mentalize the child, the child's core biological sensitivities are mobilized, such that they struggle to effectively mentalize whenever they feel emotionally overwhelmed. To lay the groundwork for this theory, let's

Mentalization. Robert P. Drozek, Oxford University Press. © Oxford University Press 2025.
DOI: 10.1093/oso/9780198916857.003.0004

start by considering how children develop the ability to mentalize, and what this all means for healthy development.

HOW DO WE LEARN TO MENTALIZE?

Recall from Chapter 3 that Peter Fonagy is the British psychoanalyst and clinical psychologist responsible for expounding our current understanding of mentalization. He explored these constructs through a series of papers published in the late 1980s and 1990s, culminating in the publication of a landmark work with several collaborators in 2002: *Affect Regulation, Mentalization, and the Development of the Self*. In this book, Fonagy and colleagues (2002) suggest that human beings are not born with the ability to mentalize. It is not innate, in the same way that breathing, hunger, or reflexes are. Rather, mentalization develops through empathic, engaged relationships with our primary caregivers.

In particular, our capacity to mentalize derives from effective parental mirroring—caregivers' efforts to "reflect back" what their children are thinking, feeling, and wanting. Caregivers do this through explicit speech as well as non-verbal communication, including tone of voice, facial expressions, eye contact, and physical movements. In the best case scenario, mirroring has two key characteristics:

- **Congruence.** The caregiver's mirroring roughly "matches" the content of the child's primary emotions. For example, if a child seems to feel dejected or disheartened, the caregiver might look at the child with a concerned expression on their face, saying in a quieter tone of voice, "You seem to be feeling sad today. Are you upset about something?"
- **Markedness.** The caregiver's mirroring clearly refers to the *child's* emotions, rather than being an expression of the caregiver's own feeling states. Markedness is not indicated through the caregiver's explicit language to the child; rather, it is expressed via the somewhat exaggerated, ironic, or "as if" quality of the caregiver's speech. So in the example of the child feeling dejected or upset, the caregiver themself does not present as extremely sad, but they speak in a slightly higher register that is different from how they would talk if they were expressing their own sadness. This approach essentially communicates to the child: *This is my effort to understand and reflect how YOU are feeling.*

When mirroring takes this shape, the child is able to SEE themself (e.g., their emotions, their desires) in the caregiver's empathic reflections. The child then "takes in" this image of the caregiver mirroring them, using the image as a representation of their own emotional experience. If this happens repeatedly and successfully throughout the child's development, the child acquires a relatively broad and robust repertoire of "emotion packages": sadness, anger, anxiety, excitement, happiness, embarrassment, desires for attention, and so on. These representations serve as the foundation for a coherent, embodied sense of self. The child knows themself, and they feel grounded in their own experience. See Figure 4.1 for an illustration of this process. These representations also lead to the ability to understand and mentalize other people's thoughts and feelings. "If I were in your shoes, I would be feeling sad right now. So perhaps you might be feeling sad, too."

This theory offers a fundamentally social, interactional view of emotional development. It means that we can only fully experience emotions in ourselves that have been seen by

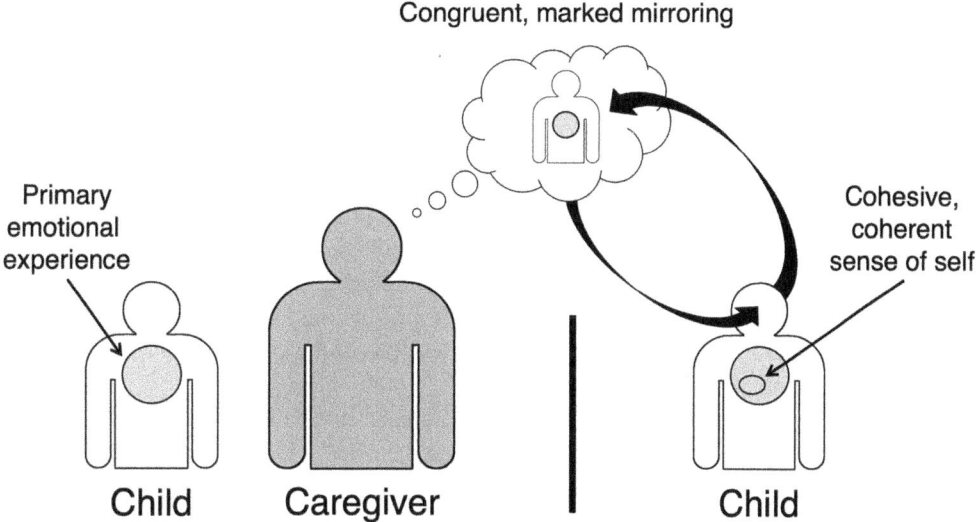

Figure 4.1 Parental mentalization and self-development. The caregiver provides congruent, marked mirroring of the child's primary emotional experience. The child internalizes these interactions, which enables them to understand their own emotions. This serves as the foundation for a cohesive, coherent sense of self.

other people and reflected back to us. In other words, in order to mentalize ourselves and others, someone needs to mentalize us first! Interestingly, now two decades after the publication of Fonagy and colleagues' (2002) book, research in developmental psychology strongly supports their seminal formulations. Caregivers' mentalizing abilities appear to be correlated with the advancement of mentalizing capacities in children (Ensink et al., 2015; Rosso & Airaldi, 2016).

Furthermore, across multiple studies, research shows that parental mentalization significantly impacts what is referred to as "attachment security," or children's sense of confidence that they are able to elicit their caregivers' responsiveness, along with an assurance that caregivers will meet their needs and preferences (Zeegers et al., 2017). As securely attached children develop into secure adults, they come to experience themselves as worthy of love and support, and other people as fundamentally trustworthy and available (Cassidy & Shaver, 2016). These findings support the idea that parental mentalization plays a central role in helping children learn how to mentalize, and in developing a solid sense of self.

WHEN MENTALIZATION GOES WRONG: HOW BORDERLINE PERSONALITY DISORDER DEVELOPS

What happens when caregivers struggle to mentalize their children? MBT suggests that these children are at increased risk of developing BPD. Continuing with Fonagy and colleagues' theory of congruent/marked mirroring, two scenarios deserve special mention.

Mirroring is not congruent enough. Here, caregivers' mirroring expresses a clear distinction between their mind and the child's mind. However, they fail to adequately reflect the content of the child's emotional experience. Examples of this include:

- Instances of emotional or physical neglect, when caregivers are so wrapped up in their own experience that they are insufficiently attuned to the child's emotions and needs.
- Scenarios when caregivers, due to their own psychological limitations, consistently "miss" specific emotional experiences of the child: sadness, insecurity, desires for validation, and so on. So while the caregiver is able to effectively mirror some of the child's emotions, there are significant dimensions of the child's subjectivity that are never "seen" or reflected back to them.
- Relatedly, some caregivers place a primary emphasis on what they think the child SHOULD be doing or feeling, rather than what the child actually is experiencing. "Don't feel sad about what that kid said to you. I'm sure he didn't mean anything by it." "How much studying did you do today? You need to do well on that test so that you can get into a good college!" "Tell me how much you love me. Mommy's had a really hard day today."

Mirroring is not marked enough. At other times, the caregiver's mirroring roughly corresponds to the content of the child's primary emotions, but there is insufficient distinction between what the caregiver is feeling and what the child is feeling. These "poor boundaries" between minds can take a variety of different shapes.

- The caregiver is quite emotionally sensitive themself, so they struggle with intense emotions whenever the child experiences intense emotions. The child is worried about something, and this makes the caregiver anxious. The caregiver gets sad because the child feels sad. The child is excited and happy about something one day, and suddenly the caregiver is in a great mood.
- At times, the caregiver can direct substantial criticism, verbal abuse, or insults toward the child. This involves not simply criticizing the child's behaviors, but *who they are* as a person. "How could you be so stupid?" "I wish you were never born." "I'm ashamed of you. You're never going to amount to anything."
- Situations of attachment trauma, where physical or sexual abuse is perpetrated by caregivers themselves. Here, the bodily integrity of the child is under threat, and the caregiver's mind *itself* is the noxious agent in the system, as it is populated by anger, rage, hatred, or the desire to use the child as an object.

The child's biological vulnerabilities can further complicate these mirroring processes. As we have discussed throughout this book, people with BPD can struggle with exquisite emotional sensitivities, which are grounded in genetics, temperament, and neurobiology. While some caregivers are able to effectively mirror their child's emotional disruptions, many caregivers struggle along these lines. Since the child's emotions are often "too big" for the situation at hand, caregivers' mirroring is not congruent enough—that is, it does not sufficiently "match" the intensity of the child's experience. And since the child's emotional instability can be emotionally overwhelming to parents, their mirroring is not marked enough—that is, there is minimal distinction between the caregivers' feelings and the child's feelings. On this view, these problems in mirroring stem from the complex interaction between the child's temperamental vulnerabilities and the caregivers' own psychological/interpersonal limitations.

All of these circumstances (e.g., of insufficient congruence or markedness in mirroring) can derail the child's ability to mentalize. Since the child's original emotional experience was never sufficiently seen or acknowledged by another person, the child does not develop the robust capacity to understand what they are feeling and wanting. Furthermore, since we usually start to mentalize other people by first mentalizing ourselves, these deficits can hinder the child's ability to flexibly understand other people's experiences as well. It is like the person lacks a basic "mentalizing roadmap" to fully understand themself and others. In circumstances of verbal, physical, and sexual abuse, children learn to not think about their caregiver's mental states, since these states are genuinely hurtful and terrifying to the child.

But these problems have even deeper implications. Given that self-mentalization serves as the bedrock for a sense of self, the child can struggle to remain fully grounded in their own experience. Rather than internalizing an image of the caregiver effectively mirroring the child's feelings, the child takes in an image of the *caregiver's* feelings and desires, which feels fundamentally incongruent with the child's experience. MBT refers to this as the *alien self*—a core sense of incoherence and incongruence in the person's sense of self (Fonagy et al., 2002). In situations of abuse and neglect, the child internalizes an uncaring or aggressive image of the caregiver into the self, which can lead to feelings of worthlessness, shame, and self-hatred. See Figure 4.2 for a pictorial representation of how the alien self develops.

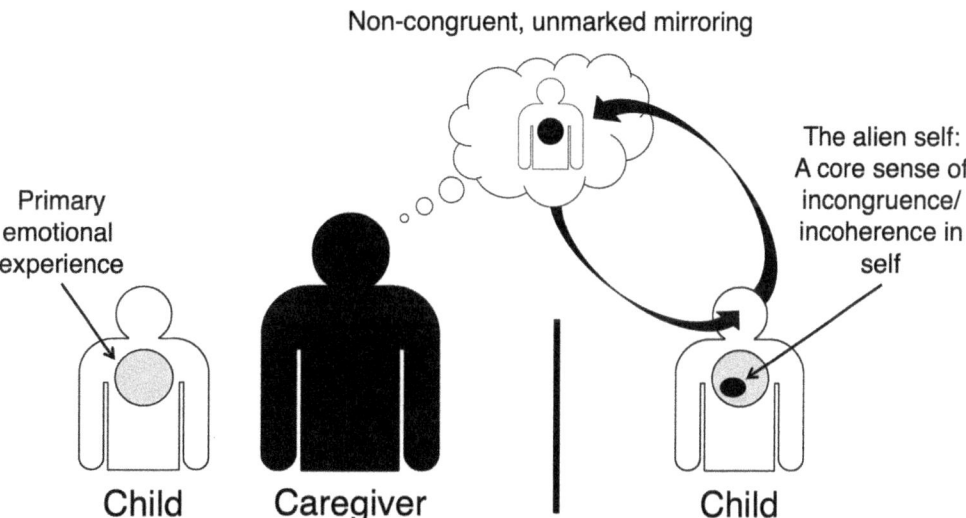

Figure 4.2 The development of the alien self. The caregiver provides non-congruent, unmarked mirroring of the child's primary emotional experience. The child internalizes an image of the caregiver's experience as part of the Self. This results in the alien self, which fails to reflect the child's primary emotional state and generates a profound sense of incongruence/incoherence in the child's sense of self.

MBT uses the above theory to explain many of the core challenges of people with BPD. Since the person was not sufficiently "seen" in their early attachment relationships, they feel especially vulnerable in current attachment relationships, especially when they are misunderstood, rejected, or abandoned by people who really matter to them. Under those conditions, their mentalizing can "go offline" in important ways:

- They fail to identify their own emotions and desires, and to understand and validate what they are experiencing.
- They can feel confused about "who they are," often finding it difficult to remain connected to themself.
- Since they internalized their caregiver's feelings growing up, they often excessively focus on *other people's* thoughts and feelings, especially how other people feel about them. There is an imbalance of "others over self."
- Consistent with MBT's construct of the alien self, people with BPD often struggle with significant instability in their experience of identity and self-esteem. This can manifest itself in pervasive feelings of fragmentation and incoherence, as well as difficulties with shame, worthlessness, and self-loathing. Since such feelings are psychologically intolerable, these individuals cope by projecting the badness *outside* of themselves: through self-injury and suicide ("My body is bad, and I need to destroy it"); through anger and resentment toward other people ("You are bad, problematic, and unacceptable in some way"); through aggressive or avoidant behavior ("You are victimizing me, so I need to get away from you, or fight back against you"); or through impulsive actions like sex, addiction, or risk-taking ("I need to take this action in order to change how I feel, right now and right away").

     While these maladaptive behaviors clearly lead to negative consequences in people's lives, they generate a momentary sense of stability and coherence in the sense of self. On this view, contrary to some stereotypes of BPD, these individuals do not take these actions in order to get attention from others, or because they want to manipulate anyone. Rather, people with BPD take these actions because *they have to*, in order to prevent a psychologically unbearable experience of self-instability, and thus to ensure the survival of the self. This theory accounts for what has been called "I hate you, don't leave me" phenomena in BPD (Kreisman & Straus, 2021), where people alternate quite intensely between directing anger/rage toward others and directing anger/hatred toward themselves. See Figure 4.3 for a visual depiction of these processes.

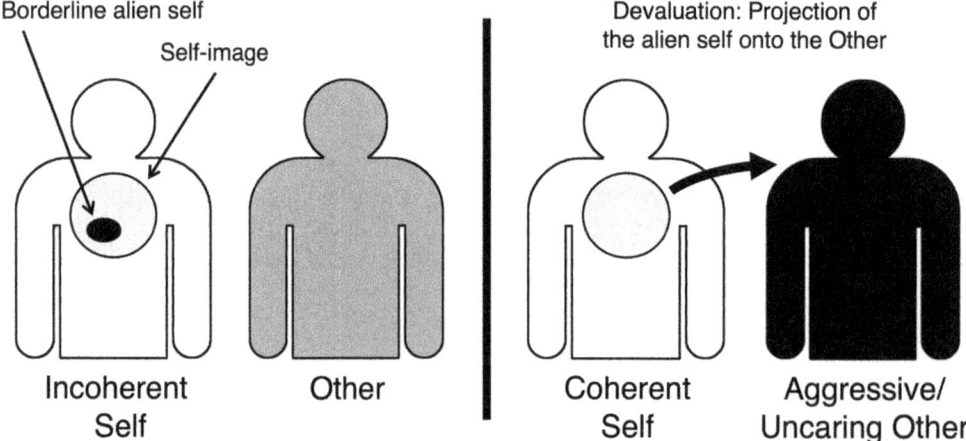

Figure 4.3 Devaluation/problem behaviors as an effort to maintain self-coherence. In BPD, people experience a profound sense of incongruence/incoherence in their sense of self, AKA "the alien self." By devaluing others and engaging in problem behaviors (e.g., aggression, self-injury, suicide), people with BPD regain a sense of coherence and stability in their self-experience.

This final aspect of MBT's theory underscores a core dilemma facing individuals with BPD. When they are feeling overwhelmed or rejected in their relationships, they need to "get the badness out of themselves" by engaging in unhelpful behaviors (e.g., aggression, self-injury, suicide), or by experiencing other people as victimizing them. This grants them a temporary sense of coherence and stability, enabling them to think again, and to avoid the terrifying experience of existential destruction. But this solution comes at a severe cost: They become highly dependent on these problem behaviors in order to feel OK in themselves, and they are forced to live in a world where they feel fundamentally unsafe and mistrustful of others. So people with BPD are able to avoid internal destruction, but only by feeling like they are continuously under threat by forces outside of themselves.

On the above theory, deficits in parental mentalizing forestall the development of the child's mentalizing, resulting in the characteristic forms of instability associated with BPD (see Chapter 2). Once again, Fonagy and colleagues' (2002) early hypotheses turn out to be extensively supported by research. Studies show that problems in parental mentalizing are associated with poorer mentalizing in children (Sharp et al., 2006), attachment insecurity (Zeegers et al., 2017), and a range of psychiatric challenges, including anxiety, difficulties regulating emotions, and behavior problems (Camoirano, 2017).

MENTALIZATION AND TRUST

Why does this ability to mentalize matter so much? Recent developments in mentalization theory center on the connection between mentalizing and what is called *epistemic trust* (Fonagy et al., 2015; Fonagy et al., 2017). MBT observes that infants are instinctively driven to receive and integrate communications from their primary caregivers. As discussed earlier in this chapter, under optimal circumstances, caregivers provide congruent, marked mirroring of the child's subjective states, resulting in the successful development of mentalization.

MBT further underscores another positive consequence of this sort of mirroring—namely, the child gains a sense of fundamental trust in their caregivers. Since the caregivers' mirroring reflects the child's subjectivity, the child feels "seen" as a unique, agentic individual. The child thus comes to trust their caregivers, experiencing them as a reliable source of knowledge: The information they impart is credible, useful, and relevant to the child as a person. In this way, all of the information related to human society and culture—involving other people, the physical environment, human history, and "how to do things" in the world—is effectively passed on from generation to generation.

However, when caregivers are unable to effectively mentalize the child, the child never ends up feeling safe and secure in their broader environment. We see this especially in family dynamics involving emotional neglect and chronic misattunement, as well as situations of verbal, physical, and sexual abuse. In addition to failing to develop a robust capacity for mentalization, the child is forced to assume a posture of epistemic vigilance: They remain closed off to communications from their caregivers, reflexively presuming the caregivers' negative intentions. They can feel misunderstood and unloved by their caregivers, or even worse, that caregivers are actively seeking to hurt them. This vigilance serves the evolutionary function of protecting the child from further trauma, since they are insulating themself from the mind of the individuals who have the power to cause them intense psychological pain.

As development unfolds, these processes can have a severe impact on the person's sense of stability and connectedness in their lives. In areas of attachment insecurity, or when under stress, the individual finds it more challenging to trust the intentions of other people. While this approach was adaptive in childhood, it can significantly limit the person's contemporary relationships, especially when the person prematurely shuts out attachment figures who are largely safe and reliable. The world feels fundamentally dangerous, leading to difficulties with anxiety, insecurity, and more tenuous connections with other people. These observations are supported by research linking childhood adversity with insecure attachment in both children and adults (Fearon & Belsky, 2016; Lo et al., 2019), along with problems in mentalizing across multiple domains (Fonagy et al., 2017; Wagner-Skacel et al., 2022).

This stance of perpetual vigilance and mistrust is highly common among people with histories of trauma, as well as individuals with BPD. They can struggle with excessively harsh, rigid views of themselves and other people (see Chapter 12). "I am bad, worthless, undeserving of love. There is something inherently wrong with me." "Other people are unsafe—they could hurt and reject me at any moment. I need to monitor them closely for the slightest sign of threat." Since the person cannot trust and apply information from others, these views cannot be easily revised based on feedback from other individuals. These beliefs remain calcified, almost frozen in time. The person becomes something of a closed system, unable to assimilate new, more benign information from the social surround.

Have you ever found yourself struggling with these sorts of difficulties with insecurity and mistrust? If so, mentalization can help. Mentalization starts to open up the pathway between yourself and other people, so that you can experience a greater sense of security, stability, and connectedness in your life.

With these ideas in mind, explore Worksheet 4.1, which invites you to consider your history through the lens of mirroring, mentalization, and trust.

Worksheet 4.1
The Theory of Mentalization

(1) *Congruent mirroring* refers to the caregiver accurately reflecting what the child is feeling. In what ways were your caregivers congruent in their mirroring of your emotional states?

(2) How did your caregivers fail to accurately reflect your feelings?

(3) *Marked mirroring* refers to the caregiver reflecting the child's emotions, rather than their own feelings. In what ways were your caregivers "marked" in their mirroring of your emotional states?

(4) In what ways did your caregivers tend to express their OWN feelings instead of mirroring yours?

[continued on next page]

(5) When have you struggled to trust other people in your life? Describe at least three specific examples, in the past or present.

(6) What made it more challenging to trust these people? These could be qualities or actions of the person in question, feelings in yourself, or situations/interactions happening in your life at the time.

(7) Are there any people in your life you have really trusted—individuals you have experienced as safe, reliable, and trustworthy? Describe at least three specific examples, in the past or present.

(8) What made you able to place your trust in these particular people? These could be qualities or actions of the person in question, feelings in yourself, or situations/interactions happening in your life at the time.

Chapter Review 4.1
The Development of Mentalization and Trust

The Successful Development of Mentalization

- *Congruent mirroring* refers to caregivers' accurate reflection of what the child is feeling.

- *Marked mirroring* refers to caregivers' reflection of the child's emotions, rather than expressing their own feelings.

- When caregivers provide congruent, marked mirroring of the child's primary emotions, the child internalizes these interactions, which teaches the child to mentalize themself and other people.

- These representations serve as the foundation for a cohesive, coherent sense of self.

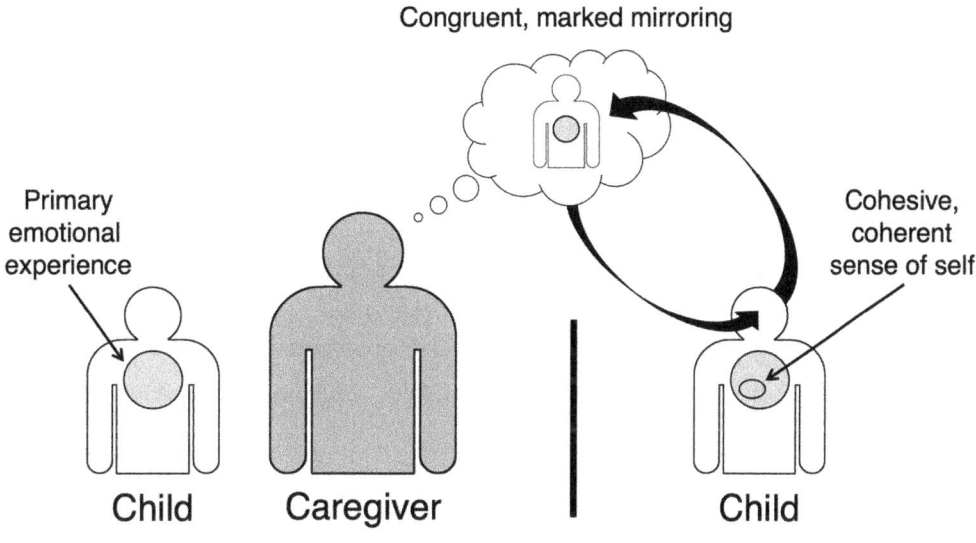

Mentalization and Trust

- *Epistemic trust* refers to an individual's ability to "take in," integrate, and apply information from other people.

- When caregivers effectively mentalize their child, the child comes to trust their caregivers, experiencing them as a reliable and useful source of knowledge.

- In situations of neglect and abuse, the child protects themself by "closing themself off" to caregivers' minds.

- The leads to the vigilance and mistrust that are highly common in BPD, resulting in difficulties with anxiety, insecurity, and tenuous connections with other people.

- Mentalization helps to open up the pathway between oneself and other people, leading to a greater sense of security, stability, and connectedness in life.

Chapter Review 4.2
How does Borderline Personality Disorder Develop?

Trauma–Vulnerability Models of Borderline Personality Disorder

- *Trauma–vulnerability* models of BPD suggest that a combination of genetic factors, neurobiology, and adverse child experiences interact to increase the likelihood that someone will develop BPD.

- At the genetic level, BPD is highly hereditary: It is more common in people with a family history of BPD, as well as among identical twins and full siblings.

- People with BPD exhibit functional and structural abnormalities in frontolimbic brain regions, which are essential in regulating emotions and behavior.

- Individuals with BPD are more likely to have suffered adverse childhood experiences, including physical, emotional, and sexual abuse, as well as physical and emotional neglect.

- According to MBT's trauma–vulnerability model, deficits in parental mentalizing forestall the development of the child's mentalizing, resulting in the characteristic forms of instability associated with BPD.

MBT's Developmental Model of Borderline Personality Disorder

- When caregivers provide non-congruent, unmarked mirroring of the child's emotions, the child internalizes an image of the caregiver's experience as part of the self.

- This impedes the development of mentalization, resulting in the formation of the alien self.

- The *alien self* fails to reflect the child's primary emotional state and generates a profound sense of incongruence/incoherence in the child's sense of self.

Non-congruent, unmarked mirroring

The alien self:
A core sense of
incongruence/
incoherence in
self

Primary
emotional
experience

Child   Caregiver   Child

[continued on next page]

- These processes explain the core challenges of people with BPD.

  - Since the person was not sufficiently "seen" in their early relationships, they feel vulnerable and insecure in current attachment relationships.

  - When the individual feels rejected and misunderstood, they experience problems in mentalizing: difficulties understanding and validating their own feelings; challenges reading and flexibly considering other people's mental states; an excessive focus on "others over self"; unstable sense of self; and negative feelings about themself, which the person manages through self-destructive, aggressive, and impulsive actions.

  - By engaging in these maladaptive behaviors (e.g., aggression, self-injury, suicidality), people with BPD get the badness "outside of themselves," temporarily alleviating an experience of fragmentation and achieving coherence and stability in their sense of self.

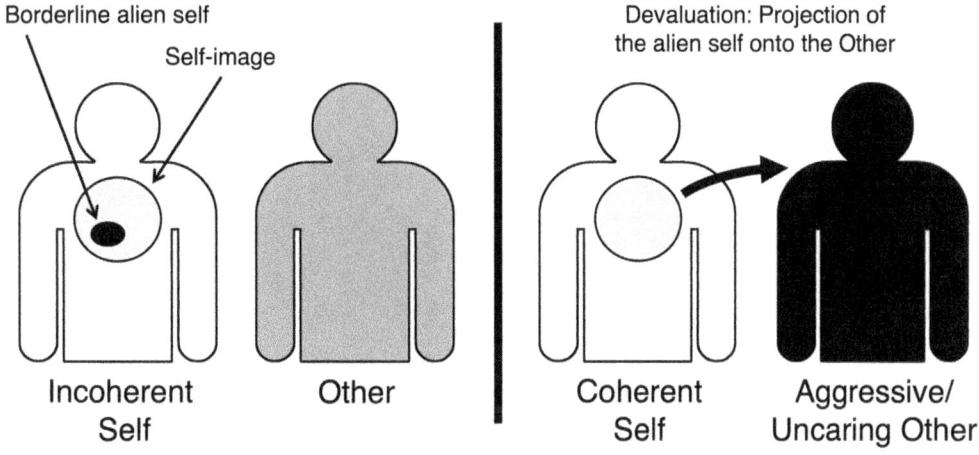

5

Mentalization-Based Treatment: The Basics

Now for the main event: mentalization-based treatment, or MBT. This chapter covers all of the fundamentals of the therapy: its background and history, the structure of the treatment, and how therapists and patients work together. In addition to orienting you to the MBT model, these core ideas will serve as the foundation for everything else we cover in the book, as we utilize MBT's principles to understand and address your symptoms of borderline personality disorder (BPD).

THE STORY OF MBT

Since MBT is all about understanding people, let's start by getting to know its two developers: Professors Anthony Bateman and Peter Fonagy. We have already reviewed the work of Peter Fonagy, the British psychoanalyst and clinical psychologist most responsible for our current understanding of mentalization. In addition to helping to research and disseminate MBT as a therapy (more on that below), Fonagy is the leading scientific researcher on the construct of mentalization, extensively studying the importance of mentalizing in parenting, child development, attachment, borderline personality disorder, trauma, epistemic trust, and psychotherapy outcomes (see Duschinsky & Foster, 2021). He has also designed an empirically validated tool for measuring mentalization, the Reflective Functioning Questionnaire (Fonagy et al., 2016). Hailed by *The Guardian* as "one of the most acclaimed child psychologists of his generation" (Doward & Hall, 2019), Fonagy has used his standing to improve public health policy in the United Kingdom, in the areas of mental health, psychotherapy, and child abuse and neglect. Check out the next page for a picture of Peter, so that you can have an image in your mind.

As a person, Fonagy is a lesson in contradictions. On the one hand, he is extremely kind, warm, and down-to-earth—simply one of the nicest people you will ever meet. On the other hand, he is a towering intellect, with an intellectual curiosity and breadth of knowledge that could almost knock you over. In MBT trainings, in response to a clinician trainee asking a question, Fonagy becomes almost visibly animated by the ideas in play, enthusiastically thinking through the topic with the person in real time, seemingly with no sense that time is passing. People feel seen by him, but also excited and humbled to be a part of (what feels like) something important happening.

Anthony Bateman is a psychiatrist and psychoanalyst from England. Bateman is the lead author and researcher who formalized the technical principles of MBT, spearheading the studies that established MBT as a leading evidence-based therapy for people with BPD. See the following page for a picture of Anthony, thoughtfully explaining mentalizing and MBT.

If Fonagy is the theoretician of MBT, then Bateman is MBT's pragmatician. He has become the primary trainer of MBT in the world, having led hundreds of trainings for tens of

Mentalization. Robert P. Drozek, Oxford University Press. © Oxford University Press 2025.
DOI: 10.1093/oso/9780198916857.003.0005

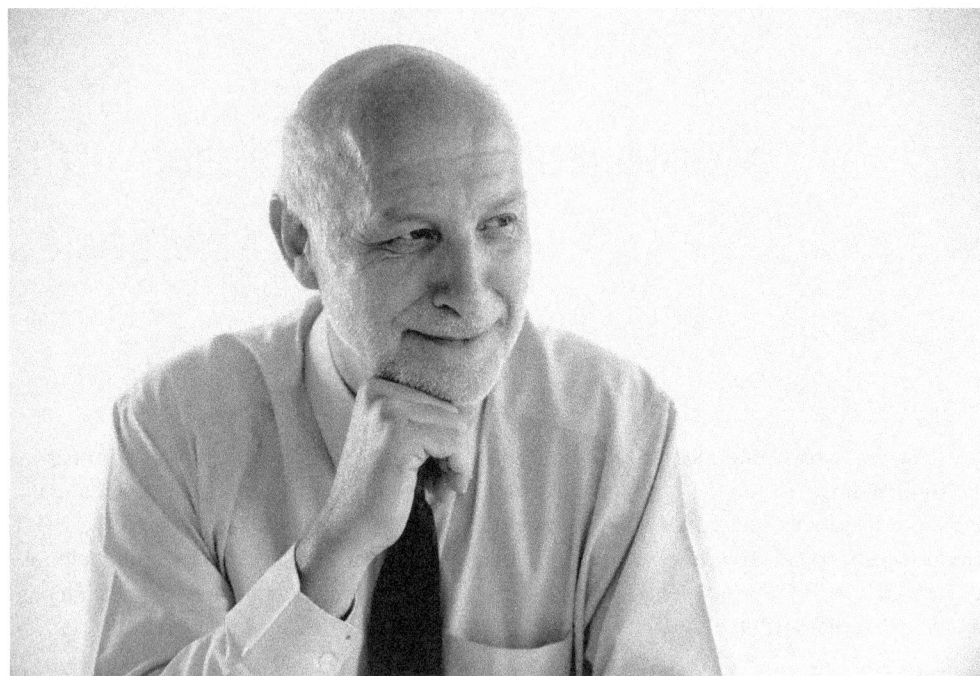

Figure 5.1 Peter Fonagy, CBE, FMedSci, FBA, FAcSS, PhD. Fonagy is the co-developer of MBT; Head, Division of Psychology and Language Sciences, University College London; and National Clinical Advisor on Children's Mental Health, NHS England. He has published over 700 papers, 300 chapters, and authored or co-authored 24 books.

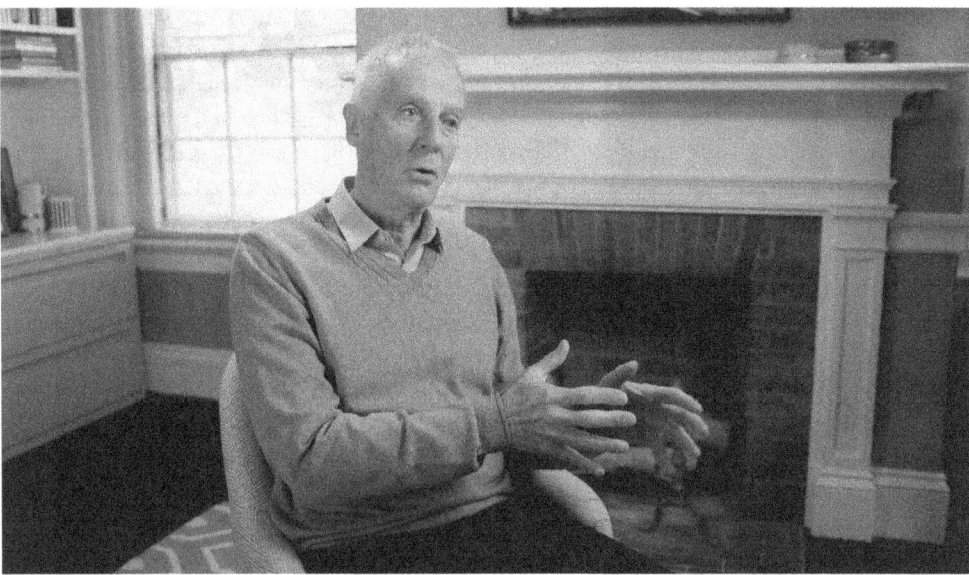

Figure 5.2 Anthony W. Bateman MA, FRCPsych. Bateman is the co-developer of MBT; consultant psychiatrist, psychotherapist, and MBT Consultant to the Anna Freud Centre in London; and Visiting Professor at University College London. He has published over 150 peer-reviewed research articles, and he has authored, co-authored, and edited 18 books.

thousands of clinicians about how to implement the treatment. Bateman has also become something of an administrative "hub" for MBT: helping to supervise groups of clinicians starting up MBT teams and programs; serving as a mentor and collaborator for researchers studying MBT's efficacy; and advancing guidelines for what makes MBT unique, compared to other forms of therapy (Bateman, 2020).

Like Fonagy, Bateman is notably unpretentious and self-effacing. If you ran into him at conference, you would probably not predict that he is one of the foremost researchers on psychotherapy in the world. You rarely see him wearing a suit and tie, and he bats away any sort of fanfare or praise. He prefers to sit back and listen, often with a slight grin as he thoughtfully considers what the other person is saying. But then when he responds, his comments are politely and subtly subversive, enabling people to rethink their original position in a new and surprising way. This has made Bateman revered as a master clinician of MBT, as illustrated by his multiple YouTube videos illustrating the technique.

So how did MBT come to be? In the 1990s, Bateman was hired into his first clinical leadership role, as the medical director of the Halliwick Day Hospital in London. Halliwick is a partial hospitalization program for patients with severe personality disorders, publicly funded through the National Health Service in the United Kingdom. Upon Bateman's arrival there, Halliwick largely operated based on principles from traditional psychoanalysis, the leading therapeutic modality at the time in England. In psychoanalysis, therapists employed a more "neutral" or dispassionate approach with their patients, working to encourage patients' insight by exploring past experience and offering interpretations about their unconscious processes. As director of Halliwick, Bateman was tasked to revamp the program—to develop an approach to care that could help these patients, while also managing the overwhelming demands for treatment that far outweighed the resources.

Halliwick's patients were struggling with debilitating symptoms, including severe levels of depression, frequent suicide attempts, regular engagement in self-injurious behavior, and recurrent inpatient admissions. In addition to having personality disorders, they faced a range of complex social difficulties: poverty, unemployment, homelessness, and legal involvement. Any treatment approach for these individuals could not reside in some ivory tower. It would have to be able to meet them where they were at.

Bateman was aware of Fonagy's recent work in mentalization, which was starting to gain traction in the London psychoanalytic scene. Bateman reached out to Fonagy to introduce himself, and they struck up a friendship. They discovered they had two important things in common: a strong interest in BPD, and a recognition that traditional psychoanalysis was likely not particularly effective at treating patients with BPD. The mental health establishment had long viewed BPD as an "untreatable" condition, but with the publication of Linehan and colleagues' (1991) landmark research on dialectical behavior therapy, a new hope for BPD was starting to dawn. Bateman and Fonagy began thinking through the practical applications of a therapeutic approach for BPD employing Fonagy's conception of mentalization. Key features included:

- A continuous focus on helping patients reflect on mental states in themselves and other people
- A "not-knowing" or inquisitive clinical stance. That is, therapists worked to stimulate *patients'* mentalizing, rather than authoritatively telling patients what they were feeling.
- A prioritization of patients' contemporary lives and functionality outside of treatment—the real-world challenges with which they were struggling

While Bateman and Fonagy worked out these principles, Bateman was able to utilize them to inform the treatment they were providing at Halliwick.

As these treatments unfolded, Bateman soon noticed that the approach seemed to be working! Halliwick's patients were functioning better, and they genuinely liked the MBT approach. Seeking to better understand what was happening, Bateman and Fonagy decided to study MBT's efficacy, completing the first randomized controlled trial of MBT (Bateman & Fonagy, 1999). The results were striking. Over the course of 18 months of treatment, while patients receiving "treatment as usual" showed minimal improvements, patients receiving MBT displayed significant reductions in self-injurious behavior, suicidal actions, inpatient hospitalizations, and depressive symptoms, as well as broader improvements in interpersonal functioning. Interestingly, follow-up studies revealed that these gains were maintained at 18 months and even *eight years* after the conclusion of MBT (Bateman & Fonagy, 2001, 2008). Bateman and Fonagy (2009) proceeded to replicate these findings in studies of outpatient MBT, once again showing that patients' progress continued 5–8 years after treatment (Bateman, Constantinou, et al., 2021).

In light of this empirical support, Bateman and Fonagy started the process of formalizing and publishing the therapeutic principles of MBT. MBT's first treatment manual was published by Oxford University Press in 2004, with subsequent editions following (Bateman & Fonagy, 2004, 2006, 2016). These publications significantly expanded the reach and impact of MBT. In addition to being intellectually captivated by the construct of mentalizing, clinicians were taken with MBT's unique blend of exploration, directiveness, egalitarianism, practicality, and emotional authenticity. Through the Anna Freud Centre in London, Bateman and Fonagy began to lecture about MBT across the world, training other clinicians in the modality. With characteristic humility, they dubbed MBT "old wine in new bottles," but therapists learning the techniques were aware that something felt *different* about this approach. MBT teams and programs sprouted up in various countries, with a notable popularity in Europe, its home continent.

In North America, Bateman and Fonagy formed training partnerships with colleagues in the world of personality disorders: John Gunderson at McLean Hospital in Belmont, Massachusetts; Jon Allen at the Menninger Clinic in Houston, Texas; and Robin Kissell at UCLA. One of the most productive of these partnerships occurred at the institution where I work, here at McLean Hospital. Bateman was close friends with John Gunderson, who in the 1970s completed much of the pioneering research that established BPD as a valid psychiatric diagnosis (Carey, 2019). On the heels of this research, Gunderson developed and directed many of McLean's treatment programs for BPD. Bateman and Fonagy began visiting these programs—to train clinicians in MBT, and also to provide guidance about how to thoughtfully integrate MBT principles into McLean's broader treatment approaches.

This inspired the origination of the MBT Training Clinic at McLean, the first adherent MBT clinic in North America. Led by psychiatrist and psychotherapist Brandon Unruh, this clinic provides insurance-based, outpatient group and individual MBT to individuals with BPD and other severe personality disorders. As a teaching center for Harvard Medical School, we have the opportunity to train young psychiatrists in MBT, in this way supporting awareness and dissemination of MBT in the broader world of mental health and psychiatry. We have also begun applying MBT's principles to treat patients with symptoms of narcissistic personality disorder, developing a modified version of MBT to address challenges regulating self-esteem (Drozek & Unruh, 2020; Drozek et al., 2023).

Taking these endeavors even further, psychiatrist and BPD researcher Lois Choi-Kain created the Gunderson Personality Disorders Institute at McLean, a training institute that educates clinicians in all of our evidence-based therapies for BPD. MBT was one of our first offerings, and Bateman, Fonagy, and other colleagues have continued these trainings for the past decade and a half, including various "adaptations" of MBT: MBT for families (MBT-F), MBT for adolescents (MBT-A), MBT for parenting (MBT-P), and MBT for pathological narcissism (MBT-N). In these ways, MBT has gained something of an academic "home base" in the United States here at McLean Hospital.

Many of these trainings have transitioned to the virtual realm in the context of COVID, enabling a wider range of clinicians from around the world to learn about MBT from the comfort of their own home. At the time of this writing, MBT is generally regarded as a first-line treatment for people with BPD (Cristea, 2017; Storebø et al., 2020), with evidence supporting its use for individuals with antisocial personality disorder (Bateman et al., 2016; Fonagy et al., 2025), and for adolescents struggling with self-injurious behavior (Rossouw & Fonagy, 2012). At the same time, clinicians are increasingly applying MBT to address psychological difficulties beyond just personality disorders, including depression, trauma and PTSD, substance use disorder, eating disorders, and psychotic disorders (Bateman & Fonagy, 2019a). The use of MBT has even expanded to help with social and cultural problems as well, such as law enforcement violence (Drozek et al., 2021), children in foster care (Midgley et al., 2017), parents undergoing divorce (Hertzmann et al., 2016), school bullying (Twemlow et al., 2005), and family members of people with BPD (Bateman & Fonagy, 2019b).

Implicit in all of this research and thinking is the foundational insight of MBT: By seeking to mentalize—that is, to "read," access, and reflect on mental states—you can work through and resolve core areas of stuckness in yourself and your relationships.

THE STRUCTURE OF THE TREATMENT

MBT has been researched and delivered in a range of different settings and formats: partial hospitalization programs, outpatient treatment, and group psychotherapy. In the midst of the COVID-19 pandemic, many MBT programs temporarily shifted to remote platforms like Zoom or telephone, revealing that MBT's utility can be preserved even in online contexts (Ventura Wurman et al., 2021). Since most readers will likely be engaged primarily in individual psychotherapy, let's review the broad structure of individual MBT, as laid out in MBT's official "treatment manual" that has been validated through scientific study (Bateman & Fonagy, 2016; see Figure 5.3). As we progress, I offer a handful of "mentalizing practice points"—ideas or recommendations about how you, as a patient in MBT, can engage in this process in a curious and thoughtful way.

Initial exploration of problems and challenges. MBT starts by exploring your experience of the problems leading you to seek treatment. As we have discussed throughout this book so far, these can include difficulties in mood, such as depression or anxiety; challenges in self-esteem (e.g., unstable or shifting sense of self; shame and self-loathing; "conditional" self-worth: "I am only worthwhile if I meet certain conditions . . . "); disruptions or lack of fulfillment in relationships; and engagement in specific behaviors that interfere with your sense of well-being and functioning (e.g., self-injury, avoidance, addiction, etc.). The therapist usually asks lots of questions at this stage, about the problem areas in question and also about your life more generally. These questions involve a mix of "fact gathering," exploration of emotions and sense of self, and examination of how you experience and engage with other people in your relationships. This conversation could occur in a single visit, or it could unfold across several appointments, depending on the topics under discussion.

Mentalizing practice point: Do your best to share as openly as you can at this stage of the process. Don't censor yourself. When your therapist has more information about how you are struggling, they will be better situated to tailor the treatment to meet your unique needs. Also, just a heads-up that your therapist may ask some questions that initially confuse or surprise you, or that you do not initially see as relevant. Feel free to express those feelings as they come up. Perhaps most importantly, take this as an opportunity to mentalize your therapist.

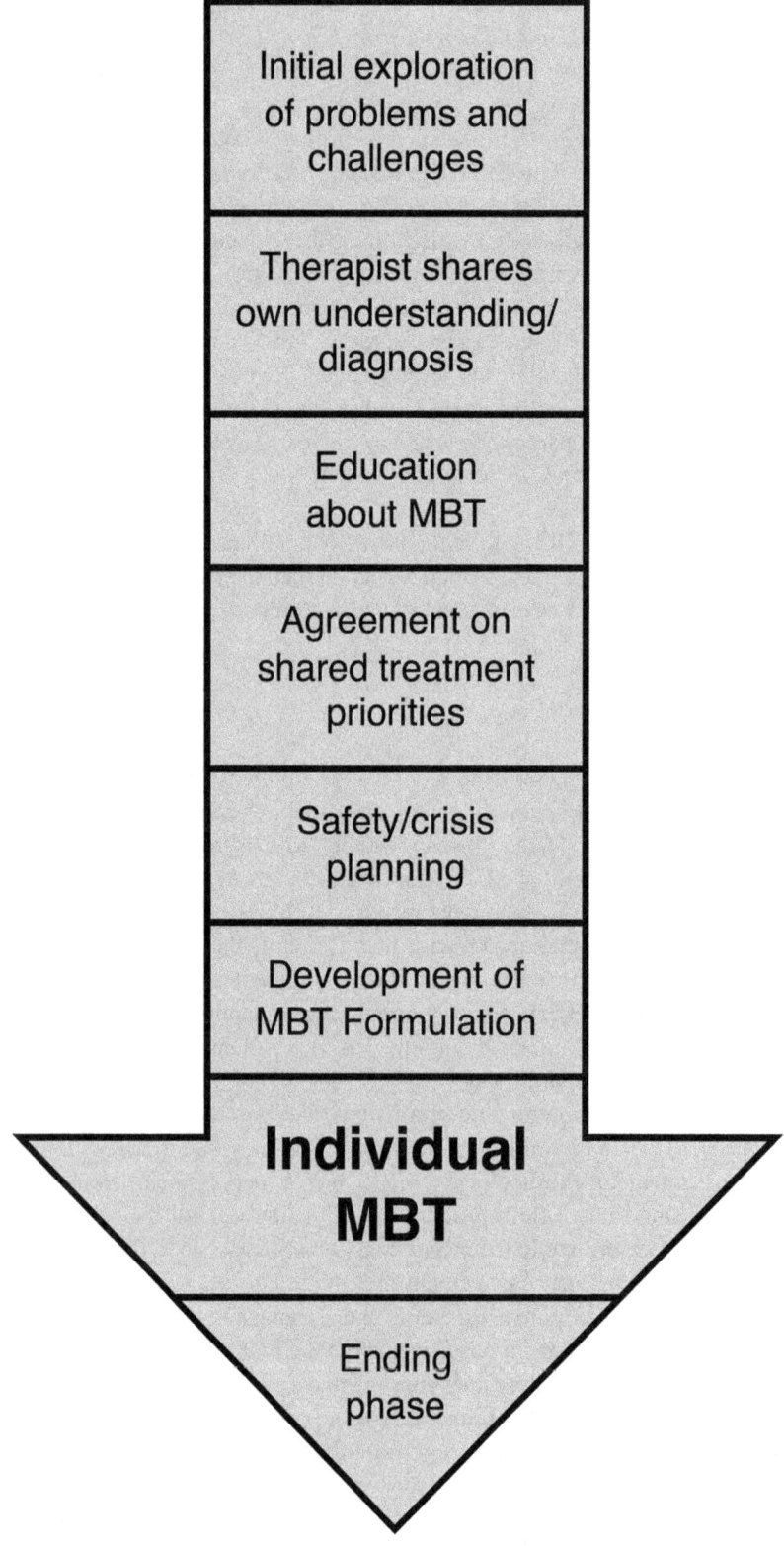

Figure 5.3 The structure of individual therapy in mentalization-based treatment (MBT). The initial phase of MBT involves several different components: exploration of patients' challenges; diagnosis-giving; education about MBT; treatment and safety planning; and development of the MBT formulation. Treatment then progresses into formal individual therapy, which variously can last 12–18 months, or can be ongoing.

"What might they be thinking, feeling, or wanting that would lead them to inquire about this particular thing?"

Therapist shares own understanding/diagnosis. Once you have reviewed your difficulties in a comprehensive way, it is your therapist's turn to convey what they think about all of this. How do they understand what you have been going through? What do they make of all this? Sometimes the therapist communicates a less formal impression, for example if they wonder if one patient's increased marital conflict could be related to him holding his wife to strict, rigid standards. Or for the patient experiencing addiction, the therapist might observe that the patient appears to be attempting to self-medicate other feelings they discussed in the meeting, such as shame about being out of work and anxiety about having to look for a new job.

At other times, the therapist could suggest that you might meet criteria for a specific psychiatric diagnosis, which MBT could be especially well-suited to treat. Obviously this book is about BPD in particular, but as we discussed in Chapter 1, many people with BPD also meet criteria for other psychiatric diagnoses as well, such as major depression, bipolar disorder, generalized anxiety, addiction, or other personality disorders (e.g., narcissistic or avoidant personality disorders). Receiving a new diagnosis can bring up diverse and complex emotions, ranging from positive feelings of hope and relief, to more challenging experiences of vulnerability, shame, and insecurity about how the therapist feels about you. Here the goal is NOT to slap a label onto you, to pathologize or stigmatize you, or to reduce you as a person to some diagnostic category.

MBT talks about the issue of diagnosis for several reasons:

- Especially in the treatment of people with BPD, there is extensive research showing that learning about the diagnosis itself has positive psychological benefits (Zanarini et al., 2018; Zanarini & Frankenburg, 2008). In fact, all of our evidence-based psychotherapies for BPD involves "diagnosis giving" as a preliminary step in the treatment (Storebø et al., 2020).
- There is a tremendous body of knowledge about different psychiatric diagnoses: their epidemiology, causes, as well as effective treatments. As you learn more about your relevant diagnoses, you can gain a greater sense of self-awareness and personal agency, as well as a feeling of relief from finally understanding patterns that have long caused you confusion and distress.
- As we will discuss further in the next section, MBT therapists try to be upfront and transparent about their feelings and opinions. For this reason, we never advocate treating patients for a diagnosis "behind their backs," an approach that could lead to dishonesty, suspicion, and confusion in the therapeutic dynamic. In contrast, by openly sharing our views about the nature of patients' challenges, we encourage a climate of trust, connectedness, and open communication in the therapy—even if patients end up ultimately disagreeing with our diagnostic impressions.

Mentalizing practice point: In considering your therapist's understanding of your problems, there is value in asking yourself: "What feelings and emotions are coming up in me as I take in this perspective? And what are these feelings about for me?" Try to ponder your therapist's ideas with an open mind, but WITHOUT losing your own perspective. "What resonates with me in what my therapist is saying? What does not quite fit for me?" Work to openly share all of these reflections with your therapist, rather than simply debating or agreeing 100% with what the therapist is saying. This helps the therapist to get to know you better: your emotions, what matters to you, and how you see yourself as a person.

Education about MBT. MBT always involves an initial "educational" component. Sometimes this happens in the context of individual treatment, for example when therapists devote several appointments to reviewing and discussing the main concepts and strategies of MBT as a therapy. In larger systems of care, this education occurs in a group format, referred to as MBT-Introductory, or "MBT-I." This book can be seen as an extended companion to MBT-I, where you can learn about the main ideas in MBT and gain practice applying these ideas to your experience.

Key topics commonly covered in MBT-I include:

- the notion of mentalizing, along with common problems in mentalizing;
- emotional experience in yourself and other people;
- the connection between attachment and mentalizing;
- understanding personality disorders and other psychiatric problems (e.g., depression, anxiety); and
- the structure, aims, and strategies of MBT.

Some patients find themselves really enjoying the educational component in MBT, while others find it "boring" or tedious, preferring to just move on and start the therapy already. The conceptual model of MBT is part of what distinguishes it from traditional exploratory, supportive, and psychodynamic psychotherapies. As you come to understand why and how mentalizing matters, you become more able to see situations as specific examples of broader processes, in your own life and even for people in general. This can help you to better "pause and reflect" in the heat of the moment, in a way that is often not possible without an organizing conceptual framework.

Mentalizing practice point: When learning about the main ideas in MBT, try to not simply approach these topics from a more abstract or intellectual perspective. Always be ready to wrestle with questions like:

- "How does this idea relate to my everyday life?"
- "What is a recent time where I have experienced this?"
- "How can I actually USE this idea, as I go throughout my day?"

The questions on the worksheets in this book will hopefully help to facilitate these forms of reflection. By making sure that the educational component in MBT remains emotionally grounded and personally relevant, you will increase the chance that MBT will be accessible and usable for you—in the moment when you actually need it.

Agreement on shared treatment priorities. Your therapist now works with you to develop what MBT refers to as *shared treatment priorities*—the areas that you both agree will serve as the common points of focus in the therapy. These usually fall into the categories of mood, self-esteem, relationships, and behavior. Most of the time, patients frame these as "problem areas," or challenges they would like to address in the treatment.

- *Mood:* "I feel depressed most of the time, and I want to work on that."
- *Self-esteem:* "I don't feel very stable in myself. If somebody doesn't like me, it is hard for me to feel OK."
- *Relationships:* "My partner and I have been growing apart, and I am worried we are going to break up."
- *Behavior:* "Whenever I get really upset, I start thinking about ways to kill myself. It makes me feel better in the moment, but I also know it is probably not healthy."

At other times, patients describe treatment priorities more as "goals," or positive things they would like to achieve through the treatment.

- *Mood:* "I want to feel happy again, the way that I was before the break-up."
- *Self-esteem:* "I would love to have better self-esteem, but I have no idea how to get there."
- *Relationships:* "I want to learn how to communicate my needs, and actually have some boundaries in my relationships with my parents."
- *Behavior:* "I need to start applying for jobs and move on with my life."

Mentalizing practice point: Developing treatment priorities is a crucial step in an MBT treatment, where you have the opportunity to ask yourself: "What are the areas of my life that I most want to improve? Where am I suffering the most? Above all else, what do I really need help with?" By identifying therapeutic goals that really matter to you, you lay the foundation for a treatment that feels relevant and meaningful to you as a person. This helps to maintain motivation for therapy when the going gets tough, as it inevitably will.

Remember that these are called *shared* treatment priorities. There might be times when your therapist feels like a certain issue should be included in the list of priorities, but you do not see the issue as a problem, or you do not feel especially motivated to address the topic. This often arises with "problem behaviors" that feel addictively compelling to you, while also interfering with your safety and functionality: self-injury, suicidal actions, substance use, restrictive eating, and so on. In such moments, try to really mentalize your therapist: "What is making my therapist feel like this issue is so important? What emotions might they be feeling about this area of my life?" Ultimately, you will both have to come to a collaborative agreement about the objectives for the therapy—a shared point of focus that can encompass your concerns, as well as your therapist's sense of what constitutes ethical and effective care. This requires a mutual process of mentalizing for both parties: "What treatment plan can we both live with? Is there a pathway that reflects BOTH of our minds and priorities?"

In light of all this, now take some time to work on the following worksheets (5.1, 5.2, and 5.3), which walk you through how to identify your personal goals and objectives for treatment. Once you complete them, feel free to discuss your answers with your therapist. This will serve as a helpful starting point for your conversation about the focus of the therapy.

Worksheet 5.1
Developing Personal Priorities for Treatment:
Mood and Self-esteem

(1) *Mood-related challenges* are emotions or feeling states that cause trouble for some
people. Circle any of the below difficulties that apply to you.

Depression or sadness	Jealousy or envy	Boredom
Emotional disconnection	Grief	Anxiety or stress
Loneliness	Guilt or regret	Self-pity
Numbness or emptiness	Anger or frustration	Panic attacks

Mood-related challenges
not listed here:

(2) If these problems are relevant for you, identify at least one mood-related goal that
you would like to achieve in therapy.

(3) *Self-esteem-related challenges* are impairments in people's sense of self and identity.
Circle any of the below difficulties that apply to you.

Shame, self-loathing, and self-hatred	Conditional self-esteem: "I am only good if . . . "
Self-criticism or self-attacks	Grandiosity and superiority
Perfectionistic standards for yourself	Unstable sense of self
Identity diffusion: basing sense of self on others' feelings and behaviors	Sense of difference or separateness from other people

Self-esteem-related challenges not
listed here:

[continued on next page]

(4) If these problems apply to you, list at least one self-esteem-related goal you would like to achieve in the treatment.

Worksheet 5.2
Developing Personal Priorities for Treatment:
Interpersonal Relationships

(1) *Interpersonal challenges* can involve difficulties in specific relationships, or broader interpersonal tendencies that cause trouble for you across various situations. Describe any difficulties you have been experiencing in your relationships with other people.

(2) Circle any of the below interpersonal tendencies that apply to you.

Social isolation and avoidance	Defensiveness
Self-focus, self-centeredness	Anger issues, reactivity
Argumentativeness or antagonism	People-pleasing
Social comparison, competitiveness	Rigidity and stubbornness
Interpersonal sensitivity	Caretaking/rescuing of others
Rebelliousness, provocativeness	Shyness, inhibition
Passivity in relationships	Difficulties trusting other people
Withdrawal, break-ups when upset	Need for dominance or control
Extensive focus on problems, illness	Poor boundaries, enmeshment
Interpersonal conflicts	Reassurance-seeking
Remaining in problematic relationships	Pessimism, complaining
Admiration- or attention-seeking	Jealousy or insecurity
Superficial relationships/lack of fulfillment	Dishonesty, misrepresentation
Apathy or indifference toward others	Judgmentalness/resentment
Talking too much/not asking others questions	Seeking out emotionally unavailable people

[continued on next page]

Excessive dependency, reliance
on others

Criticizing or devaluing others

Problems initiating new relationships in
valued domains (e.g., sexual, friendships)

Challenges with assertiveness,
self-expression, making requests

Maladaptive interpersonal tendencies
not listed here:

(3) If any of the above problems apply to you, specify at least one interpersonal goal you
would like to achieve in the therapy.

Worksheet 5.3
Developing Personal Priorities for Treatment:
Behaviors and Functionality

(1) *Behavioral challenges* are actions an individual takes (or avoids taking) that interfere with their ability to function effectively in their lives. Circle any of the below difficulties that apply to you.

Addiction/substance use

Perfectionism or workaholism

Poor self-care, activities of daily living

Impulsivity/risk-taking

Suicidal actions

Self-injurious behavior

Cheating, plagiarism

Procrastination

Legal issues (e.g., theft, violence, destruction of property)

Maladaptive eating (e.g., binging, restricting, purging)

Addictive behaviors not connected to substances (e.g., involving sex, gambling, spending, exercise, technology, video games)

Compulsive/safety behaviors related to anxiety management (e.g., avoidance, checking compulsions, ruminations)

Avoidance or inconsistency in valued domains (e.g., involving work, school, relationships, hobbies)

Behavioral challenges not listed here:

(2) If any of the above problems apply to you, define at least one behavioral goal you would like to achieve in the treatment.

Safety/crisis planning. I just mentioned the idea of "problem behaviors," defined broadly as actions you take that can interfere with your health, well-being, and stability in your life. While sometimes these are directly related to safety (e.g., in the case of self-injury or suicide), problem behaviors can also be more related to interpersonal relationships and overall functionality, for example when you have angry outbursts, request excessive reassurance from others, or avoid taking actions that would help you meet personal goals. MBT is especially effective in treating these sorts of challenges. To that end, one important tool is MBT's Crisis Plan, a personalized set of strategies for how you can "pause and reflect" when you feel drawn to engage in maladaptive behaviors. At the start of the therapy, your therapist collaborates with you to develop a written Crisis Plan, and you use it throughout the treatment in order to initiate and maintain effective mentalization.

In particular, the crisis plan helps you to identify the "warning signs" that you are headed down a dangerous path, where you might be tempted to engage in your identified problem behaviors. These might be particular thoughts ("I am worthless and unlovable," "Nobody cares about me," "I am never going to get better anyway, so what's the point of even trying?"), emotions (e.g., sadness, panic, hopelessness, feelings of emptiness and separation from yourself), or behaviors (e.g., curling up in a ball in your bed, rereading old text messages from past romantic partners, pacing around your apartment).

If you start to notice these warning signs, MBT suggests that you actively work to engage in behaviors that you have historically found helpful in managing your intense emotions, whether those be self-directed coping skills (e.g., watching TV, going for a walk, listening to upbeat music, taking a hot shower, eating your favorite type of candy); communicating with other people, either to provide distraction from your challenges or to directly discuss and receive support around your difficulties; or if you continue to feel like you are going to engage in your problem behavior, reaching out to treatment providers in order to receive additional support and guidance.

Many crisis plans also include ideas about what steps to take "if all else fails," in order to alter the environment and ensure that you are unable to take action on your destructive impulses (e.g., throwing away your razors in the dumpster outside, asking your partner to hide your psychiatric medications, wearing latex gloves to prevent yourself from scratching yourself). This particular format for the Crisis Plan is based on the version developed by the Veterans Health Administration to address suicide risk among military veterans (Stanley & Brown, 2008), adapted here to apply to maladaptive behaviors more generally.

Mentalizing practice point: There is no "one size fits all" approach to developing an effective Crisis Plan. The content and format of different crisis plans vary significantly, depending upon your particular problem behaviors, the coping strategies that you happen to find most helpful, and your therapist's preferences and recommendations. In MBT, what matters most is that (a) you HAVE a written crisis plan; (b) you genuinely USE this plan when you feel like you are moving toward engaging in your problem behaviors; and (c) you work closely with your therapist to develop a plan that is tailored to your unique challenges and strengths.

Some patients starting out in MBT will feel like they are "beyond" utilizing a crisis plan in order to manage their harmful impulses. "I know all of the skills already, but none of them actually work to keep me safe. If they did, I wouldn't need MBT!" I hear you, and MBT would agree that simply "using skills" is ultimately insufficient to help you achieve greater functionality and fulfillment in your life. That's why we have all of the mentalizing strategies outlined in this book. However, all of the research on MBT involves crisis planning as an essential component. Too many people with BPD have a long history of receiving ineffective treatment, and we need to ensure that we are providing the version of the therapy that science has shown to be the most useful in addressing your challenges.

In addition, the Crisis Plan is an essential tool in helping you to mentalize surrounding your maladaptive behaviors. Regardless of the particular skills and strategies contained in your plan, whenever you intentionally pause to *follow* the plan, you are actively trying to "hold on to your mind" in the moment of emotional unrest—in other words, you are mentalizing! Each step in the Crisis Plan involves reflecting on mental states, whether that be reflecting on your own mental states *[Step 1]*, considering your behaviors that are likely to positively impact your mental states *[Steps 2 and 6]*, engaging with other people's mental states *[Step 3]*, or utilizing other people's mental states in order to address your own distressing feelings and impulses *[Steps 4 and 5]*.

If you end up faltering and falling into your problem behaviors, try not to be too hard on yourself. Even though you might feel disappointed in yourself, this is a highly common and understandable occurrence in the treatment of BPD. Just do your best to let your therapist know as soon as possible, making sure to "put it all out there" and include as much information as possible about what unfolded for you. If you are engaged in an MBT treatment, your therapist will likely want to examine these events with you in some detail. This involves conducting what we call a "mentalizing functional analysis" (Bateman & Fonagy, 2016, pp. 227–233), where your therapist "stops and rewinds" to explore how you ended up engaging in the problem behavior. This involves:

1. gathering the basic facts of the situation, including the circumstances leading up to the behavior;
2. exploring your mental states (e.g., emotions, desires, feelings about yourself) at various points in time throughout the episode;
3. identifying your deficits in mentalizing (e.g., rigid or externally focused thinking, disconnectedness from yourself or others) potentially contributing to you taking the action in question; and finally
4. carefully working with you to address these problems in mentalizing, utilizing the strategies summarized throughout this book.

If you neglected to use your crisis plan during your challenging experience, your therapist will probably want to mentalize *that* with you. What got in the way of you utilizing your plan? Moving forward, how might you bring in the plan earlier in the process, in order to work toward a different outcome? By reflecting in these ways in therapy, you will increasingly start to remember your plan outside of sessions, and to take steps to "reflect rather than reflex" when you are tempted to engage in your problem behaviors.

With all of these ideas in mind, draw up your own MBT Crisis Plan, utilizing the bare bones format outlined in Worksheet 5.4 on the following page. Once you have a first draft of the plan, share it with your therapist, for additional discussion, feedback, and revision.

Worksheet 5.4
Your Mentalization-based Treatment (MBT) Crisis Plan

Step 1: Recognize signs that lead to your maladaptive behaviors.

Thoughts:

Feelings/emotions:

Behaviors:

Step 2: Utilize coping strategies without assistance from others. Outline at least five helpful strategies here.

Step 3: Get in touch with friends or family members, in order to just "chat," talk about light topics, or discuss their lives and experience. List at least five different friends/family members who would be helpful in this way, along with their contact information.

[continued on next page]

Step 4: Reach out to friends or family members, in order to discuss your current difficulties and how you are struggling. Identify at least five safe and reliable supports, along with their contact information.

Step 5: Contact professionals. Detail relevant clinicians and/or healthcare organizations here, along with their contact information.

Step 6: Take steps to make your environment safe. Describe anything you can do "if all else fails," in order to ensure that you are 100% unable to engage in your problem behaviors.

Note. The steps in this worksheet are adapted from the Safety Plan: VA Version, as presented in Stanley, B., & Brown, G. K. (2008). *The safety plan treatment manual to reduce suicide risk: Veteran version.* United States Department of Veterans Affairs.

Development of the MBT formulation. The formulation is essentially the "treatment plan" in MBT. After meeting with you for several visits, the therapist writes up a document that summarizes what they have gathered about your main problems in mentalizing. You review and discuss this with your therapist, collaboratively revising the formulation until you both feel like it reflects your core challenges. Sometimes therapists initially develop the formulation on their own and later present it to patients for feedback; in other cases, therapists and patients map out the formulation together, in real time. While the structure and content of formulations vary depending on the particular therapist, patient, and program, topics commonly covered include

- strengths in mentalizing;
- core challenges in mentalizing, including any tendencies toward certainty, concreteness, reactivity, and emotional disconnection;
- "attachment strategies," or your customary manner of managing closeness and connectedness in your relationships (see Chapter 8); and
- possible ways these patterns might play out in the therapeutic dynamic.

As we will discuss in Chapter 6, one main aim of this book is to help you review these areas for yourself, and to consider how they relate to your everyday experience. This is a cornerstone of MBT, and a key element in helping you to actually *practice* mentalizing when you need it most. As treatment progresses, you and your therapist will often revisit the formulation, updating and revising it to reflect new developments in how you understand your unique problems in mentalizing.

Mentalizing practice point: Patients can sometimes relate to the MBT formulation primarily as an intellectual document—an abstract "evaluation" that describes and explains their challenges. However, while most formulations will shed some new light on your difficulties, that is not their main purpose. The aim of the formulation is simply to itemize areas where your reflectiveness tends to get shut down. By being aware of the shape that your non-mentalizing takes, you will be more able to catch yourself in those moments, and to reflect in new, more adaptive ways that lead to better outcomes in your life.

We can think about our lives as being something of a minefield. There are safe areas to walk, and then there are places where, if we are not careful and make a misstep, we could really hurt ourselves and experience tremendous pain and suffering. The problem is that we cannot know the locations of the land mines in advance, so our ability to move around the field is significantly constrained. Now imagine that someone gives us a map of the field, which identifies all of the locations underneath the ground where the mines are hidden. If we had such a map, we could walk around the field with a greater sense of freedom and safety. As we approached the "danger zones" where the land mines are buried, we just need to keep our wits about us—to walk with a level of caution and intentionality, in order to make sure that we do not lose our footing. The MBT formulation is like a map through your own personal "mind field." (Get it? MIND field. I am really proud of that one.) It recounts your unique vulnerabilities in mentalizing, so that you can "reflect rather than reflex" surrounding your core areas of vulnerability.

Bring your formulation with you everywhere you go. Take a picture of it on your phone, so that you can review it and start to catch yourself when you are tempted to respond more reflexively in your life. But when you start to catch yourself, what do you do instead? This book will delineate a range of strategies along these lines—ways to expand your repertoire of effective pathways for mentalization.

Individual MBT. With all of these preliminary steps completed, you and your therapist proceed into the main phase of MBT, which constitutes the bulk of the treatment. Most patients meet with their therapist for once-weekly appointments, but some therapists see patients for twice-weekly visits, depending on the specific treatment setting and the severity of patients' challenges.

Each session begins by "setting an agenda" for the meeting. The agenda involves 1–2 scenarios from your current life, usually related to your shared treatment priorities, as well as mentalizing difficulties covered in your formulation. These could be experiences where you struggled emotionally or interpersonally; where you noticed progress in some problem area; or where you encountered confusion or uncertainty, and would like greater clarity around the issue. Since treatment priorities always involve contemporary challenges in well-being and functionality, agenda items tend to focus on experiences in your recent, current, or future life, rather than events in the distant past. Examples include:

- some recent experience, situation, or interaction;
- an ongoing experience, situation, or interpersonal relationship; or
- some future or potential event, about which you are having an emotional response.

Ideal agenda items are specific rather than abstract. This ensures that sessions do not become too "heady" or intellectualized, and that you are able to fully access and experience your emotions and desires—an essential element in effective mentalizing (see Chapter 14). For example, we would steer clear of agenda items like:

- "I have an unstable sense of self, given my history of past trauma."
- "I have bad boundaries with people."
- "I need tools for working on my anxiety."

While these topics are valid and important areas of difficulty, they are one step removed from patients' lived, contemporary experiences. More grounded and clear-cut agenda items might be:

- "I got into a big fight with my boyfriend this week, and I felt really bad about myself afterwards."
- "My parents were pressuring me to come over and hang out with them on Saturday night. I didn't want to go, but I couldn't really say no to them."
- "I was really anxious at my internship yesterday. I felt so worried that I was doing a bad job, and that everyone could see how insecure I am."

Agenda-setting usually takes no more than five minutes. Once you and your therapist have established and prioritized the agenda items for the appointment, you work together to "mentalize" the areas in question. Usually this follows the domain-based trajectory of mentalizing reviewed in Chapter 3: first exploring the content of the experience (the "what"); then considering its broader context (the "why"); and finally addressing any problems in mentalizing involved in the situation (the "how").

Your therapist will probably ask you to outline the details of the situation under discussion: what happened, who was involved, what was said, and what actions were taken. You and your therapist then consider relevant mental states in the scenario: what you were feeling and wanting; what other people might have been feeling and wanting; how you are feeling and thinking about it now, and so on. When this process goes well, your experience of the matter gradually becomes more elaborated and complex. You notice emotions and desires that did not initially occur to you; you consider connections between feeling states and other aspects of the circumstance (e.g., events, behaviors, other psychological processes); or you take a broader perspective on the situation, focusing on factors that were not as prominent in your original experience.

Often your therapist will give you feedback about some problem in mentalizing they might be observing in you. Perhaps you are feeling quite certain about something; you may be prioritizing "external" aspects of the scenario, focusing less on internal processes; or you could be more "in your head" about the issue, rather than authentically connecting to your or others' emotions. You collaborate with your therapist to address the problem in question, progressively moving to a stance of greater flexibility, curiosity, humility, connectedness, and psychological mindedness around the experience.

Appointments close with five to ten minutes of "session wrap-up." Here you and your therapist consider relevant "take-aways" from the discussion, any areas of improvement, and topics for further inquiry in upcoming meetings.

Mentalizing practice points: The success of individual MBT depends significantly on the relevance of the agenda items that you bring to your appointments. By mentalizing topics that really matter to you, you will feel more engaged in the therapy, and your progress in sessions is more likely to lead to actual change in your everyday life. So before coming to session, really try to ask yourself:

- "What moments over the past week were most impactful for me?"
- "If I had to identify the single time since my last visit where I felt the most pain or distress, what would that be? What about the most pleasure or excitement?"
- "Consider my treatment priority of _____. When did I struggle the most in that area? Where did I see the most positive growth?"

If you struggle to remember relevant moments from your week, try keeping an open "Mentalizing Moments" note on your phone. Here you can record important experiences and interactions, so that you have them ready at the start of your therapy appointments.

Ending phase. The duration of individual MBT can vary significantly, depending on the treatment setting, specific MBT provider, and the needs of the particular patient. In the randomized controlled trials supporting MBT's effectiveness, patients received MBT for approximately 18 months (Bateman & Fonagy, 1999, 2009). Here in the MBT Clinic at McLean Hospital, the therapy course follows the academic calendar and lasts 12 months. Research is currently underway comparing the efficacy of traditional MBT to "short-term" MBT, which takes place over 20 weeks (Juul et al., 2019). For many of us who provide MBT in private practice, treatment has no predetermined end date, continuing based on continued progress in the shared treatment priorities. As patients achieve their goals and maintain their progress over an extended period of time, we often decrease the frequency of appointments, gradually moving toward a formal conclusion of the treatment.

WHAT TO EXPECT IN MBT SESSIONS: "TWO MINDS IN THE ROOM"

We have already reviewed the broad structure of MBT appointments: first agenda-setting, then mentalizing, and finally session wrap-up. Throughout these appointments, your therapist will likely be utilizing MBT's distinctive "therapeutic stance," or broad attitude that cuts across their specific comments and interventions. Above all, MBT therapists tend to be quite inquisitive and "not-knowing" in their clinical approach. In other words, they are going to be asking a lot of questions about your feelings and about other people's feelings. **In fact, MBT therapists are explicitly prohibited from making assumptions and proclamations about your mental states.** This can be confusing to some patients, who think, "Why is my therapist asking me how I felt when my boss insulted me? Isn't it obvious?!" However, remember that MBT believes that it is most helpful for *you* to be mentalizing in therapy. So we recommend that therapists spend their time trying to think up a good question, rather than trying to generate clever ideas or hypotheses about what is going on inside of you.

MBT therapists also tend to be quite active and directive in therapy appointments: setting and pursuing the session agenda; guiding your attention to specific aspects of your experience; asking lots of questions, and then continuing to ask these questions if you do not fully answer them; not allowing extended silences; doggedly encouraging you to consider certain topics; sharing their understanding of what you are saying; communicating their own feelings and ideas about what you are discussing; and sometimes even interrupting you to ask you to say more about something, or to consider some other matter entirely. This active stance can be jarring at first, especially if you are accustomed to therapists who tend to "follow your lead" in a more neutral or passive way.

There are several reasons why MBT therapists utilize this more active approach.

- As an evidence-based psychotherapy, MBT truly prioritizes your functional improvement. We are not satisfied with the status quo, and we genuinely want your life to get better. That means that we often vigorously pursue topics that, in our view, are directly related to your goals for treatment.
- While we avoid explicitly "filling in" your feelings, behind the scenes, we are always asking ourselves the question: "To what extent is this patient reflecting on mental states in a flexible, curious, and engaged manner?" And we are willing to do whatever we can to ensure that this happens. This often entails steering the discussion away from areas that we see as unhelpful, and then asking a question or making a comment that will hopefully stimulate more adaptive mentalizing about some other thing.
- Among MBT therapists, a motto of the therapy is "Two minds in the room." Our assumption is that it is genuinely helpful for patients to be in a relationship with a therapist who engages in the treatment as a real human being. This means not necessarily sharing tons of information about their personal lives, but rather transparently expressing a full range of thoughts, emotions, and desires as they arise in the therapy sessions, in an authentic yet boundaried way. As you experience and connect to your therapist as a three-dimensional person, you gain essential "practice" mentalizing in complex, emotionally charged interpersonal relationships.

So how are YOU supposed to participate in your therapy sessions? Above all else, we recommend that you actively work to maintain a *mentalizing stance* in MBT. In other words, try to remain curious about, and connected to, mental states in yourself and other people, including your therapist. Let's consider these elements in turn.

When mentalizing yourself, actively work to really understand your own internal processes. This can involve considering several facets of experience:

- *The past:* "In that situation, what was I feeling and wanting? How was I feeling about myself?"
- *The current moment:* "As I am talking about all of this, what emotions and desires am I experiencing?"
- *The therapeutic relationship:* "In this interaction with the therapist, what is coming up for me? Do I notice any emotions, wishes, feelings toward the therapist, or feelings about myself?"

- As you notice and identify these feelings in yourself, endeavor to communicate them openly to your therapist. This enables your therapist to understand what is happening internally for you—a necessary condition for them being able to help you with your challenges.

In psychotherapy, many patients can cognitively "know" what they are feeling, but they can struggle to *feel* the emotion in question. They worry that it is somehow "weak" to experience their feelings, or they feel embarrassed to show or express their emotions to another person. For other patients, emotions are like a muscle that has never been flexed—they do not quite know how to access them. Accordingly, when you are working to mentalize yourself in therapy, strive to actually *experience, access, and inhabit* your emotions and desires. We refer to this process as mentalized affectivity—the ability to access an emotion while also reflecting on it at the same time (Jurist, 2018). We are going to spend a lot of time in this book trying to help you do this in a robust and meaningful way. By strengthening this muscle in yourself, you will develop a stronger sense of self, while also cultivating deeper, more authentic connections with other people.

Similarly, when you are mentalizing other people in MBT sessions, seek to maintain a spirit of genuine curiosity and empathy towards them. Try to really put yourself in the other person's shoes—to temporarily see the world from their perspective. We utilize several "mentalizing prompts" to help with this:

- "What is this person feeling and wanting? How are they feeling about themself?"
- "How might this other person be experiencing this situation?" As a follow-up, consider how it could be completely understandable and valid for them to see things in this way. (This can be tough, especially if you are in a conflict with the person.)
- In addition to recognizing what the other individual might be feeling, attempt to actively resonate and empathize with their emotions and desires—to care about what they are going through.

This brings us to the final component in the mentalizing stance mentioned earlier, involving your therapist. I have to disclose something to you along these lines—something that I personally know about your therapist, but they might not have told you yet. So please discreetly look around and make sure that no one is listening, and maybe move your face closer to the page for dramatic effect.

Your therapist is a person, too.

I know, it is an intense idea. This means that you have to apply all of these same principles of mentalizing in the clinical interaction itself. Especially as you get to know your therapist better and the therapeutic process evolves, you might feel drawn to relate to your therapist in a range of reflexive ways:

- Debating or "arguing" with your therapist, telling them why they are wrong, or trying to change their mind
- Without sharing about it openly, internally *focusing* on the problems with your therapist's position or behavior
- Responding defensively or reactively to your therapist's comment or question
- Criticizing something that your therapist has said or done, including some question they have asked you

All of these approaches are inherently anti-mentalizing. Rather than attempting to *understand* your therapist's perspective, they ignore or negate that perspective. This is not to say that your therapist is always correct, or that you should blindly agree with your therapist's view. Remember, MBT is always about TWO minds in the room. In MBT, we urge both parties—therapists *and* patients—to actively seek to understand the other person's experience, while simultaneously remaining grounded in their own experience. We delight in different perspectives, respecting and appreciating those differences without trying to get both people "on the same page." As we will discuss further in Chapter 15, this paves the way for what MBT refers to as *we-mode*—a state of mutual understanding, shared curiosity, reciprocity, and genuine connectedness to Self and Other in the therapeutic relationship.

So how exactly do you mentalize your therapist? Try keeping in mind a handful of mentalizing practice points.

- When your therapist imparts their perspective about something, really try to give it a fair hearing, *without* blindly assuming that this perspective is definitively true. This could involve asking your therapist further questions about what they are thinking, and why they are seeing things in this way. Once you have a clearer sense of their outlook, work to examine your own feelings about it: "What resonates for me about what my therapist is saying? Could they be getting at something here?" Take a moment to really consider this. And then: "What does NOT ring true for me about my therapist's view? How does my experience potentially contradict what my therapist is saying?"
- If you ever find yourself disagreeing with something your therapist says or does (I promise, this *will* happen), "press pause," and try to refrain from criticizing or arguing with them. Instead, really consider the question: "What is my therapist thinking or feeling that is leading them to take this position? What could *their* view be?" Taking this one step further: "Is there anything valid, reasonable, or understandable in this way of seeing things?"
- You can apply these same mentalizing principles to the therapeutic relationship itself. At any given moment in the treatment, but especially if you are experiencing tension or conflict with your therapist (again: It's gonna happen!), try wondering, "What is my therapist thinking, feeling, or wanting in their interaction with me?" Then contextualize these feelings: "How might this be related to them—their lives outside of the therapy, their personality, and who they are as a person? To what extent could they also be reacting to *me*—who I am as a person, how I am treating them, and what I am going through?"

In this section, we have considered a range of questions that will hopefully help you to maintain a mentalizing stance in your therapy sessions. Just to be clear: The purpose of these questions is not to determine "the truth" about what you or others are feeling. Rather, as you authentically wrestle with these prompts, you are adopting a posture of curiosity and openness to mental states in yourself and other people. In MBT, we care more about the *practicing and trying* than about "getting it right." The more that you genuinely practice mentalizing in your therapy appointments, the easier it will be for you to do this in the areas where you struggle in your everyday life. That is how change happens in MBT.

Chapter Review 5.1
Mentalization-Based Treatment: The Basics

Background of Mentalization-based Treatment

- Mentalization-based treatment, or "MBT," is a structured, exploratory, and highly collaborative psychotherapy with roots in psychoanalysis, attachment theory, and developmental psychology.

- MBT helps people to mentalize—to reflect on mental states in themselves and other people—in areas of their life where they tend to get "stuck."

- MBT was developed and researched in the 1990s by Drs. Anthony Bateman and Peter Fonagy, and originally implemented in the National Health Service in the United Kingdom.

- MBT is an evidence-based therapy for people with borderline personality disorder (BPD), with emerging research supporting its use for individuals with antisocial personality disorder, and for adolescents struggling with self-injurious behavior.

The Structure of MBT: From Start to Finish

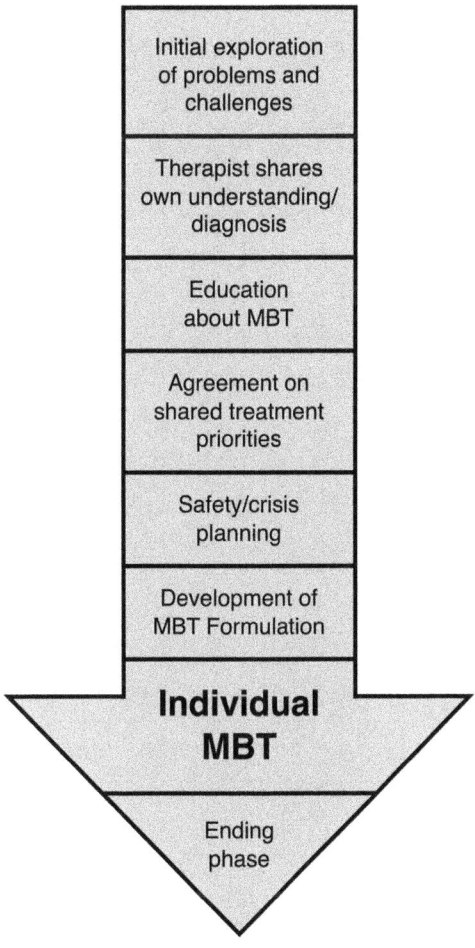

Initial exploration of problems and challenges

Therapist shares own understanding/ diagnosis

Education about MBT

Agreement on shared treatment priorities

Safety/crisis planning

Development of MBT Formulation

Individual MBT

Ending phase

[continued on next page]

What to Expect in MBT Sessions

- MBT sessions start with agenda-setting, progress to mentalizing, and end with session wrap-up.

- The agenda involves 1–2 specific scenarios from your current life, usually related to your goals for treatment and ongoing areas of difficulty.

- You and your therapist "mentalize" each situation: first exploring the content of the experience (the "what"); then considering its broader context (the "why"); and addressing problems in mentalizing involved in the situation (the "how").

- MBT therapists utilize a "not-knowing" or inquisitive therapeutic stance—asking lots of questions about mental states in you and other people.

- Their job is to help YOU to mentalize, so they are not allowed to make assumptions or proclamations about your mental states.

- MBT therapists are active and directive in their exploratory approach: encouraging you to consider certain topics; sharing their understanding of what you are saying; communicating their own feelings and ideas; and even interrupting you to ask you to elaborate on something.

Chapter Review 5.2
Mentalizing Practice Points: How to Engage in Therapy Sessions

The Mentalizing Stance in MBT

MBT recommends that you adopt a *mentalizing stance* in therapy sessions—that is, remain curious about, and connected to, mental states in yourself and other people, including your therapist.

Mentalizing Yourself

Actively work to really understand your own internal processes. This can involve considering several facets of experience:

- *The past:* "In that situation, what was I feeling and wanting? How was I feeling about myself?"

- *The current moment:* "As I am talking about all of this, what emotions and desires am I experiencing?"

- *The therapeutic relationship:* "In this interaction with the therapist, what is coming up for me? Do I notice any emotions, wishes, feelings toward the therapist, or feelings about myself?"

- Do not simply try to "figure out" what you are feeling in these contexts. Strive to actually *experience, access, and inhabit* your emotions and desires.

Mentalizing Other People

When mentalizing other people in MBT sessions, seek to maintain a spirit of genuine curiosity and empathy toward them.

- "What is this person feeling and wanting? How are they feeling about themself?"

- "How might this other person be experiencing this situation?" As a follow-up, consider how it could be completely understandable and valid for them to see things in this way.

- In addition to recognizing what the other individual might be feeling, attempt to actively resonate and empathize with their emotions and desires.

[continued on next page]

Mentalizing Your Therapist

Your therapist is a person too, and mentalizing them is an important part of how YOU make progress in the treatment.

- "What resonates for me about what my therapist is saying? What does not ring true for me about my therapist's view?"

- "What is my therapist thinking or feeling that is leading them to take this position? Is there anything valid, reasonable, or understandable in this way of seeing things?"

- "What is my therapist thinking, feeling, or wanting in their interaction with me? How might this be related to them, and who they are as a person? To what extent could they also be reacting to me—who I am as a person, how I am treating them, and what I am going through?"

6

How to Use This Book

We have been reviewing the difficulties involved in borderline personality disorder (BPD; Chapter 1), as well as how mentalization-based treatment (MBT) understands and addresses them (Chapters 2–5). With these elements in place, we can consider the aims and purpose of *this* book about MBT. For this all to make sense, let me tell you a little bit about myself: how I got started with MBT, and what has led me to write this book.

MY STORY IN MBT

I first learned about MBT in 2009. I was working as a psychotherapist at the Veterans Administration (VA) in the Boston area, primarily utilizing a psychoanalytic approach with my patients. While most of my patients responded well to this modality, some of them did not seem to be getting much better. These were the patients who met diagnostic criteria for BPD and other personality disorders, struggling with symptoms of suicidality, self-injurious behavior, unstable sense of self, and significant impairments in social and vocational functioning. Many of them were homeless, unemployed, and living in poverty, while simultaneously experiencing other psychiatric challenges like substance use disorder and PTSD. I did not know it yet, but these patients shared many similarities with the patients treated at the Halliwick Day Hospital in London, where MBT was first developed and researched.

At the time, I was completing a fellowship at a local psychoanalytic institute. After presenting one of my challenging cases for supervision one evening, one of the analysts there asked me, "Have you ever heard of mentalization-based treatment? You might want to try it with this person." I immediately purchased and devoured Bateman and Fonagy's (2006) treatment manual, doing my best to internalize the techniques on my own. The timing was right: Anthony Bateman and Peter Fonagy were about to visit the United States for one of McLean Hospital's first 3-day trainings in MBT, and I was able to secure a spot. In an incisive way, the training started with some observations about how therapists often provide psychotherapy. Quite naturally, therapists gravitate toward developing and communicating their own ideas about patients' experiences: what patients seem to be feeling about a particular situation; "why" they do what they do; how their problems developed in early family relationships; how their thinking might be distorted, or at odds with reality; and more "effective" strategies patients could be implementing in order to improve their lives. MBT observed that, while these techniques make therapists feel good about themselves, the techniques are often not very helpful to patients with BPD. Patients either take issue with the ideas, explaining why the ideas do not apply to them. Or they passively "absorb" these formulations ("Yeah, I guess that makes sense, when you put it that way"), and yet their challenges continue in their lives outside of session.

This "diagnosis" of my practice deeply resonated with me. In fact, I was doing versions of all these things with my patients who were not getting any better! MBT's alternative approach—namely, directing all of our interventions to stimulating patients' *own* reflectiveness about mental states in themselves and other people—made intuitive sense to me.

Mentalization. Robert P. Drozek, Oxford University Press. © Oxford University Press 2025.
DOI: 10.1093/oso/9780198916857.003.0006

I appreciated the inherently egalitarian nature of this stance, which prioritized patients' own agency in the therapeutic process. This model naturally set limits on therapists' own narcissism—our impulses to be the star of the therapeutic show. I did not know how to do all of this yet, but I felt strongly that there was something important to learn here.

This training happened over the weekend, and these principles were put to the test on Monday morning. I met with my first patient of the day, a Marine Corps veteran with BPD, who was hospitalized on an inpatient unit due to suicidal thinking and impulses. I worked to channel all of the principles I had learned at the training, to see if I could make them my own, and if they would be helpful to the patient. After meeting for about ten minutes, the patient paused the appointment to say, "Something is different about you today. I can't quite put my finger on it, but you really seemed to be *listening*." I felt like the universe was speaking to me: *MBT is onto something.* I started folding MBT's recommendations into my other treatments as well, with notable effects. My patients really liked MBT, and as I hewed to the strategies, our sessions flowed more smoothly. Perhaps most importantly, my patients genuinely seemed to be getting better: exhibiting decreased depression, suicidality, self-injury, anger issues, impulsivity, and inpatient hospitalizations, and also experiencing increased stability and connectedness in their relationships with others.

In these early stages of me learning MBT, Anthony Bateman graciously provided support to me over e-mail: answering questions, clarifying aspects of the technique, and providing consultation about clinical challenges as they arose. With his help, and with the encouragement of the VA, I started up a one-person, unofficial MBT program for veterans with personality disorders and difficulties with emotional regulation. At its height, I was seeing 15–20 patients for weekly MBT, while also facilitating three longitudinal MBT psychotherapy groups. We had to keep creating new groups, in order to accommodate the level of interest from veterans.

While I felt highly fulfilled by all of this work, it was also somewhat isolating. To my knowledge, I was the only clinician at the VA providing MBT. While attending further trainings at McLean Hospital, I would see scores of staff from various McLean programs, who spent all of their time delivering and teaching our evidence-based therapies for personality disorders: dialectical behavior therapy, mentalization-based treatment, transference-focused psychotherapy, and good psychiatric management. I felt a longing to be a part of this larger community, where I could engage with and learn from other clinicians who were devoted to using these treatments to help these patients.

At the time, there were no formal "jobs" available in the MBT Clinic at McLean, as the program was small and staffed mostly by trainees. So I decided to volunteer my time there, in order to gain further experience providing MBT as part of a broader team. Developed and led by the psychiatrist Brandon Unruh—himself a trainer in MBT through the Anna Freud Centre in London—the program provided adherent individual and group MBT to patients with symptoms of personality disorders, which essentially means significant challenges in self-esteem and relationships. Before Zoom was even a thing, Anthony Bateman would join Rounds virtually from London every week, to provide continued MBT clinical supervision for the patients we were treating.

My first patient in the Clinic was named Jonathan, a talented visual artist in his 40s. Having been in four-times-weekly psychoanalysis for 16 years, Jonathan had largely regressed in that treatment. He struggled with debilitating anxiety and depression, inability to work, profound social isolation, and suicide attempts, resulting in multiple inpatient hospitalizations. We accepted Jonathan for a pared-down treatment with us: once-weekly individual MBT with me and once-weekly group MBT with Brandon Unruh—the same treatment package shown to be effective in randomized controlled trials of MBT. As I have described in detail elsewhere (Drozek, 2019, Ch. 7), Jonathan's response to MBT was remarkable. By the end of his year in the MBT Clinic, he was experiencing significantly improved mood, no suicidal thinking, no inpatient admissions, and consistent fulfillment in his work and social relationships. At the time of this writing, all of these gains have continued and proliferated. Perhaps most movingly, Jonathan is now in a stable, loving romantic relationship—the first in his adult life.

This treatment floored me. How was it that we had provided Jonathan *less* treatment than he had been receiving, and yet his response was so much better? This only reinforced the value of the MBT approach in my mind, also underscoring an almost ethical imperative of ensuring that patients who are suffering can access evidence-based treatment, which can genuinely improve their lives. I was ultimately hired as a staff psychotherapist and supervisor in the MBT Clinic, where I now serve as the Clinical Director. This commenced a period of highly productive work in MBT. Inspired by Anthony Bateman and Peter Fonagy's pedagogical approach, I became especially interested in the question: "How can we write and teach MBT in a manner that makes it as accessible as possible to therapists, so that they can easily learn the techniques and deliver them to patients?" Collaborating with colleagues, I helped to develop the *domain-based* theory of mentalizing reviewed in Chapter 3: a streamlined, step-by-step approach to assessing mentalization and delivering MBT (Drozek et al., 2023; Drozek & Henry, 2021).

I had the honor of becoming an official "trainer" in MBT, helping Anthony Bateman and Peter Fonagy to lead MBT trainings for clinicians across the world. Brandon Unruh and I began offering online supervision in MBT, while continuing to train and supervise clinicians here at McLean through the MBT Clinic. We also worked to spearhead new applications of MBT: MBT for pathological narcissism, or people who struggle with disruptions in self-esteem (Drozek & Unruh, 2020; Drozek et al. 2023); MBT-informed psychoanalytic psychotherapy (Drozek, 2019; Drozek, 2022); and MBT as a method to address law enforcement violence (Drozek et al., 2021).

This all brings to me to why I am writing this book. In my current role at the hospital, much of my work involves completing diagnostic assessments for patients, where we discuss the relevance of the personality disorder diagnosis and consider effective forms of treatment. When I recommend MBT as a form of therapy for patients, the most common question I receive is, "Are there any books that I can read about what MBT is, and how it works?" Unfortunately, as I mentioned in Chapter 2, all of the books about MBT are written by and for clinicians! In my view, this has significantly hamstrung people's awareness of MBT as a therapeutic modality that can potentially help them. My hope is that this book can serve as an accessible introductory text about MBT, so that individuals with BPD can learn more about this evidence-based treatment.

For many years, I have facilitated the MBT-Introductory groups discussed in Chapter 5, or "MBT-I." After I led MBT-I group sessions, patients would often ask me, "Is there anything else I can read to learn more about this? Or even a worksheet that I can complete, like they have in DBT?" In light of this, I developed a short "workbook" for patients, which introduced the main ideas in MBT, including worksheets to help patients apply these concepts to their everyday lives. Patients have really appreciated this resource, explaining that it has helped make MBT more pragmatic and "experience-near" for them. The Anna Freud Centre, the centralized training institute for MBT, now distributes this workbook at their trainings. Therapists have begun using the workbook as a tool in individual and group MBT, to help guide patients through the introductory phase of the therapy. The present book is an expanded version of that workbook, aimed to make these worksheets available on a wider scale.

In my private psychotherapy practice, my main focus is providing individual MBT to patients with personality disorders, trauma and dissociative disorders, and addiction. In my sessions with patients, I actively utilize MBT's techniques to help patients address their challenges with mood, self-esteem, relationships, and functionality. As we work on these issues together, patients will often ask me, "But HOW do I mentalize about this issue? What does that even look like?" This has made me realize that, while we have myriad illuminating treatment manuals for MBT, there are no books reviewing how patients *themselves* can apply these techniques to address their challenges. As a stopgap remedy for this problem, I have developed patient-centered "translations" of MBT's therapeutic interventions, writing these up in Word documents so that patients can independently apply these techniques in their lives outside of sessions. This book strives not simply to expose people to the abstract concepts of MBT, but to formulate MBT's strategies in a clear, accessible manner for people who are suffering.

THE FORMAT OF THIS BOOK

This book is divided into three parts. We are just now finishing up Part 1, "Mentalization and Borderline Personality Disorder." Part 2, "Keeping Mentalization Online," covers all of the problem areas that we target in MBT, as well as mentalizing techniques that you can use to address these difficulties in your life. Part 3, "Bringing It All Together," synthesizes all of the principles reviewed in the book into a handful of core strategies, geared toward helping you develop a life of greater purpose, fulfillment, and trust—in yourself and in your relationships.

From here on out, each chapter reviews one fundamental concept in MBT, ranging from "What is Your Attachment Style?" (Chapter 8) to "How to Recognize 'What' People are Feeling" (Chapter 9) to "Addressing Problems with Externalization and Concreteness" (Chapter 13). All chapters follow roughly the same structure. They always open with a **case example**—a brief vignette about a patient whose experience illustrates the ideas under discussion. By grounding MBT's concepts in people's everyday lives and challenges, I hope to keep things accessible and experience-near. While each case example contains elements from real patients I have treated, they are really more like amalgamations, synthesizing several people's experiences in order to express a central difficulty MBT can be helpful in addressing. So when you read about someone in the book, rest assured that they are disguised, and their privacy is being protected.

Structure of Each Chapter

- *Case example:* a brief story about a patient whose experience illustrates the ideas under discussion

- Summary of MBT's core concepts about the topic area of the chapter

- *Mentalizing warm-up:* one to two questions asking readers to consider the case in light of the concepts just reviewed

- *Mentalizing practice points:* practical recommendations about how to reflect on mental states surrounding the topic under discussion

- *Mentalizing cool-down:* a single question encouraging readers to apply MBT's strategies to the case that started the chapter

- *Worksheets:* questions about the subject matter covered in the chapter, encouraging readers to relate these constructs to their everyday experience *(can appear throughout the chapter)*

- *Chapter reviews:* brief summary sheets of the chapter's main ideas *(always appear at the end of the chapter)*

The chapters then present the main ideas related to the topic under discussion, highlighting information that will hopefully enable you to "see yourself" somewhere in the subject matter.

In my experience, whatever is happening in my life at any particular time, there are always at least *parts* of these topics with which I can identify, if I am looking for it. All chapters are relatively brief, including just enough information to help you get started in MBT. Above all else, this book aims to be pragmatic and usable for you.

After we consider the main conceptual information in the chapter, you have the opportunity to relate these ideas to the case example from the beginning of the chapter. This is called a **mentalizing warm-up**: one to two questions inviting you to reconsider the case in light of the new information just reviewed. These warm-ups help you to internalize and wield the theory covered in the book—taking it for a "test drive" by applying it to someone else's life, before linking it to your own experience. Sometimes it is easier to mentalize ourselves if we mentalize someone else first!

Chapters ultimately progress to what I call **mentalizing practice points**, or practical recommendations about how to reflect on mental states in the area in question. You have already seen some examples of these in Chapter 5, when we were reviewing the structure of the treatment. Remember: In MBT, we are not trying to change your thoughts, or to teach you behavioral skills. We are simply trying to help you to mentalize, in the areas where you tend to struggle. Mentalizing practice points sketch out the shape and direction of these forms of reflectiveness, attempting to answer the question: "What would it actually look like for me to 'reflect rather than reflex' in the situation I am going through right now?"

As a clinical social worker by discipline, I explain to my patients that of course I am not qualified to prescribe medications. But there is one thing that I am licensed to prescribe: mentalization! *[Ba-dum ching.]* Whereas DBT has behavioral skills, MBT has mentalizing practice points—the "mentalizing prescriptions" that illustrate how to apply the techniques of MBT in your everyday life. After reviewing these suggestions, chapters transition into a **mentalizing cool-down**: one question encouraging you to apply these principles to the case that started the chapter. We then close out each chapter by considering how the patient progressed when they sought to mentalize around their core areas of vulnerability.

Worksheets consist of questions about the topic areas covered in each chapter, encouraging you to consider how these constructs relate to your everyday experience. Worksheets can be seen as self-directed tools to stimulate mentalizing—to reflect on your feelings, other people's feelings, and patterns in relationships. While worksheets sometimes appear at the end of the chapter, often they occur immediately after the section in question. This can help you to apply these concepts directly to your life, while the reading is still fresh in your mind.

Chapter reviews are brief summary sheets of the main ideas in the chapter. Think of them as the SparkNotes for each chapter—the absolutely essential information that MBT wants you to take away about the concepts under discussion. While some chapter reviews detail basic facts about MBT, others compile the mentalizing practice points outlined throughout the chapter. In this way, you can have a "one-stop shop" that recaps the key practical recommendations throughout the book. Since they sum up key information, chapter reviews always appear in the final pages of the chapter. Feel free to browse the chapter reviews to get a sense of what each chapter has to offer, or to refresh your memory about key topics covered.

THE AUDIENCE FOR THIS BOOK

This book is geared toward four primary audiences:

- people with BPD and other psychological challenges, who are interested in using MBT to address their emotional or interpersonal difficulties;
- clinicians seeking to learn more about MBT, or to teach their patients about the therapy;

- family members of people with BPD, who want to gain information about MBT as a resource; and
- members of the general public, who are curious about mentalizing and MBT.

Let's consider these groups of readers in turn.

People with borderline personality disorder and other psychological challenges

In Chapter 1, we reviewed all of the diagnostic criteria for BPD. If you identified with these symptoms, or if you have been formally diagnosed with BPD by a clinician, then this book is for you. You might also be experiencing symptoms of other personality disorders:

- needs for admiration, sensitivity to shame/humiliation, difficulties with resentment and interpersonal conflicts, and an externally focused, "conditional" self-esteem associated with narcissistic personality disorder (Drozek & Unruh, 2020; Drozek et al., 2023);
- rigidity, perfectionism, rumination, disconnection from emotions, and excessive focus on work/productivity linked with obsessive compulsive personality disorder;
- irresponsibility, dishonesty, aggression, lack of financial autonomy, or law-breaking or unethical behaviors related to antisocial personality disorder; or
- avoidance, isolation, inhibition, social anxiety, fear of being humiliated, and a sense of inferiority and inadequacy connected with avoidant personality disorder.

Or perhaps you are experiencing psychological challenges not obviously related to issues of personality: anxiety, depression, posttraumatic stress disorder, psychosis, addiction, eating disorders, or problems in your relationships.

If you have been struggling in any of these ways, I want to let you know that we successfully employ MBT to treat all of these concerns (Bateman et al., 2023). I am hopeful that this book will offer you some clarity in these matters, and that you will be able to chart a new path forward in your life. As we discussed in Chapter 5, a foundational component in mentalization-based treatment is the MBT Formulation, a document that summarizes patients' core challenges in mentalizing. **We are going to use this book to help you develop your own, personalized MBT Formulation.** Throughout the book, you will learn about all of the different shapes that problems in mentalizing take, utilizing the worksheets to pinpoint specific examples of these problems in your core areas of difficulty. When completed and assembled together, these worksheets will contain all of the information that we would normally include in an official MBT Formulation.

But we are not just going to "identify" your problems in mentalizing. As we explore these challenges throughout the book, we will consider MBT's strategies for getting mentalization back online, once it has become disrupted. These are the mentalizing practice points mentioned earlier, which are summarized in the chapter reviews throughout the book. As you learn how to practice mentalizing in the situations where you struggle, you will start to experience improvements in mood, self-esteem, relationships, and functionality. That is how MBT works.

A word of warning about the book: *It is long.* Sorry about that, but as the first book for patients about MBT, I wanted to make sure to cover all of MBT's core concepts and strategies. In light of this, if you feel at all overwhelmed by the amount of information in these pages, I suggest that you "pick and choose" the chapters that feel most interesting and relevant to you. While each chapter builds on the one before it, most of the chapters in Parts 2 and 3 remain relatively freestanding and self-contained, so hopefully you can understand the main ideas even if you have skipped over the previous chapters. At the very least, if you want to prioritize taking in the "big picture" of a chapter, I recommend simply reviewing (a) the two-part case example that bookends the chapter, and (b) the chapter reviews (immediately following the conclusion of the case example), which summarize the relevant theory and strategies covered in much greater detail throughout the chapter.

If you are currently engaged in a psychotherapy, I encourage you to bring in the worksheets from this book to share them with your therapist, so that you and your therapist can start to discuss your idiosyncratic troubles in mentalizing. If you are specifically involved in individual MBT or an MBT-informed psychotherapy, your therapist can then use your responses on these worksheets to inform or update the MBT Formulation they develop with you.

And if you do not have a therapist—wait, you don't have a therapist?! While the ideas and principles in this book will hopefully be useful for you in and of themselves, they tend to work best when they are folded into a psychotherapeutic treatment. Plus you should NOT have to be going through these challenges all on your own. So put this book down for a moment, and try googling "How do I find a therapist?" online. Since I do not know you, I cannot offer advice here in any great detail. But consider investigating the following resources, which many patients find helpful when seeking to get connected to a new therapist.

- Your primary care doctor
- If you attend college, your school's student health department
- Your insurance company
- The "Find a Psychologist" tool from the American Psychological Association
- Your local chapter of the National Association of Social Workers
- The National Alliance on Mental Illness "NAMI Helpline"
- Virtual psychotherapy, or one of the many therapy apps on your phone. This type of treatment is offered in a range of different formats (e.g., video, phone, text), by organizations with different services, availability, and cost. Some of these companies are legitimate and others are not, so make sure to read reviews before proceeding.
- If you are a person of color, or a member of another oppressed or marginalized group, there are various services that specialize in "matching" you with culturally competent psychotherapists who are members of your community, or who have clinical experience working with people in your community.

If you are interested in finding a therapist who provides individual MBT, try visiting the website for the Anna Freud National Centre for Children and Families. They maintain a database of official "MBT practitioners" across the world, or clinicians who have received extensive training and supervision in MBT. They also publish an online list of accredited MBT supervisors—clinicians who are certified trainers in MBT, and who of course specialize in offering MBT themselves. Since they train and supervise therapists in MBT, MBT supervisors can often introduce you to other therapists in their community who are competent providers of MBT. If you live outside of the United States, you can also try googling "mentalization-based treatment in *[insert the name of your country of residence]*." Many countries have "associations" of MBT providers based in the country, along with websites for the organizations that include profiles and contact information for their members.

If you live in the Northeastern United States, check out MBT Boston, an association that Brandon Unruh and I started to help train clinicians in MBT, and to connect patients to psychotherapists whom we have personally supervised. Our website has contact information for these therapists, so that you can reach out to them directly. If you are interested in more intensive services, McLean Hospital has several programs that offer MBT and MBT-informed psychotherapy. The Gunderson Residence is a residential program that provides all of the evidence-based therapies for personality disorders, including MBT. Similarly, the Gunderson Outpatient Program is an intensive outpatient program that delivers all of these evidence-based therapies. I personally run the MBT group component of this program, and several of us provide twice-weekly individual MBT for some patients in the program.

On the west coast of the United States, the Mentalizing Initiative is a non-profit organization dedicated to educating clinicians about MBT. Led by Robin Kissell, one of the first MBT trainers in the United States, the faculty there are all expert MBT therapists, many of whom maintain private practices where they offer MBT.

OK, well hopefully that is enough information to help you get started in finding a therapist. Now feel free to move on to Part 2 of the book, where you can begin considering your personal problems in mentalizing, and how to address them.

Clinicians seeking to teach their patients about MBT, or to learn more about it themselves

You might also be engaging with this volume as a mental health clinician—a psychotherapist or psychopharmacologist who is interested in learning more about MBT, or teaching your patients about it. If this is the case: bravo and welcome! There is far too much therapy out there that is not informed by research and science, and thus that has the potential to be iatrogenic, harming patients rather than helping them. By taking the time out of your schedule to learn about one of our evidence-based therapies, you are investing in the lives of your patients. That displays a level of humility on your part—the recognition that you are only seeing part of the picture, and that you need to learn more in order to better serve your patients. That attitude is the beating heart of MBT.

As a clinician, there are several different ways for you to use this book. If you are working with patients individually, you can invite them to purchase the book and collaboratively work your way through the text together: giving the chapters as reading assignments; instructing patients to complete the worksheets; and discussing the chapters and completed worksheets in sessions, all to the end of exploring with patients how these ideas relate to their challenges outside of sessions. You can do this at the outset of an MBT treatment, or you can fold these exercises into an established psychotherapy, in order to introduce patients to the MBT model. If patients cannot afford the book, feel free to photocopy the worksheets and chapter reviews for them. You can then use session time to provide initial psychoeducation about BPD and MBT, utilizing the book as a guide for the content and sequencing of session topics. For example, one appointment could cover the topic of "Mentalization: What is It?" (Chapter 3), the next visit could focus on "How does Borderline Personality Disorder Develop?" (Chapter 4), and so on.

If you are leading MBT-I groups as part of your practice, this book is meant to serve as a companion to such groups. While the current chapter is more editorial and specifically related to this book as a text, the other 14 chapters cover all of the main elements involved in an MBT treatment—the essential information that patients need in order to get started in MBT. Feel free to tailor the structure and sequence of the group sessions to meet the needs of your practice or organization, and to the interests of the particular patients you are treating. You can lead 14 different group sessions, covering one chapter per week and following the order outlined here. You also could use a more "buffet style" approach: reviewing chapters that you see as most essential and interesting, and skipping over chapters that feel less relevant to your patients. When some chapters contain more information, you might choose to spread those out over several weeks. This opens up additional time for discussion and questions, especially if your patients have more to say about certain worksheets and chapter reviews.

Some of you might also be leading longer-term MBT groups, or groups that accept patients on a rolling admissions basis. Here you can periodically fold in 1–2 sessions of psychoeducation from the book, to ensure that new and existing patients are well-versed in the information that is central to MBT's efficacy. At times, you might notice that a particular problem in mentalizing could be taking hold in the group, and so you can "press pause" to facilitate a session on a relevant chapter from the book. For example, if patients seem consistently disconnected from their emotions, you could facilitate a group session where you read and discuss Chapter 14, "Addressing Problems with Disconnection and Dissociation." Or if group members appear to be consistently blaming other people for their problems, you can lead a session on Chapter 12, "Addressing Problems with Certainty and Rigidity." This infuses mentalizing principles into the group process, fostering a group culture of reflectiveness and helping members to get "unstuck" from maladaptive patterns.

A word of caution about the scope of this book. This book can be seen as a patient-centered introduction to the concepts and techniques of MBT, something akin to the *DBT skills training handouts and worksheets* (Linehan, 2015a), but for MBT. In this way, the text is intentionally didactic and content-focused: We have some information to get across! However, while MBT contains educational components (especially in its earliest phases), it is not primarily a didactic therapy. MBT is a patient-centered and *process-based* psychotherapy, which aims to stimulate patients' mentalizing around their unique concerns and functional challenges. So I recommend that you employ this book to supplement and reinforce the therapy you are already providing, not as a therapeutic approach in and of itself.

To learn more about how to structure and deliver all components of MBT, consider purchasing the main MBT treatment manual, Bateman and Fonagy's (2016) *Mentalization-based treatment for personality disorders: A practical guide*. This is the definitive presentation of the comprehensive treatment package of MBT, the one source to which I always return in order to remain grounded in the model. Bateman and colleagues (2023) also recently published a highly accessible "primer" on MBT, complete with visual illustrations of therapist–patient interactions, along with guidelines for applying MBT across different settings, diagnoses, and patient populations.

Another helpful book is our own *Mentalization-based treatment for pathological narcissism: A handbook*, written by myself, Brandon Unruh, and Anthony Bateman (Drozek et al., 2023). While that volume focuses on helping patients who struggle with instability in self-esteem, it also introduces what we call the *domain-based* model of mentalizing: a simplified account of MBT's therapeutic techniques that can be useful for clinicians who are just getting started with MBT in general. This model parallels the tripartite conception of mentalizing introduced in Chapter 3 of this book: first exploring the content of patients' experiences (the "what"), then placing these experiences in a broader context (the "why"), and finally addressing any problems in mentalizing that emerge throughout that process (the "how"). By thoughtfully integrating these techniques with the patient-centered strategies contained throughout this book, you will be encouraging your patients' own sense of agency in implementing the therapeutic principles of MBT.

Family members or loved ones of someone with borderline personality disorder

Research suggests that MBT is especially helpful for family members of individuals with BPD (Bateman & Fonagy, 2019b), resulting in

- decreased adverse incidents between family members and the person with BPD;
- improvements in family members' depression, anxiety, and overall burden of the person with BPD's illness; and
- improved functioning, empowerment, and sense of well-being in the family.

If you are a family member or loved one of someone with BPD, this book can serve as a useful introduction to the problems in mentalizing associated with BPD, as well as the strategies that research suggests are particularly effective at addressing the symptoms of BPD. While of course your role as a family member is not to teach your loved one therapeutic techniques (that's what therapists are for!), these chapters will help you gain a broader understanding of this leading evidence-based treatment for BPD, so that you can steer your loved one in the right direction (e.g., to MBT therapists, to this book) when they are struggling.

As other books have illustrated (Manning, 2011; Mason & Kreger, 2020), loving someone with BPD can be a tumultuous endeavor, leading to feelings of fear, sadness, anger, and emotional exhaustion. MBT has an aphorism that is relevant here: "Non-mentalizing begets non-mentalizing." When your loved one is struggling to reflect on mental states in themself and other people, quite understandably, you might reflexively fall into difficulties with non-reflectiveness yourself. This could include:

- becoming emotionally dysregulated and reactive in your interactions with your family member;
- focusing extensively on *their* feelings rather than your own;
- "blaming" your loved one for your challenges—that is, failing to reflect on your own contributions in complex family dynamics; and
- feeling certain that you have to fix, save, or rescue the person with BPD.

While this book is written to and for people with BPD, all of MBT's tools are equally applicable to your *own* challenges that arise in your relationship with the person with BPD. So I encourage you to read and digest the ideas in these chapters, and to consider how they might relate to where you struggle in your everyday life. Complete the worksheets if you like, and try implementing the mentalizing practice points while you are interacting with your family member.

As the research on MBT for families and BPD illustrates, when you are able to effectively practice mentalizing in your relationship with your loved one with BPD, you will start to feel better in these dynamics, and the quality of these relationships will improve over time. This is all to say that the converse of the aforementioned aphorism is also true: *Mentalizing begets mentalizing*, in yourself and with the people that matter to you most.

Members of the general public who are curious about mentalizing and MBT

Finally, you might be reading this book as a member of the general public who simply wants to learn more about mentalizing, or MBT. Perhaps you came across this book on Amazon, or saw it on the shelf in the bookstore. Maybe you read an inspiring, 5-star review of the book in some esteemed literary magazine! (A guy can dream, can't he?) You might have a friend or family member who faces psychiatric challenges, and you are wondering if MBT could help. You could work or study in an academic discipline where mentalization was mentioned (e.g., neuroscience, philosophy, history, sociology), and you are curious about the concept and its applications.

If any of these descriptions apply to you, then you have come to the right place. This book aims to be an accessible entry point to mentalization and MBT, geared toward readers who have no previous knowledge of these ideas. And in terms of how to use this book, the answer is simple: any way that you like! Take the liberty to just read the chapters in the book, skipping over the worksheets if you are not interested in them. However, if you feel up to it, take a crack at completing the worksheets as well. Think of the worksheets as practical tools for learning the theoretical concepts in the book. That has definitely been my experience: When I consistently relate the constructs of MBT to my everyday life, I am able to wield them, and to understand them at a greater depth and complexity.

If you really want to take things to the next level, try out some of the mentalizing practice points as you go. Who knows? They just might help. As we discussed in Chapter 3, mentalizing is a fundamentally human capacity, an essential element in what it means to be a social being in the world. Similarly, problems in mentalizing are ubiquitous across human experience. Whenever we are stressed, anxious, or upset about something, there is usually some trouble in mentalizing in play for us, whether or not we meet criteria for any psychiatric diagnoses. In my experience, when I apply the principles of MBT in my personal life, I tend to feel better about myself, and I am able to be more emotionally present, empathic, and flexible in my relationships. Even if you do not feel like you are struggling in any significant way, mentalization can lead to a greater sense of fulfillment, connectedness, and self-esteem in your everyday life and interactions. I hope that this book can serve as a helpful introduction to these ideas—at an intellectual level and also a personal one.

PART 2

Keeping Mentalization Online

7

Identifying Your Triggers

Chloe had a long history of unstable relationships with romantic partners, marked by jealousy, arguments, and frequent break-ups. That all changed when she met her girlfriend Elizabeth. Elizabeth was unlike anyone Chloe had ever dated. In addition to being "totally hot," Elizabeth was kind, stable, and highly empathic. She had a good job as an accountant, and she made a lot of money. (Usually Chloe had to support all of her girlfriends financially!) Rather than going out and partying all of the time like Chloe's exes, Elizabeth preferred to hang out at home for the night: getting take-out, watching Netflix, and cuddling on the couch together. Elizabeth was also highly affectionate and complimentary of Chloe, which made Chloe feel safe, cared for, and comforted. She knew she had found her person.

The relationship progressed quickly, and they decided to move in together. Chloe loved this, as they were able to spend *all* of their time together, never having to be apart. But living together also brought new complications into their relationship. Elizabeth worked mostly from home, and after her work day ended, she liked to unwind by playing video games for an hour or two. Chloe would make dinner for them while Elizabeth played, but she started to get annoyed by how often Elizabeth was playing these games. When they spent time together on the couch in the evenings, Elizabeth would often scroll Instagram and Reddit on her phone, rather than cuddling and focusing on Chloe. Whereas previously they had sex every day, now this was happening only 2–3 times per week, since Elizabeth was supposedly "tired and worn out."

Chloe started to feel increasingly insecure, and worried about the relationship. She had thought that Elizabeth was different, but clearly Elizabeth's feelings for her were fading. Elizabeth seemed more invested in video games and social media than in their relationship! This all led to arguments and conflicts between them, with Chloe accusing Elizabeth of not caring about her, and Elizabeth calling Chloe "unreasonable" and (on one occasion in their worst fight) "needy." These words hit Chloe like a sledgehammer. This was her biggest fear: being needy and "too much" for other people, and Elizabeth had already seen this side of her. Chloe started to retreat to their bedroom, trying to escape from all of this under the covers. But Elizabeth's words continued to play in a continuous loop in Chloe's mind. How could the relationship go on if Elizabeth was seeing her this way? Chloe started to feel more hopeless and desperate, even thinking that it might be better if she were not around. Here she was in the same position she always was: feeling rejected by a romantic partner, and trapped in a relationship where she was more invested than the other person, with no clear way to get out. What could she do to break this unchanging pattern?

WHAT IS A "TRIGGER" IN MBT?

The term *trigger* has become almost ubiquitous in contemporary culture. As normally understood, a trigger is an event or situation that provokes an intense, distressing emotional reaction in someone, such as fear, anger, or panic. While sometimes triggers are connected to an individual's past traumatic or stressful experiences (e.g., in the case of traumatic reminders

Mentalization. Robert P. Drozek, Oxford University Press. © Oxford University Press 2025.
DOI: 10.1093/oso/9780198916857.003.0007

associated with posttraumatic stress disorder), in other cases, they could simply be related to contemporary experiences that generate painful emotions in people. With references to "trigger warnings" and "getting triggered," most discussions about triggers center on our responsibility to be responsive to other people's feelings: recognizing our power to upset and impact others; refraining from taking actions that could cause others distress; and preemptively alerting other individuals that we are about to communicate something that might upset them. In other words, thinking about triggers reminds us to mentalize other people!

Mentalization-based treatment (MBT) outlines a slightly different conception of a trigger. In Chapter 2, we saw that BPD involves an inverse connection between attachment and mentalizing: When you feel threatened or insecure in a particular relational domain, you might struggle to flexibly reflect on mental states in yourself and other people. In light of this theory, MBT is especially interested in helping you to identify your *attachment-related* triggers—that is, the external factors that precipitate your insecurities about yourself and others, or that activate your characteristic manner of engaging with other people. By being aware of your attachment-related triggers, you will be more able to "hold on to your mind" as you encounter them. This enables you to make different choices in the areas where you tend to get stuck in your life.

In order to help you recognize your triggers, let's review a few key points about how MBT understands them. First, triggers should always be external elements in the world around you, such as events or circumstances, others' actions or qualities, or things that other people say. We would never list as a trigger something happening *inside* of another person (e.g., someone else judging you), or something happening inside of you (e.g., you feeling insecure that someone is judging you). Once you get "inside" in these ways, the problem in mentalizing has often already occurred! For example, you feel *convinced* that someone is judging you, or you feel quite certain that you deserve to be judged (Chapter 12). So we suggest that you rewind the movie of your life to the moment just BEFORE you started to feel upset, excited, or worked up. "Press pause" at that moment, and ask yourself the question: "What were the things happening around me that led things to unravel?" It is sometimes not easy to answer this question, so keep reading to learn more about the different shapes that triggers can take.

Second, while triggers in MBT can be factors that generate painful emotions in you, they also can be seemingly "positive" factors in your life, which lead you to feel excited, enthusiastic, or hopeful that some particular thing will happen. *Anything that makes you feel emotionally stimulated qualifies as a trigger in MBT.* When we are excited about something, we feel motivated to pursue it, and we have something to lose. Our field of vision starts to narrow, and we focus on the thing that matters to us: some person that we care about, some response that we crave from someone, or some event that we really want to happen, such as getting a good grade on a test or being promoted at work. The stakes feel high, and it becomes difficult to reflect in a flexible, thoughtful way. As the psychoanalyst Stephen Mitchell (1993) proposed, human motivation encompasses both hopes and dreads: "expectant, optimistic longings and fearful, gripping terrors" (p. 9). A trigger is anything that stimulates dread, but also anything that arouses hope. For the sake of clarity, I will refer to aversive or upsetting experiences as *distressing* triggers, and pleasurable or enticing experiences as *exciting* triggers.

Third, triggers can be framed in terms of situations in general, as well as specific scenarios that impact you. For example, general triggers could be "Any time that I receive constructive feedback from an authority figure," or "Whenever I start up a new romantic relationship, and I am spending a lot of time with the person." More specific triggers might be "My father criticizing my political beliefs," or "My best friend taking a long time to respond to a text message." While recognizing general triggers enables you to see yourself from a "big picture" perspective ("I tend to struggle when . . . "), noticing specific triggers helps you to attend to the minutiae of everyday experiences and interactions. By identifying *both* general and specific triggers in your life, you are able to keep your balance when you know that one of these scenarios is coming your way.

Finally, you can use a helpful rule of thumb to pinpoint triggers in your life. By and large, triggers are external factors that provoke one or more of the following three responses in you:

- Any intense emotional state, painful or exciting;
- The appearance of your typical attachment patterns, or characteristic manner of managing closeness in your relationships (more on this coming up in Chapter 8);
- Any difficulties in mentalizing: challenges considering mental states in yourself or other people; disconnection from your emotions; tendencies toward certainty, impulsiveness, reactivity, and so on.

So start with any of the above reactions that resonate with you, which you can easily notice in your experience. Then "work your way backwards" to the external element that typically prompts these reactions in you. What tends to make you feel that way? That "thing" would likely qualify as a trigger in MBT.

Mentalizing Warm-up

With all of these ideas about triggers in your back pocket, take a look back at Chloe's story at the start of the chapter, on page 109. What are Chloe's triggers, and how do they impact her?

TYPES OF TRIGGERS

Now that we understand what a trigger is in MBT, let's review six different "types" of triggers. By understanding the shape that triggers can take, you will be in a better position to inventory your own personal triggers, and how they impact you. The following list is not meant to be comprehensive, but hopefully it covers many of the domains that feel relevant to you.

Six Types of Triggers

- Interpersonal interactions
- Valued interpersonal interactions NOT happening
- Interpersonal situations
- Valued interpersonal situations NOT happening
- Events or circumstances
- Valued events or circumstances NOT happening

Interpersonal interactions. The most common types of triggers are interpersonal interactions themselves, most notably what people say to you and how they treat you. When it comes to distressing interpersonal triggers, examples include someone criticizing you, giving you constructive feedback, or making a comment that you find offensive or upsetting. Examples of exciting interpersonal triggers might be someone giving you a compliment, expressing their love for you, or initiating a sexual interaction with you. When identifying your triggers related to interpersonal interactions, always make sure to describe the comments or actions that are likely to activate you. You can specify these interactions at various levels of abstraction, as illustrated by the following examples:

- *Specific interactions with particular individuals, or groups of people:* "Getting into an argument with my significant other"; "My father telling me he is proud of me"; "My kids making a lot of noise when I am trying to do work"; "Talking with my boyfriend about our plans for the future"; "My sister ditching me to hang out with her boyfriend"
- *Types of interactions that you find emotionally activating, regardless of the person:* "Whenever anyone raises their voice at me"; "Receiving positive feedback about my intelligence"; "People cutting me off in traffic"; "If someone touches me without asking me first"
- *Interactions with certain kinds of people, or people in specific roles:* "People in authority behaving in an immoral, unjust manner"; "In romantic relationships, the other person talking about their exes"; "When really attractive people show me attention"
- *People taking actions that are not directly related to you, but still impact how you feel:* "My partner loading the dishwasher incorrectly"; "My boss making decisions that are bad for the company"; "My dad continuing to drink alcohol, even though it is bad for his health"

To apply some of these ideas, let's return to our discussion of Chloe at the start of the chapter. For Chloe, examples of distressing interpersonal triggers could be Elizabeth playing video games after work, scrolling Instagram and Reddit on her phone, and calling Choe "unreasonable" and "needy" in the context of their arguments—all of which led Chloe to feel insecure, rejected, and hopeless in the relationship. If Chloe wanted to frame her triggers in more general terms, she might say "Romantic partners engaging in other activities, rather than spending all of their time with me" or "Other people expressing constructive feedback to me, especially the idea that I am 'too much' for them." Examples of Chloe's exciting triggers might be Elizabeth being highly affectionate and complimentary of Chloe, as well as Chloe and Elizabeth having daily sexual interactions. More general versions of these triggers could be "My girlfriends providing extensive one-on-one attention to me, especially at the start of the relationship" or "In romantic relationships, when my partner and I have lots of sex and intimacy with each other."

Valued interpersonal interactions NOT happening. Especially when you value or crave a particular response from another person, you can also feel quite upset when you do NOT receive those responses in your relationships. For many people, the *absence* of a positive interpersonal interaction can be just as triggering as the presence of a negative one! Examples of such scenarios include:

- Someone does not give you positive feedback about something you have done, who you are, or your personal qualities
- Someone fails to relate to you in a specific manner that you desire: they do not provide you with care, support, or admiration; they cease offering reassurance; they are not affectionate with you; they do not give you sexual attention; they do not seek you out, or share openly with you; they do not rely or depend on you, in the way that you really enjoy

- Someone refrains from taking actions that are not directly related to you but still impact how you feel: they do not perform specific tasks that you value (e.g., your kids forget to clean up after themselves); they do not treat other people in certain ways (e.g., your sibling avoids setting a boundary with your parents, with whom they have an enmeshed relationship); they do not engage in activities or contexts that you value (e.g., your significant other skips a work event that would have been good for their career)

As noted previously, you can frame these sorts of triggers at various levels of abstraction: noting the specific person or group that triggers you ("My friends not reaching out to check on me, when they know I have been struggling"); specifying the types of interactions that you find upsetting, independent of the parties involved ("People not thanking me when I do something nice for them"); or describing the type of person and interaction that distresses you ("Treatment providers taking a long time to respond to my e-mails").

In Chloe's relationship, examples of these sorts of triggers were Elizabeth not cuddling and focusing on Chloe when they were spending time together, as well as Elizabeth decreasing the frequency of her sexual engagement with Chloe. In broader terms, Chloe might say: "In romantic relationships, my partners not showing me physical, emotional, and sexual attention."

Interpersonal situations. So far, we have been discussing how distressing and exciting interactions with other people can trigger you. But simply *being* in some relationships or situations can raise your overall level of emotional arousal, regardless of how things end up unfolding in the interactions in question. You might feel especially emotionally sensitive when spending time with your parents, or an ex-romantic partner. You could feel anxious and on edge when you attend staff meetings at work, given the possibility that you might have to speak in front of your colleagues. Or you may feel excited and overwhelmed going on a first date. This person seems really cool, but there is just so much uncertainty. *Are they going to like me? Am I going to like them? Am I going to say something foolish and embarrass myself?*

In the above scenarios, observe that the situations are triggering even before something bad happens, or before something good happens. Sometimes triggering situations are primarily distressing, for instance when you are worried about potential negative outcomes in the scenario (e.g., someone criticizing, rejecting, or judging you). At other times, the situations are more exciting, as in when you feel confident that something clearly positive will happen there (e.g., someone complimenting or admiring you). In many other cases, the situations are *both* distressing and exciting, simultaneously—you feel worried about the worst case scenario, but also hopeful about the best case one!

Examples of triggering interpersonal situations include:

- *Relationships with certain individuals or groups of people:* friends, family members, colleagues, sexual partners, significant others, treatment providers
- *Specific interpersonal circumstances or time periods:* starting a new romantic relationship, visiting your family for the holidays, going to a party with your friends
- *Interpersonal situations oriented around particular activities or tasks:* work projects, sexual performance, speaking in public
- *Relationships with particular types of individuals, or people in certain roles:* authority figures, romantic partners, people you perceive to be "intelligent" or "successful"

In Chloe's experience, triggering interpersonal situations are likely romantic relationships in general, given her significant emotional investment in them, and the powerful feelings she tends to experience (e.g., hope, excitement, longing, anxiety) simply *being* in these relationships. With Elizabeth in particular, Chloe's triggering situations might include (a) this emotionally intense period at the start of their new relationship, (b) the experience of moving in together, as well as (c) the circumstance of "spending time together around the new apartment," which seems to generate significant anxiety in Chloe.

Valued interpersonal situations NOT happening. When you truly value a particular relational experience, you can encounter strong painful emotions (e.g., sadness, loss, anger, hopelessness) when that experience does not unfold in your life. Perhaps you long for a stable, loving romantic relationship, but after years of trying the dating apps, you are still alone. You might be estranged from your family of origin, so you end up feeling sad whenever the holidays approach, thinking about what you are missing in those relationships. Or perhaps you are quite socially isolated. You spend Saturday nights by yourself, scrolling the Internet and imagining all of the people out there in the world, hanging out with their friends and enjoying themselves.

These examples underscore how, for many people, the *absence* of interpersonal relationships can be even more upsetting than the presence of painful or problematic ones. We see this especially for people who struggle with social anxiety, social isolation, and avoidant personality disorder. However, even if you feel quite connected and engaged in your life, there still might be some areas where you are triggered by a lack of robust connectedness with others.

Identifying your triggers along these lines is relatively straightforward. Simply ask yourself: "Are there any relationships or connections that I wish I had, where I get upset when I focus on the fact that I do not have them?" These could be relationships with certain individuals or groups of people, including friends, family members, colleagues, sexual partners, significant others, or treatment providers. In Chloe's case, after ending a romantic relationship but before starting up another one, she would often feel sad, lonely, and despondent. In addition to missing her last partner, she was also acutely aware of how alone and isolated she felt when she was not in a relationship. This made her more likely to "jump in" to new relationships with partners who were not always right for her, in order to help her feel grounded and connected to herself again. On this view, "not being in a romantic relationship" was one of Chloe's primary attachment-related triggers.

Events or circumstances in the world. Not all triggers involve relationships or interactions with other people. You care about lots of things in your life, including events or circumstances that can significantly impact how you feel, and how you feel about yourself. Examples of distressing events include

- Getting fired or laid off from a job
- Financial losses, or loss of possessions
- Getting into an accident
- Struggling with medical illness or physical ailments
- Poor grades, or other negative evaluations of your performance in a work/academic setting
- Moving, getting evicted, or changing your living situation
- Challenging things happening in your immediate involvement, for instance involving weather, noise or sound, or being in a location (e.g., a public place, hospital, or dangerous setting) that you find upsetting
- Certain times of day, times of year, or anniversaries of past events
- Stressful conditions in broader society and culture: politics, war, violence and societal unrest, school shootings, the COVID-19 pandemic
- Encountering objective factors (e.g., sounds, smells, visual stimuli) that remind you of past traumatic or distressing experiences

Exciting triggers are essentially the mirror image of these experiences, such as receiving a promotion, acquiring more money or possessions, getting good grades, or buying an incredible new home.

You can also be triggered by these sorts of events when they unfold in other people's lives, especially if you really care about the person. Your family member is diagnosed with cancer, and you are worried you are going to lose them. Your partner gets laid off, which creates financial stress for your family. Your best friend is accepted to graduate school, but it is halfway across the country, so they are going to have to move. When summarizing your triggers, make sure to include *all* triggering circumstances that impact you: in your life, in the lives of your loved ones, and in broader society, culture, and the world. All of these things can make it more challenging to mentalize in a flexible, emotionally grounded manner in your everyday experience.

Valued events or circumstances NOT happening. When you truly value a particular state of affairs, you can feel quite destabilized and upset when that thing does *not* happen. You were hoping for that promotion, but your boss gave the job to your colleague instead. You put in an offer on your dream house, but the sellers accepted another offer, which was way over the asking price. You have been working out and watching your diet, but when you weigh yourself, you have not lost a single pound!

Valued events usually involve work, academics, finances, possessions, health and body, or living situation. To itemize these triggers, ask yourself the question: "Are there any events or circumstances that I really want to happen, which tend to upset me when they do not happen?" As above, these could be things that you hope will unfold in your life, in other people's lives, or in broader society, culture, and the world.

Now that you have a clear understanding of the different types of triggers, you are ready to apply these ideas to your own life. Worksheet 7.1 helps you to identify your own personal triggers, in the six categories we just discussed.

Worksheet 7.1
Understanding Your Triggers

(1) *Triggering interpersonal interactions* are things that other people do or say that make you feel any intense emotional state—painful or exciting. Describe at least three interpersonal interactions that tend to cause you distress, anxiety, or emotional pain.

(2) Now describe at least three interactions that make you feel intense emotions of excitement, hope, pleasure, or happiness.

(3) You also might feel upset when particular interpersonal interactions do not unfold in your life. For example, someone you care about fails to treat you in a certain way, or to say a certain thing to you. List at least three interactions where you become triggered when they do NOT happen.

(4) *Triggering interpersonal situations* are relationships or circumstances where you feel distress or excitement simply *being* in the scenario, regardless of how the situation unfolds. Examples include relationships with individuals or groups, or situations where you/others are engaged in some activity together. Outline at least three such situations, as well as how they impact you.

[continued on next page]

(5) You also might feel distressed when you do not have certain interpersonal relationships or connections in your life. Describe any such relationships that you lack, which tend to upset you when you focus on not having them.

(6) *Triggering events* are objective circumstances in the world that impact how you feel, and how you feel about yourself. They do not directly involve personal relationships or interactions, instead concerning issues like profession, health, finances, or living situation. List at least three events that tend to cause you distress, anxiety, or emotional pain.

(7) Now describe at least three events that make you feel intense emotions of excitement, hope, pleasure, or happiness.

(8) You might also feel upset when certain valued events do NOT happen in your life. For example, you do not get that promotion at your job, or they do not accept your offer on your dream house. Describe any events where you feel distress if they do not unfold for you.

MENTALIZING PRACTICE POINTS: MENTALIZING YOUR TRIGGERS

Now that you have a better sense of what your attachment-related triggers are, what do you actually *do* with this information? MBT recommends a handful of different strategies to help you effectively respond to triggering experiences.

Reflect on the emotional meaning of the trigger. As we have discussed, triggers are always external events, situations, or interactions. In the moment of emotional activation, it can feel like you are experiencing this intense emotion *because* the external thing is so problematic or wonderful, as the case may be. Under those conditions, your emotions just end up just getting "tugged around" by the world around you, depriving you of a full sense of agency in your life.

In contrast, MBT suggests that there is something happening in *you* that is making you vulnerable to the trigger's influence. Throughout this book, we will explore these processes together in detail, considering how MBT understands and addresses your core psychological vulnerabilities. In the meantime, when you find yourself struggling with a particular trigger in your life (e.g., your partner making an insensitive comment, your professor giving a difficult assignment, spending time with certain challenging family members), try shifting the focus from "other people's outsides" to your *insides*. Ask yourself the question:

"What is going on in ME that makes me feel so emotional about this thing?"

When wrestling with this query, if your mind continues to focus on the external issue ("Well, she really should not be treating me this way . . . "; "I just do not have enough time to finish this paper"; "They are such ignorant people, so I cannot have a relationship with them"), make an effort to reorient back to internal processes in you, namely your emotions, desires, and feelings about yourself that could be leading you to feel more activated by the trigger in question. Feel free to journal about these feelings, so that you can see them written out in front of you in black-and-white. While these explorations do not necessary "resolve" or alleviate the mental states in question (more on that in Chapters 12 and 13), it is an essential step in fostering a mentalizing process in therapy. As you appreciate the emotional meaning that your triggers hold for you, you will experience a greater sense of autonomy and self-control when you see them coming your way.

Forecast the trigger. Have you ever gotten into a physical altercation with someone? If you know that you are about to get punched and there is no way to avoid it, the recommendation is that you brace yourself for the impact: Keep your head steady, clench your jaw, tighten your core, and hold your breath. This process of "steeling yourself" can surprisingly decrease the damage of the attack.

Similarly, when you know that you are about to encounter one of your triggers, there is value in explicitly "forecasting" it to yourself—that is, taking some internal action that reminds you of the coming storm. Strangely, taking this extra step can often temper the impact that your triggers have on you, endowing you with a "mentalizing buffer" in intense, stressful situations. You can forecast your triggers in several ways:

- *Make some private comment that acknowledges the situation, the trigger, and the impact it might have on you.* "I am about to go out on a date, where I will probably feel quite anxious and insecure. I cope with this by getting very invested, very quickly." "Visiting with my parents, they often make some comment about my weight. I usually get defensive, and I respond by criticizing them."
- *Try writing these statements down on a piece of paper, or in your journal.* When you see your triggers written out in front of you—visually separated from you in

physical space—you can often experience some degree of *emotional* distance from the trigger itself.

- *Identify and cue up a "warning soundtrack" in your mind.* When you are watching a horror movie, there is often that scene where one of the side characters hears a noise somewhere in the house, making that excellent decision to investigate by walking by themself down the stairs into the dark basement. What could go wrong? As they take that first step down the stairs, the soundtrack changes: Slow, foreboding music rises in the scene. While the character remains haplessly unaware, *we* start to feel on edge, bracing ourselves for the danger that is about to leap out of the shadows.

    But what if this character had the ability to hear their own background music? Would things proceed any differently for them? Most likely they would pause, just as their foot is about to fall on the next step. They would look up, listening. *Something doesn't seem to be right here. Maybe it's NOT the best idea for me to go by myself into this basement, given all of the people that have just been brutally murdered in this house.* And then hopefully they would have the presence of mind to turn around, and walk back up the stairs.

    Now that you aware of your triggers, you do not need to go by yourself down into the basement anymore. If you were that character in the movie, what would you want your warning soundtrack to be? Think about it for a moment, and then write down the name of the song here:

    _____

    Next time that you are entering a triggering situation, bring up this song in your mind. This will be your "warning soundtrack," helping you to keep your wits about you, when there is trouble on the horizon.

- *Try visual foreshadowing of the impending trigger.* Perhaps you are more of a visual thinker, where you process information through images or pictures. In that case, create some pictorial signifier for the potential disruption. You could imagine experiencing the situation through a yellow filter, indicating that there are hazards approaching. If you like comic books, visualize jagged lightning bolts above your head—a mentalizing "Spidey-sense" letting you know that danger is brewing. Or you might picture one of those triangular road signs with an exclamation mark, suggesting that you should proceed with caution.

If this approach appeals to you, take a moment to sketch out some image reminding you that you might be entering a "danger zone" on the highway of your life.

Next time you are entering some situation or interaction that might be activating for you, call this image up in your mind—a signpost for impending triggers.

"Press pause" on the triggering moment. How do you respond when you actually *encounter* your triggers in everyday life? Your boss tells you that you have been underperforming, and you have to shape up. Your significant other accepts your proposal (phew!), but now you have to plan an entire wedding in less than a year! Your mother has started showing signs of depression: sleeping in late, losing weight, and not responding to phone calls and text messages. You have never had to deal with this before, and you do not know what to do.

Let's continue with the metaphor of "life as a movie." There is an effect in movies called "bullet time." First popularized in *The Matrix*, bullet time involves slowing down time in the middle of the action, such that high speed movements usually invisible to the naked eye (e.g., the movement of bullets) are visible to the audience. While the characters in the action come almost to a standstill, and the camera pans around them at a normal pace, achieving an almost panoramic perspective on the event. Similarly, in MBT, we recommend that you attempt to "press pause" on the triggering moment, so that you are able to take a deep breath and stop the process of escalating emotional intensity. Now you get to play the role of the *camera* in the movie—the action stops, but you still possess the presence of mind to observe and investigate the situation, without having to jump into the fray.

This is the first part of "reflecting rather than reflexing"—trying to not reflex, react, or respond impulsively in the moment of emotional vulnerability. From a pragmatic perspective, this can involve several components.

- *Work to not engage in any of your problem behaviors.* You have probably heard the aphorism, "When in doubt, do nothing." Or similarly: "Don't just do something, sit there!" In Chapter 5, you already started to identify your personal "problem behaviors"—actions that you reflexively take that undermine your emotional stability, interpersonal relationships, and personal values. If you need a refresher, just turn back to your responses on Worksheets 5.2 and 5.3, or just ask yourself: "What do I do that tends to make the situation worse, that I often regret afterwards?" So in the moment of "pause," try to do everything in your power to

NOT do those things. Of course, this is all easier said than done, which is why there
are eight more chapters in this book!

- *"Fast-forward" the movie of your life.* If you are having trouble not engaging in
  your problem behaviors, take a moment to "fast-forward" beyond the current scene.
  Imagine yourself taking those actions. How would you feel afterwards? How might
  other people feel, and how would they respond in return? What would the overall
  consequences be in the situation? By "playing the whole tape through" in this way,
  you can often strengthen your fortitude to refrain from acting on your immediate
  impulses. This stops you from creating additional wreckage through your problem
  behaviors, while also opening up space for adaptive mentalizing to take place.

Reflect rather than reflex. Once you have pressed pause on the triggering situation,
what do you do next? Many readers will be hoping for a behavioral skill at this point: deep
breathing, muscle relaxation, distraction, self-soothing, and so on. While we are not opposed
to these sorts of strategies in MBT, we tend to put the emphasis in a different place: reflection about mental states. This whole book is devoted to illustrating in detail the different
mentalizing strategies that you can employ in your areas of emotional vulnerability. For now,
in your moments of emotional unrest, consider some of our most basic mentalizing questions
about psychological processes in yourself and other people:

- "What emotions am I feeling right now?"
- "What am I wanting in this situation?" More specific versions of this question
  include:
  - "What do I want to happen?"
  - "What do I want the other person to do?"
  - "How do I want the person to feel? How do I want them to think and feel
    about me?"
- "How am I feeling about myself? Where is my self-esteem in all of this?"
- If there is another party involved in this situation, try putting yourself in their shoes:
  - "What is the other individual feeling or wanting?"
  - "What is their perspective on the situation?"
  - "Even if I disagree with the person, can I notice anything potentially valid about
    their way of seeing things? Do they have a point about ANYTHING?"

As you know by now, MBT is all about stimulating a process of reflection about mental
states. If you genuinely wrestle with these questions, you are engaging in that process, regardless of what you "come up with" in your considerations. *The process is the destination.*
All of the research on MBT supports the idea that reflection *itself* is the key ingredient in how
people get better, when directed toward their areas of emotional and interpersonal difficulty.

If necessary, consider staying away from (or leaving) the triggering situation. We
have discussed how, as human beings, it is difficult to mentalize effectively when we are
under more emotional stress. So it is entirely possible that, at this point in your life and treatment, there are some triggers that are perhaps too overwhelming to experience. You might
feel too emotionally fragile to spend time with an ex-romantic partner, or too on edge to visit
your hometown, where you have a significant history of trauma. In MBT, we want you to be
engaging in your life in a productive, meaningful way, but we also recognize that there are
limits to what a vulnerable mind can endure. If you are feeling concerned about having to
encounter a certain trigger, the following recommendations might be helpful for you.

- *Conduct a mentalizing inquiry of your ability to engage with the triggering
  experience.* Try asking yourself: "If I were to encounter this thing, how confident
  am I that I could 'press pause' on the situation—to reflect rather than reflex? If

I could effectively engage in the scenario, what would that do to me emotionally afterwards? Would I still be able to function in my life, and to stay safe?" If you are significantly concerned about your ability to function either within or following the experience, it is completely reasonable to skip or postpone the interaction. As time moves on in treatment, you will gain a range of mentalizing strategies that will strengthen your ability to effectively engage in scenarios that might be upsetting to you.

- *Explore the experience with your therapist or a trusted friend.* As we will discuss in Chapter 8, many people struggle with tendencies toward *avoidance*—that is, staying away from experiences that trigger uncomfortable feelings, in a manner that prevents them from living a full and meaningful life. In light of this, when you are considering sidestepping a triggering situation, you might find it difficult to distinguish between unhelpful avoidance and sensible self-care. So consider bringing these issues into therapy, or discussing them with a trusted friend, who themself is not just likely to tell you what you want to hear. Work on exploring the question: "Am I staying away from this situation because I truly cannot handle it, or am I lowering the bar for myself, in way that is keeping me stuck?" Note that this question is not simply focused on behaviors ("Should I stay, or should I go?"), but on your *mental states* surrounding the desire to avoid. By calling upon other people's independent perspectives about these matters, you are often able to better understand your own motives and desires in the triggering situation.

- *Give yourself permission to leave the triggering situation, if necessary.* While encountering your trigger in the moment, there are times when you might feel extremely overwhelmed and potentially unstable. You could feel quite strongly that, if you stay in the situation, you are going to engage in your problem behaviors (e.g., lashing out, hurting yourself, becoming visibly emotional in front of people), in a way that could be harmful to yourself or others. Under these circumstances, you should feel free to leave the scenario, and to conduct an "after action review" of the experience once things have settled down a bit.

Mentalizing Cool-down

Now that you have learned about MBT's recommendations for addressing triggers, return to Chloe's story at the start of the chapter, on page 109. What would it look like for Chloe to apply these strategies in her interactions with Elizabeth?

RETURNING TO CHLOE

When we last saw Chloe, she was feeling quite insecure in her romantic relationship, as well as hopeless in her life more generally. Concerned about her worsening suicidal thinking, Chloe decided to seek out individual therapy, finding a therapist who had some training in MBT. Together, Chloe and her therapist explored not simply Chloe's external triggers, but the emotional meaning these triggers held for her. Chloe began to see that she had a pattern of basing her sense of self and psychological well-being on the attentiveness of her romantic partners. When her partners engaged in visible behaviors that she associated with "care" (e.g., physical affection, compliments, sexual interactions), she felt like they loved her. But when Chloe's partners failed to take these concrete actions, Chloe thought they were pulling away from her, and in fact were going to abandon her. This then threw Chloe into something of an existential panic, as had been happening recently with Elizabeth.

Chloe did not really know what to *do* with any of this information yet. However, as Chloe recognized that her own assumptions were likely influencing how she experienced her relationship with Elizabeth, Chloe felt a bit less sensitive when Elizabeth focused on other things. Chloe and her therapist identified the stretch of time after Elizabeth finished her work day—while Chloe cooked dinner and Elizabeth played video games—as a key period of emotional vulnerability for Chloe, when she was at risk for feeling like Elizabeth was rejecting and abandoning her. In an effort to "forecast" this distressing experience, Chloe would articulate this trigger to herself: "Whenever Elizabeth plays video games while I am cooking dinner after work, I feel insecure and desperate, and I worry that she does not care enough about me." Chloe's favorite song was "Blank Space" by Taylor Swift ("Got a long list of ex-lovers, they'll tell you I'm insane"), and she started playing this while she made dinner for them. This personalized "warning soundtrack" helped to keep Chloe on her toes, reminding her that she was susceptible to taking things personally while Elizabeth was occupied in this way.

Chloe's increased reflectiveness continued as they hung out together on the couch later in the evening, while Elizabeth scrolled Instagram and Reddit on her phone. Chloe worked to "press pause" on these moments, refraining from either criticizing or withdrawing from Elizabeth, as she was often tempted to do. Instead, Chloe endeavored to mentalize both herself and Elizabeth in these interactions. She remained in touch with her fears that Elizabeth was bored with her, while also accessing her desire to be Elizabeth's only focus while they spent time together. Chloe also appreciated Elizabeth's emotions of stress and anxiety from working all day, as well as her tendency to cope with these feelings by distracting herself with electronic devices. Chloe wondered if perhaps Elizabeth's distractedness had very little to do with her, and more with Elizabeth's own approach to managing her distressing emotions.

In a gentle way, Chloe expressed her wish to have more quality time with Elizabeth at the end of the day, rather than both of them sitting alongside each other with their respective electronic devices. Elizabeth was highly receptive to this, and they started trying to turn off their laptops and cell phones from 8 PM onward, so that they could have more time directly engaging and communicating with each other. Over time, Chloe increasingly felt more secure in the relationship, experiencing a newfound confidence that Elizabeth loved her, cared about her, and was committed to their relationship. Their sex life improved, although still probably not to the level that Chloe would have preferred. Chloe felt less depressed, and her suicidal thinking began to subside.

Now experiencing decreased emotional and interpersonal instability, Chloe and her therapist were able to work together in earnest on Chloe's broader challenges in her sense of self.

Utilizing the strategies you will learn in the upcoming chapters, Chloe developed a greater sense of agency and groundedness in her own experience, independently of how other people were relating to her in any given interaction or relationship.

Chapter Review 7.1
Identifying Your Triggers

What is a Trigger in MBT?

- In MBT, a trigger is an external factor that precipitates your insecurities about yourself and others, or that activates your characteristic manner of engaging with other people.

- Triggers are always **external** in nature: events or circumstances, other people's actions or qualities, or things that other people say.

- MBT distinguishes between **distressing** triggers and **exciting** triggers. Distressing triggers generate painful emotions in you, while exciting triggers are "positive" factors in your life, which lead you to feel excited, enthusiastic, or hopeful that some particular thing will happen.

- Triggers can be framed in terms of situations in general ("Any time that I receive constructive feedback from an authority figure"), as well as specific scenarios that impact you ("My best friend taking a long time to respond to a text message").

- *A helpful rule of thumb to identify your triggers:* What are the things that happen around you that provoke one or more of the following three responses?

  - Any intense emotional state, painful or exciting

  - The appearance of your typical interpersonal patterns

  - Any difficulties in mentalizing

- By being aware of your triggers, you will be more able to "hold on to your mind" as you encounter them. This enables you to make different choices in the areas where you tend to get stuck.

Six Types of Triggers

- **Interpersonal interactions:** what people say to you and how they treat you

- **Valued interpersonal interactions NOT happening** (e.g., someone not giving you positive feedback, support, or attention)

- **Interpersonal situations:** relationships with certain individuals or groups, or relational scenarios oriented around particular activities (e.g., work projects, sexual performance, speaking in public)

- **Valued interpersonal situations NOT happening** (e.g., in cases of social isolation, estrangement from some individual, or not having a certain type of relationship)

- **Events or circumstances in the world:** involving work, academics, finances, possessions, health and body, living situation, time of day/year, current events, or your immediate environment

- **Valued events or circumstances NOT happening** (e.g., not receiving a job, home, promotion, award, or financial profit)

Chapter Review 7.2
Mentalizing Practice Points: Mentalizing Your Triggers

Reflect on the Emotional Meaning of the Trigger

Shift the focus from the outside thing to YOUR internal states, namely your emotions, desires, and feelings about yourself that could be leading you to feel more activated by the trigger in question. "What is going on in ME that makes me feel so emotional about this thing?"

Forecast the Trigger

Take some internal action that reminds you of the coming storm.

- Make a private comment that acknowledges the situation, the trigger, and the impact that it might have on you. "Visiting with my parents, they often make some comment about my weight. I usually get very defensive, and I respond by criticizing them."

- Try writing these statements down on a piece of paper, or in your journal.

- Identify and cue up a "warning soundtrack" in your mind.

- Try visual foreshadowing of the impending trigger. Imagine or draw some pictorial signifier of the potential disruption.

"Press Pause" on the Triggering Moment

- Work to not engage in any of your problem behaviors. Remember: "When in doubt, do nothing!" Or: "Don't just do something, sit there!"

- "Fast-forward" the movie of your life. If you took those actions, how would you feel afterwards? How might other people feel, and how would they respond in return? What would the overall consequences be in the situation?

[continued on next page]

Reflect Rather than Reflex

Attempt to mentalize yourself and other people in the situation.

- "What emotions am I feeling right now?"
- "What am I wanting in this situation?"
  - "What do I want to happen?"
  - "What do I want the other person to do?"
  - "How do I want the person to feel? How do I want them to think and feel about me?"
- "How am I feeling about myself? Where is my self-esteem in all of this?"
- Try putting yourself in the other party's shoes:
  - "What is the other individual feeling or wanting?"
  - "What is their perspective on the situation?"
  - "Even if I disagree with the person, can I notice anything potentially valid about their way of seeing things? Do they have a point about ANYTHING?"

Consider Staying Away from (or Leaving) the Situation

- Conduct a mentalizing inquiry: "If I were to encounter this thing, how confident am I that I could 'press pause' on the situation—to reflect rather than reflex? If I could effectively engage in the scenario, what would that do to me emotionally afterwards? Would I still be able to function in my life, and to stay safe?"

- Explore the experience with your therapist, or with a trusted friend: "Am I staying away from this situation because I truly cannot handle it, or am I lowering the bar for myself, in a way that is keeping me stuck?"

- Give yourself permission to skip or leave the triggering situation, if you feel too overwhelmed, vulnerable, or reactive.

What is Your Attachment Style?

Alan had always seen himself as a highly "sensitive" person: extremely worried about what other people thought of him, easily insulted and embarrassed in social interactions, and prone to anger if he ever felt like others were judging him. Alan coped with these feelings by always having one person with whom he could spend all of his time, with whom he felt safe, connected, and unconditionally loved. When he was young, this person was his mother, but gradually he shifted his focus onto best friends, and ultimately romantic relationships.

In college, Alan met Maggie, and they fell madly in love. Maggie was everything he could want in a partner: warm, nurturing, and always ready to highlight his positive qualities. As their relationship developed, Alan felt more frustrated with his family of origin, whom he saw as critical and self-centered, especially compared to Maggie. He distanced himself from his family, and Maggie became his safe haven—the single person to whom he could go whenever he was feeling worried or insecure.

Soon after graduating college, Alan and Maggie got married, and Alan started his career as a software developer. While he enjoyed writing code, those old feelings of anxiety began to arise in his interactions with his co-workers. He felt highly uncomfortable in group situations with colleagues (e.g., meetings, social outings, making small-talk in the break room), and especially in his relationship with his boss Larry. Larry was "all business," all the time. He did not smile, he did not give compliments, and he became impatient at the slightest sign of mistakes or inefficiency. Alan tried to do whatever he could to garner Larry's approval: working longer hours, volunteering for additional projects, and checking and re-checking his code to make sure things were "perfect."

These feelings all came to a head after Larry gave Alan constructive feedback about one of his coding projects, for a program that was experiencing some glitches. Alan felt humiliated by this, and resentful that Larry was blaming him for something that was clearly not his fault. Alan was fed up with this situation: Larry was a narcissist and a control freak, and his colleagues were superficial and inauthentic, always ready to lie down and let Larry walk all over them. After work meetings, Alan would hide in a bathroom stall and cry, scratching himself to try to make himself feel better—something he had not done since high school.

Alan started becoming defensive and argumentative with Larry, and his work suffered: He would avoid working on the project, ignore colleagues' e-mails, and call in sick whenever he was feeling too upset about how he was being treated. While Maggie tried to comfort him in his distress, this could not quell Alan's feelings of anxiety and rage. He felt like this work situation was clearly "toxic," but he could not figure out what to do about it.

AN INTRODUCTION TO ATTACHMENT THEORY

Attachment theory is a school of thought in psychology that focuses on how children navigate interactions with their caregivers in order to maintain a sense of security, trust, and safety. Originally developed by the British psychiatrist and psychoanalyst John Bowlby in the 1960s and 1970s, attachment theory has become a widely accepted (and scientifically supported)

Mentalization. Robert P. Drozek, Oxford University Press. © Oxford University Press 2025.
DOI: 10.1093/oso/9780198916857.003.0008

model that is able to explain child development, personality functioning, and mental health challenges (Cassidy & Shaver, 2016; Herstell et al., 2021; Mikulincer & Shaver, 2012).

What are the core ideas of attachment theory? Attachment theory suggests that infants need an emotionally attuned relationship with at least one primary caregiver for their successful development, especially in order to learn how to regulate emotions in relationships. The theory suggests that children are evolutionarily drawn to seek out and maintain proximity and connectedness with their caregivers. When caregivers are consistently available and responsive to the child, the child feels secure and confident in the caregivers' accessibility, leaving them free to confidently explore their environments. The child thus develops a largely positive sense of self, while simultaneously experiencing other people as safe, reliable, and trustworthy.

However, as we learned in Chapter 4, when caregivers are more aggressive, rejecting, or emotionally neglectful, the child feels *insecure* about the caregivers' availability and responsiveness. These interactions are "internalized" by the child, resulting in a negative sense of self-esteem, as well as an experience of other people as threatening, unreliable, and unable to meet the child's needs.

In these ways, children come to develop what attachment theory calls attachment "strategies" or "styles." These styles constitute our characteristic manner of experiencing and regulating closeness in our relationships—*our core ways of feeling and being with ourselves and other people*. Attachment styles tend to persist throughout the course of development, such that we "carry with us" our interpersonal templates from childhood into our contemporary relationships (Kim et al., 2021).

ATTACHMENT STYLES IN MBT

Attachment plays a pivotal role in the symptoms of borderline personality disorder (BPD). In Chapter 2, we saw that BPD is significantly associated with insecure attachment styles (Smith & South, 2020; Zhang et al., 2022), and attachment-related insecurities are the primary driver of problems in mentalizing. If you feel insecure and rejected in your relationships, you are more likely to

- feel confused about what you are feeling;
- jump to conclusions about what other people are feeling;
- hold rigid beliefs about yourself and other people;
- feel the need to *take action* in order to change how you are feeling; and
- blame other people for your challenges, while reflecting less on how YOU are engaging in your relationships.

As you learn how to identify your personal attachment styles in relationships, you will start to "catch yourself" before engaging with people in unhelpful ways. This will give you a greater freedom of choice in how you relate to other people, interrupting the problems in mentalizing that lead to so much suffering in BPD.

Let's consider some key points about mentalization-based treatment's (MBT) specific approach to attachment styles. First, attachment styles encompass both internal *and* behavioral processes—that is, the way that we feel in our relationships (e.g., confident, desperate, afraid, judgmental), as well as how we relate to other people in our interactions with them (e.g., with autonomy, dependency, avoidance, or dismissiveness; see Mikulincer & Shaver, 2016). If you only focus on your emotions in relationships, without sufficiently considering what you do with other people, you are likely to misclassify your unique attachment style.

For example, you might feel quite anxious, insecure, and preoccupied with rejection in your relationships, but this does not automatically mean that you have a "preoccupied" or anxious attachment style. If you primarily respond to these feelings by keeping to yourself and avoiding other people, then you might have more "avoidant" attachment tendencies. However, if you cope with these feelings by seeking out frequent contact and communications with other people, then you probably employ more preoccupied attachment strategies. So when identifying your personal attachment styles, make sure to consider both "the inside and the outside"—your emotions as well as your behaviors.

Secondly, most people do not employ only a single attachment style, demonstrating it "across the board" in all situations and relationships. Rather, most of us exhibit what psychologists call "dimensional" attachment styles—exhibiting different interpersonal approaches to a greater or lesser degree, depending on the specific relationship or "type" of relationship (Fraley et al., 2015). For instance, you might feel secure and comfortable in your interactions with family members, while feeling more insecure and avoidant in situations (e.g., work, school) where your performance is being monitored and evaluated. Or perhaps you feel bored and emotionally removed in most romantic relationships, but then with certain people you date, you find yourself feeling more self-conscious and "needy," for reasons you do not fully understand.

Accordingly, MBT encourages you to examine your attachment styles as they manifest themselves in the diverse spheres of your life. This follows the broad approach outlined in Chapter 7, where you identified your personal triggers in certain relationships, circumstances, and types of interactions. While it is possible that you utilize the same interpersonal approach in all of your relationships, it is also likely that you employ *different* interpersonal approaches, depending on the specific relational context. See here for examples of these different relational contexts, along with how you might start to specify your attachment patterns along these lines.

- *Relationships in specific life domains:* with friends, family members, colleagues, sexual partners, significant others, treatment providers. "In my romantic relationships, I tend to. . . ."
- *Relationships with particular individuals in these domains:* your parent, your current romantic partner, your boss, your best friend, your therapist, your co-worker who sits right next to you, and so on. "With my therapist, I often. . . ."
- *Relationships with people who have specific qualities or characteristics:* personality traits, level of intelligence, socio-economic status, degree of attractiveness, demographic characteristics (e.g., age, gender, race, ethnicity), or status and power in the aforementioned "life domains." "When interacting with people whom I see as more intelligent and accomplished, I usually. . . ."

Attachment strategies can also be especially sensitive to *what happens* in the above contexts. Specifically, your attachment strategies can shift based on whether people are treating you in ways that you value (or devalue). Perhaps you really crave your parents' admiration and approval. In that case, you will likely be drawn to pursue and actualize that in your interactions with your parents: by telling them things you think will impress them, by not discussing things that might lead them to judge you, and by relating to them in ways that you know they appreciate (e.g., laughing at Mom's jokes, complimenting Dad's cooking). As long as your parents treat you in a more "neutral" or approving manner, you probably would be more attachment *seeking* with them—that is, behaving in ways that facilitate these forms of connectedness. However, if your parents start to show their disapproval or frustration with you, your attachment strategy might "switch" to a more avoidant approach. You could feel less interested in spending time with them; you start cancelling plans; or you could be more withdrawn and standoffish in your interactions with them.

So when identifying your unique attachment styles, consider how you engage with other people under several key circumstances:

- People acting more "neutral" or ambiguous in their way of being with you—that is, it is not immediately clear to you if they are seeing/treating you in the way you would most want. "If I feel uncertain how a sexual partner feels about me, I tend to. . . ."
- People engaging with you in a manner you truly value: giving you positive feedback, attention, admiration, affection, and so on. "When my friends offer me emotional support, I usually. . . ."
- People NOT relating to you in the manner you desire: They fail to give you positive feedback, attention, admiration, or affection. "If my children seem to be ignoring me, I often. . . ."
- People relating to you in a manner to which you ascribe negative value: They criticize, reject, abandon, threaten, or attack you. "When my wife dismisses and invalidates my perspective, I feel compelled to. . . ."

Finally, when identifying your typical attachment strategies in MBT, consider *how* you connect and relate to other people, rather than simply "why" you developed your idiosyncratic attachment styles. Once the treatment starts, MBT does not devote significant therapeutic attention to exploring your childhood, or figuring out "what happened in the past" that led to your challenges. The reasons for this are severalfold:

- There is no research showing that "past-focused" treatments are especially effective at alleviating the symptoms of BPD. You might have some direct experience with this: You could have a lot of ideas of how your experiences in childhood shaped who you are, and yet these intellectual formulations have not yet been able to help you live your life in a different way *today*.
- Extensive research suggests that the most effective therapies for BPD focus on patients' current experiences and functionality in their everyday lives (Stoffers-Winterling et al., 2022). Accordingly, as reviewed in Chapter 5, MBT sessions tend to focus on your recent areas of challenge and instability, especially your attachment-related experiences in contemporary relationships.
- Many people with BPD find themselves regularly thinking and ruminating about the past, in ways that often just make them feel more upset and overwhelmed. In this way, "focusing on the past" can actually interfere with you living your life fully in the present! If you happen to have *both* BPD and posttraumatic stress disorder (PTSD), there is emerging research suggesting that certain psychotherapies, including MBT, are helpful in addressing your symptoms of PTSD (Slotema et al., 2020; Smits et al., 2022). Consider researching these forms of therapy, or asking your therapist if they might be applicable for you. While MBT's techniques can be useful in treating PTSD, this topic is outside the scope of the present book, which focuses on treating BPD in particular.

In light of all these points, when working to identify your attachment styles in MBT, we recommend that you examine certain key factors in your contemporary life, including:

- your own internal states (e.g., emotions, desires, feelings about yourself) that you experience in your relationships;

- your most common manner of behaving and engaging with other people; and
- similarities and differences in these processes across different relationships, situations, and life domains.

GETTING STARTED: ATTACHMENT ANXIETY VERSUS ATTACHMENT AVOIDANCE

With all of these points in mind, let's get started in identifying your particular attachment strategies. In contemporary research on insecure attachment, the most fundamental distinction is between attachment *anxiety* and attachment *avoidance* (Crowell et al., 2016). Broadly speaking, attachment anxiety can be seen as a "pull" form of connectedness ("I need you! Come closer!"), whereas attachment avoidance is more of a "push" approach ("I can't deal with you. Get away!"). My 10-year-old son loves playing with magnets, and he has come up with a helpful analogy to explain these categories: "One *[attachment anxiety]* is like the way that a magnet pulls metal toward it, while the other *[attachment avoidance]* is like when the magnet pushes other magnets away from it."

Attachment anxiety is accompanied by a range of internal processes, including a negative view of yourself, the tendency to idealize certain other people, intense desires to be close to others, fears of rejection and abandonment, discomfort with being alone, and feeling angry or upset when others are insufficiently responsive to you. Attachment anxiety is the attachment style most commonly seen in BPD (Smith & South, 2020; Zhang et al., 2022), where you often cope with distress by *moving closer* to other people. Behaviors along these lines include:

- Consistently seeking out relationships, interactions, and communications (e.g., via phone, text, or DMs) with other people
- Always having a "favorite" or primary person (e.g., romantic partner, best friend, family member) with whom you are spending your time
- Dependency issues: regularly seeking out support or reassurance from other people, or relying on them in order to feel emotionally stable
- In romantic relationships, going from one relationship to another, with minimal time in between. (This sometimes involves promiscuity, infidelity, or having numerous sexual partners.)
- Progressing from "zero to 60" in relationships: quickly becoming attached to another person, and pursuing forms of connectedness (e.g., sex, spending all of your time together, saying "I love you," moving in together) that are more advanced than the actual stage of the relationship
- Difficulties ending relationships, or remaining in relationships even when the other person is not treating you in the way that you deserve.

As you might already know from personal experience, these forms of attachment anxiety can lead to significant negative consequences in your life. You might feel deeply anxious and insecure in your relationships—about yourself but also how people feel about you. You could feel less capable of managing life on your own, and so you "lower the bar" and avoid opportunities (e.g., in work, academics, hobbies) that require greater agency and autonomy. You may inadvertently alienate other people, coming across as "needy" or "too much" through your efforts to seek out support and connectedness. These tendencies can lead to arguments, break-ups, and estrangement in your relationships. You also might place yourself in unsafe and psychologically damaging situations, all in an effort to receive the love and validation you need in order to feel OK.

Attachment avoidance can entail a variety of internal experiences: interpreting other people as scary, threatening, or problematic; desire to avoid other individuals, or reluctance to engage with them; anxiety in social interactions and close relationships; reticence around directly expressing your feelings; and discomfort surrounding "asking for help" and relying on others. It is important to note that, if you experience attachment avoidance, you might also struggle with attachment anxiety, as manifested by a highly negative view of yourself, as well as fear of others' criticism, disapproval, and rejection. Or you could feel largely "secure" in yourself, but you avoid other people for other reasons: You are more of a loner; you are quite self-reliant; or you might even disparage or look down on other people in certain ways, seeing them as more trouble than they are worth.

If you struggle with attachment avoidance, you cope with your distress not by moving closer to other people, but by moving away from them. Relevant behaviors here include:

- Staying away from situations that involve significant interaction with other people: work, school, friendships, dating relationships, or group events
- Inhibition and restraint in close relationships
- Shyness in new relationships
- Tendency to withdraw from other people
- Social isolation, or spending significant time alone
- If you also struggle with attachment anxiety, you could avoid activities, contexts, or situations where you feel scrutinized or judged.

Much like attachment anxiety, attachment avoidance comes with notable negative consequences. Everything in life feels like work: You experience stress, anxiety, and pressure simply navigating the social world. Things that seem relatively straightforward to other people (e.g., going to the store, applying for a job, using dating apps) require a tremendous amount of emotional energy for you. Perhaps the biggest problem with an avoidant attachment style is a sense of stagnation and paralysis. You feel like you should be able to move yourself forward in your life, but you are unable to summon the willpower to realize your full potential (e.g., in work, school, friendships, romantic relationships). Other people might feel hurt or angry about your inconsistencies, or alienated by you. Over time, they rely on you less, expect less of you, and pull away from you. This leaves you feeling more isolated and alone.

Mentalizing Warm-up

Now that you understand the distinction between attachment anxiety and attachment avoidance, turn back to Alan's story at the start of the chapter, on page 127. Where do you see characteristics of attachment anxiety in Alan's experience? Where do you observe a more avoidant attachment style?

By now, hopefully you are already identifying with some of the characteristics of attachment anxiety or attachment avoidance. In social psychological research on attachment, the most widely used self-report measure of insecure attachment is the Experiences in Close Relationships scale (Brennan et al., 1998; Crowell et al., 2016; Mikulincer & Shaver, 2016). Worksheet 8.1 includes some of the questions from that questionnaire, which I have modified from the research version for use with the general public. So while the results are not "official," they should still help you to explore your own tendencies toward attachment anxiety versus attachment avoidance.

Worksheet 8.1
Attachment Anxiety versus Attachment Avoidance

(1) Consider the statements below that relate both to attachment anxiety and attachment avoidance. Place a check mark next to all of the statements with which you identify.

ATTACHMENT ANXIETY

☐ I worry a lot about my relationships.

☐ I feel anxious that other people won't care about me as much as I care about them.

☐ I want to get very close to others, and this sometimes scares them away.

☐ I worry about being rejected or abandoned.

☐ I need a lot of reassurance that people really care about me.

☐ Sometimes I try to force others to show more feeling, more commitment to our relationship than they otherwise would.

☐ If I can't get people to show interest in me, I get upset or angry.

☐ I feel distressed if other individuals are not available when I need them.

☐ When I don't have others around, I feel anxious and insecure.

☐ I find that other people don't want to get as close as I would like.

☐ When others disapprove of me, I feel really bad about myself.

☐ I worry about being alone.

☐ I resent it when people who are important to me spend time away from me.

ATTACHMENT AVOIDANCE

☐ I prefer not to show others how I feel deep down.

☐ I feel uncomfortable being close to other people.

☐ When people start to get close to me, I find myself pulling away.

☐ I get uncomfortable when someone wants to be very close with me.

☐ I don't feel comfortable opening up to other individuals.

☐ I feel uneasy sharing my private thoughts and feelings with others.

☐ I try to avoid getting too close to other people.

☐ I find it difficult allowing myself to depend on others.

☐ I don't share much with the people in my life.

☐ I try to refrain from asking others for comfort, advice, or help.

☐ I don't usually discuss my problems and concerns with other individuals.

☐ I don't like depending on others.

☐ I avoid turning to other people in times of need.

[continued on next page]

(2) Now tally up the total number of statements you selected in each category. This should give you a sense of the extent to which you employ each strategy in your relationships. If your numbers are roughly equivalent, then you likely possess a "mixed" attachment profile, involving elements of both anxiety and avoidance.

Attachment anxiety:_____   Attachment avoidance:_____

(3) What does attachment anxiety look like for you? Please provide at least one example.

(4) What does attachment avoidance look like for you? Please provide at least one example.

Note. The statements in question (1) above are drawn and adapted from the Experiences in Close Relationships (ECR) scale, with permission from P. R. Shaver. The ECR is presented in Appendix E of Mikulincer, M., & Shaver, P. R. (2016). *Attachment in adulthood: Structure, dynamics, and change* (2nd ed., pp. 533–534). Guilford Press. See also Brennan, K. A., Clark, C. L., & Shaver, P. R. (1998). Self-report measurement of adult romantic attachment: An integrative overview. In J. A. Simpson & W. S. Rholes (Eds.), *Attachment theory and close relationships* (pp. 46–76). Guilford Press.

MODELS OF SELF AND OTHER: SECURE, PREOCCUPIED, FEARFUL, DISMISSIVE

Other attachment researchers have proposed a theory of attachment styles that highlights our internalized models of relationships—that is, our beliefs, expectations, and interpersonal patterns surrounding Self and Other (Bartholomew, 1990; Bartholomew & Horowitz, 1991; Griffin & Bartholomew, 1994). This approach allows for a more nuanced description your unique attachment styles, as they manifest in important life domains.

The theory centers on the different types of *value* that you ascribe to yourself and other people. If you have a *secure* attachment style, then you ascribe a positive value to yourself and others—that is, you have a sense of your own inherent worth and self-esteem, and you see other people as generally accepting of and responsive to you.

If you have a *preoccupied* attachment style, you assign negative value to yourself and positive value to others. You might struggle with feelings of self-hatred and worthlessness, and you only feel good about yourself when you receive validation and care from other people, whom you see as "better" than you in some way (e.g., more likable, kind, attractive, stable).

If you have a *fearful* attachment style, you ascribe negative value to yourself and negative value to others. You see yourself as deficient and unlovable, and you also expect that other people are going to see you in the same way. So you avoid close relationships with people, protecting yourself from rejection, criticism, and abandonment.

Finally, if you have a *dismissive* attachment style, you endow positive value to yourself and negative value to other people. You could have a largely stable and positive sense of self-esteem, but you view other people as more problematic, leading to tendencies toward self-reliance, invulnerability, superiority, even arrogance at times. See Table 8.1 for a summary of these different attachment styles, including their related emotional and interpersonal processes.

As discussed throughout this chapter, while it is possible that you only employ one attachment style in your interactions with others, it is more likely that your attachment styles vary somewhat in different life domains (e.g., family, friendships, intimate relationships, work relationships), or in specific relationships. For example, you might feel largely secure and confident in your work relationships, more anxious and preoccupied in romantic relationships, and dismissive/argumentative in your interactions with your parents and siblings. As you develop a more nuanced appreciation of your personal attachment style, you are better equipped to anticipate your key areas of interpersonal vulnerability, and to utilize mentalization to chart out new pathways for connectedness in your relationships.

Mentalizing Warm-up

Now that you appreciate the distinctions between the four specific attachment styles, revisit Alan's story at the start of the chapter, on page 127. What attachment styles (e.g., secure, preoccupied, fearful, dismissive) does Alan utilize in the different areas of his life? What life events trigger shifts in Alan's attachment tendencies in these domains?

The Relationship Style Questionnaire (RSQ) is a useful, empirically validated measure that can help you identify your predominant attachment style (Griffin & Bartholomew, 1994). Worksheet 8.2 contains some questions from the RSQ, as well as other prompts inviting you to consider how the various attachment styles (e.g., secure, preoccupied, fearful, dismissive) manifest themselves in different domains of your life.

Table 8.1 MODELS OF SELF AND OTHER IN ATTACHMENT THEORY. EMOTIONAL, INTERPERSONAL, AND FUNCTIONAL PROCESSES INVOLVED IN THE FOUR DIFFERENT ATTACHMENT STYLES: SECURE, PREOCCUPIED, FEARFUL, AND DISMISSIVE.

		Model of Self	
		Positive View of Self	Negative View of Self
Model of Other People	Positive View of Others	*Secure Attachment* • Positive sense of self-esteem, positive view of others • Comfortable with intimacy and independence • Flexible balance between independent and attachment-seeking behaviors • Tends to be associated with emotional stability and consistent, stable relationships	*Preoccupied Attachment* • Negative sense of self, idealization of others • Extensive focus on relationships • Need for other people to regulate your emotions and self-esteem • Behaviors include seeking relationships, constant communication, "neediness" and dependency • Often leads to emotional instability, unstable and intense relationships
	Negative View of Others	*Dismissive Attachment* • Positive sense of self-esteem, negative view of others • Marked by self-reliance, invulnerability, decreased interest in others, resentment and superiority, and focusing on others' defects • Behaviors include self-sufficiency, engagement in solitary activities, haughtiness, defensiveness, and argumentativeness • Leads to alienation from others, estranged relationships, and interpersonal tensions and conflict	*Fearful Attachment* • Low sense of self-esteem, experience of others as judgmental and threatening • Associated with social anxiety, loneliness, discomfort forming new relationships, and strong aversion to humiliation and embarrassment • Behaviors include avoidance of social/work situations, "shyness," cancelling plans, restraint and inhibition in interpersonal interactions • Leads to social isolation and stagnation/paralysis in work, school, friendships, and romantic relationships

Worksheet 8.2
Models of Self and Other

(1) Consider the statements below that relate to four different attachment styles. Place a check mark next to all of the statements with which you identify.

SECURE ATTACHMENT

☐ I find it easy to get emotionally close to others.

☐ I do not worry about being alone.

☐ I feel at ease depending on other people.

☐ I am comfortable having people depend on me.

☐ I do not worry about having others accept me.

PREOCCUPIED ATTACHMENT

☐ I am not sure that I can always depend on others to be there when I need them.

☐ I want to be completely emotionally intimate with other individuals.

☐ I feel uncomfortable when I do not have close emotional relationships.

☐ I worry that others don't value me as much as I value them.

☐ I find that people are reluctant to get as close as I would like.

DISMISSIVE ATTACHMENT

☐ It is very important for me to feel independent.

☐ I am comfortable without close emotional relationships.

☐ It is very important for me to feel self-sufficient.

☐ I prefer not to have other people depend on me.

☐ I prefer not to depend on others.

FEARFUL ATTACHMENT

☐ I find it difficult to depend on people.

☐ I worry that I will be hurt if I allow myself to become too close to other individuals.

☐ I struggle to trust others completely.

☐ I am uncomfortable being close to others.

☐ I feel anxious that, if I put myself out there, other people will judge and criticize me.

(2) Now tally up the total number of statements you selected in each category. This should give you a sense of the extent to which you employ each strategy in your relationships.

Secure attachment:_____   Preoccupied attachment:_____

Fearful attachment:_____   Dismissive attachment:_____

[continued on next page]

(3) *Secure attachment* involves a flexible balance between independence and connectedness with others. Circle the life domains where you experience attachment security.

Family relationships   Friendships   Work/school relationships

Romantic/sexual   Relationships with   Other life domains:
relationships   treatment providers

(4) What does attachment security look like for you in those domains? If relevant, provide at least three examples.

(5) *Preoccupied attachment* involves using relationships with valued others to regulate your emotions and self-esteem. Circle the life domains where you experience attachment preoccupation.

Family relationships   Friendships   Work/school relationships

Romantic/sexual   Relationships with   Other life domains:
relationships   treatment providers

(6) What does preoccupied attachment look like for you in those domains? If relevant, provide at least three examples.

(7) *Fearful attachment* involves avoiding rejection/criticism from others through social avoidance and withdrawal. Circle the life domains where you experience fearful attachment.

Family relationships   Friendships   Work/school relationships

Romantic/sexual   Relationships with   Other life domains:
relationships   treatment providers

[continued on next page]

(8) What does fearful attachment look like for you in those domains? If relevant, provide at least three examples.

(9) *Dismissive attachment* involves distancing yourself from others through self-reliance, invulnerability, devaluation of others, and argumentativeness. Circle the life domains where you experience dismissive attachment.

Family relationships   Friendships   Work/school relationships

Romantic/sexual   Relationships with   Other life domains:
relationships   treatment providers

(10) What does dismissive attachment look like for you in those domains? If relevant, provide at least three examples.

Note. The statements in question (1) above are drawn and adapted from the Relationship Style Questionnaire (RSQ), with permission from D. W. Griffin. The RSQ appears as presented in Griffin, D. W., & Bartholomew, K. (1994). The metaphysics of measurement: The case of adult attachment. In K. Bartholomew & D. Perlman (Eds.), *Advances in personal relationships: Attachment processes in adulthood* (Vol. 5, pp. 17–52). Jessica Kingsley.

MENTALIZING PRACTICE POINTS: EVOLVING YOUR ATTACHMENT STYLE

How do you change and evolve your attachment style? This entire book reviews a wealth of strategies to do just that. By using the techniques of mentalizing, you start to see yourself and other people in different ways, which naturally impacts how you engage in your relationships. Since most of these techniques focus on mentalizing internal processes (e.g., thoughts, expectations, beliefs, emotions, desires, feelings about yourself), in this chapter, you will learn strategies to shift *behaviors* connected to your attachment patterns. MBT recommends several approaches to address your attachment-related challenges.

Identify attachment-related behaviors that you want to change. It is important to note that not all of your attachment-related behaviors are "bad," maladaptive, or problematic. For example, if you have traits of preoccupied attachment, you might really value spending time with people, and so you probably do a good job of maintaining contact with your friends, family, and romantic partners. Or if you utilize a more dismissive attachment style, you draw a sharper boundary between yourself and other people. You thus could be quite effective at "saying no" when someone asks you to do something that contradicts your values and preferences.

Accordingly, when attempting to modify your longstanding attachment patterns, the first step involves recognizing specific attachment-related behaviors that cause trouble for you in your life. This can include actions, interpersonal tendencies, or broader relational patterns that negatively affect

- how you feel (e.g., in yourself, about yourself, about your relationships);
- how other people feel (e.g., in themselves, about you);
- your ability to function effectively in your relationships; and
- your capacity to achieve and maintain the kinds of relationships that you want.

For example, if you struggle with fearful attachment, your problem behaviors could include avoiding social situations, or not speaking freely and openly when you are around other people, out of fear that you might embarrass yourself. If you are more preoccupied in your approach, one of your maladaptive behaviors could be jumping into relationships too quickly, without sufficiently considering if the other person is a good fit for you. If you tend to be more dismissive of others, your target behaviors could include argumentativeness, defensiveness, and criticizing other people.

The good news is that you have already started identifying your maladaptive attachment-related behaviors earlier in the book, back in Chapter 5 when you were developing your personal priorities for treatment. Turn back to Worksheet 5.2 on page 78 for a list of interpersonal tendencies that could potentially interfere with your life and well-being. Write those down here, along with any additional attachment-related behaviors that you want to change in your treatment.

Maladaptive Attachment-related Behaviors

_____

_____

_____

_____

Stay on the lookout for your attachment-related impulses. In Chapter 7, we discussed the importance of forecasting your triggers, so that you can have greater self-control when challenging situations come your way. MBT recommends that you use a similar approach when working on your attachment-related problem behaviors. While it can sometimes feel like your problem behaviors simply *happen* to you, with the help of mentalizing, you can get a "sneak peek" into these behaviors—before they are released to the public. Outside the heat of the moment, when you are not at all tempted to take these actions, try reflecting upon your own mental states immediately leading up to the behavior in question.

- "What do I feel in my body before I engage in the behavior? What physical sensations do I experience?" This could include increased heart rate, a tightness in your chest, tensing your muscles, or flushing of your face.
- "Are there any thoughts, ideas, or images that go through my mind, when I am really wanting to do this thing?"
- "What emotions do I experience before taking the action? How do I feel about myself?"
- "What does the impulse *itself* feel like? Can I put words on it in any way?"

For example, if one of your problem behaviors is reassurance-seeking from romantic partners, you might observe that before taking this action, you experience a tightness in your chest, feelings of panic and desperation, and a strong sense of insecurity and shame, like there is something wrong with you. The impulse itself feels like an intolerable pit in your stomach, which you need to get rid of by asking how the other person feels about you.

Once you have contended with the above questions, keep these reflections in your back pocket, and carry them around with you as you are living your life. Stay on the lookout for them, as internal signposts of your urge to engage in the problem behavior. When you notice these feelings arise, work to privately articulate the impulse in question: "I am experiencing the desire to _____" or "I am feeling the strong wish to _____." As you mentalize in these ways, you develop the increased ability to notice these desires *before* you engage in the problem behavior. This opens up a tiny bit of space between impulse and action, creating a greater sense of self-control surrounding the interpersonal approaches that have been getting in your way.

Mentalize your attachment-related motives. If you have BPD, you might reflexively describe the motives for your actions in more externally focused terms: "I yelled at him because he was criticizing me" or "This situation wasn't right, so I had to stand up for myself." In addition, you may justify maladaptive behaviors by focusing on your altruistic motives ("I can't break up with him right now because he has so much going on in his life. It would create too much stress for him"), or by invoking seemingly "neutral" or innocuous desires ("I was just trying to speak my truth"). Interestingly, when you mentalize your motives in these sorts of terms (i.e., as externally caused, altruistic, or harmless), you are much more likely to engage in the maladaptive behavior under consideration. At an intellectual level, you recognize that the behavior is ineffective or unwise, but at an emotional level, you still *feel* quite justified in taking the action. Consequences be damned! Accordingly, you continue to engage in your problem behaviors, and you remain "stuck" in the same unhelpful attachment styles.

In contrast, MBT suggests that you reflect on your *attachment-related* motives surrounding your problem behaviors in relationships. These motives always involve some future event that you want to take place in the relationship. Such "events" could be the other person relating to you in a certain way (e.g., validating you, sharing about their problems, joking around with you), or even you or others experiencing particular feeling states. By considering your personal motivational investment in your attachment-related behaviors, you will gain an increased sense of agency surrounding them: You will feel more able to refrain from taking these actions, and to adopt new behaviors that facilitate greater intimacy and connectedness with others.

So when you are drawn to engage in one of your attachment-related problem behaviors, try reflecting on the following questions:

- "What do I want to happen by engaging in this behavior?"
- "What do I wish to feel by taking this action? Are there emotions from which I am trying to distance myself?"
- "If I take this action, how am I hoping to feel about myself? Are there benefits I am seeking, at the level of my self-worth and self-esteem?"
- "Could there be any avoidance at play for me here? Am I trying to prevent negative events from happening? Am I attempting to avoid certain feelings in myself, or to stop other people from seeing me in a particular way?"
- *When the behavior directly involves an interpersonal interaction:*
  - "If I take this action, how do I want the other person to feel? How do I want them to feel about *me*? How do I want them to view me?"
  - "If I engage in this behavior, what do I want the other person to do? How am I hoping they will respond to me, or engage with me?"

Reflect on the negative consequences of the attachment-related behavior. Motives always concern the best case scenario—what you are wanting and hoping for by taking the action. However, before engaging in your attachment-related problem behaviors, MBT recommends that you consider the *worst* case scenario as well—the unintended consequences of utilizing the interpersonal approach in question. For example, you might wrestle with the following questions:

- "Are there any downsides to taking this action? What is the worst case scenario if I move forward with this?"
- "Could doing this lead to any negative consequences in me? How might this affect my emotions, mood, and self-esteem?"
- "Could taking this action negatively affect other people at all: their emotions, desires, and feelings about themselves?"
- "If I engage in this behavior, could that ever make me want to engage in *other* problematic behaviors, which may cause more trouble for me or other people?"

For instance, if you are tempted to text an ex-romantic partner who really hurt you, you might attempt to imagine the worst outcome from you reaching out in this way. Perhaps they do not respond to your text right away, and you feel even more hopeless, desperate, and alone. You then might text them again several more times, and finally they block you just like they used to do. You end up feeling humiliated and powerless—the same way that you always have with them.

As you mentalize in these ways, you are flexibly considering a range of perspectives on your problem behaviors—not simply the "pros" of the behaviors, but their "cons" as well. This can grant you the presence of mind to refrain from taking the actions that are holding you back in your life.

Consider alternative attachment-related behaviors. As you probably already know all too well, it is extremely difficult to just *not* do something that you really want to do. It can feel like you are getting sucked into the void, and no amount of willpower can make you hold your ground. MBT suggests that you *fill* that void with mentalization, and specifically mentalization about other ways of being with other people, which are more consistent with how you want to be in the world.

Earlier in the chapter, you learned how insecure attachment is associated with negative views of yourself (as we see in preoccupied and fearful attachment) and negative views of other people (as we see with dismissive and fearful attachment). In contrast, secure attachment involves ascribing *positive* value to Self and Other, such that you are able to flexibly remain connected to other people while also maintaining your autonomy and independence. In light of this, when you are working to not engage in your problem behaviors in relationships (e.g., dependency, enmeshment, argumentativeness, avoidance), consider what it might look like for you to engage with others in a manner more consistent with your own self-worth, as well as the worth and value of other people.

- "In this situation, how could I conduct myself with a greater sense of integrity and self-respect? What would allow me to maintain my dignity—to affirm my inherent worth as a person?"
- "What actions could I take that are more consistent with other people's worth and value? How could I treat them with respect and care, in the manner they most deserve?"
- "Are there any behaviors that could *simultaneously* reflect my own value and the value of other people? What would it look like for me to engage with others in that way? What would that be like for me, and for other people?"

To illustrate: if you are trying to alter your attachment-related behavior of "talking about your medical or psychiatric issues in social situations," you could reflect on what alternative behaviors could express your *own* value in the situation. "Maybe I could share about some of the *good* things happening in my life right now: my new job, our upcoming vacation, or the fact that I finally started doing yoga. My whole life is not just problems—I sometimes forget that." Or if you want to curb your attachment-related behavior of "defensiveness whenever anyone gives you constructive feedback," you might pause to consider how you could affirm your care for the person in question. "Perhaps I could ask them more questions about their view of me—to really try to understand the point they are trying to make before arguing with them. This would show them the respect that they deserve."

As always in MBT, the aim here is not to get you to do or say anything in particular. Rather, the point is reflection *itself*, and specifically reflection on ways of being in your relationships that are in keeping with your own worth as a person, as well as other people's worth. By "interrupting" your problem behaviors with these forms of mentalizing, and by trying to live out these new behaviors in your life, you will gradually develop a more secure, engaged attachment style—one that leads to greater fulfillment, stability, and meaning in your relationships.

Mentalizing Cool-down

Now that you know more about MBT's strategies for addressing insecure attachment, consider Alan's story at the start of the chapter, on page 127. What would it look like for Alan to apply these techniques in his recent interpersonal challenges?

RETURNING TO ALAN

Prompted by his recent challenges with emotional and interpersonal instability, Alan made the decision to seek out psychiatric support, ultimately connecting with a therapist who specialized in MBT. Alan and his therapist worked together to develop an MBT formulation (see Chapter 5), which examined Alan's typical manner of navigating closeness in his relationships. Alan learned that he employed a combination of anxious and avoidant attachment strategies. He noticed attachment anxiety in his dependency on his wife Maggie, his insecurities in social and professional situations, his approval-seeking at work, and his tendency to utilize Maggie's validation and support to regulate his emotional states. He observed attachment avoidance in his estranged relationship with his family of origin, as well as his recent tendencies toward isolation, withdrawal, and non-responsiveness in his work relationships.

Alan's MBT formulation also outlined the more nuanced attachment patterns proposed in the "models of Self and Other" theory of attachment. See here for an excerpt of Alan's MBT formulation covering these areas:

You can feel highly worried about how other people see you (e.g., in social and work interactions, especially with your boss Larry), anticipating criticism from them and feeling badly about yourself if you ever feel like they are judging you *[fearful attachment]*. You cope with these feelings by "trying harder" on your work assignments in order to gain others' approval, and by receiving unconditional love and support in your relationship with your wife Maggie *[preoccupied attachment]*.

When other people validate and admire you, you feel temporarily secure in yourself, like you are finally able to breathe and relax into yourself. However, if people give you *negative* feedback, that is highly destabilizing to you, and you end up "switching" to a more antagonistic stance: feeling superior to others, focusing on their negative qualities, becoming defensive and argumentative, and pushing other people away from you (e.g., through missing work, not communicating with colleagues, ignoring your family of origin) *[dismissive attachment]*.

At the outset of therapy, Alan identified his highest priority problem behaviors as his defensiveness and argumentativeness with Larry, and his avoidance of work-related responsibilities. Alan worked with his therapist to explore his relational motives surrounding these actions. He recognized that he felt ashamed and humiliated whenever Larry gave him constructive feedback. By criticizing Larry in these moments, Alan felt more "in control" and powerful, and these feelings of shame temporarily faded into the background. Alan also discovered that, by engaging in his avoidant behaviors (e.g., hiding in the bathroom, calling in sick, not responding to e-mails, procrastinating on his project), he was trying to escape from his stress and anxiety that he was doing a bad job at work, and that other people were judging and rejecting him for his poor performance. And while it embarrassed him to admit this, Alan saw that there was a tiny part of him that actually wanted people to *notice* his decreased engagement—so that they would worry about him, reach out to him, and give him the support and validation that he desperately craved.

Alan tried to notice his impulses to argue and avoid, as they arose in him throughout his workday. With his therapist's help, he recognized certain "warning signs" of his behavior of sending critical e-mails to Larry. Experiencing a mixture of powerlessness and rage, Alan would shake his head, clench his fists, and rehearse all of the things that he wanted to say to Larry to "put him in his place." As Alan caught himself *before* taking these actions, he reflected upon the negative consequences of these behaviors. Larry had been patient with him so far (Larry was aware of Alan's psychiatric issues), but this could not go on forever. If Alan continued being argumentative, missing work, and neglecting his assignments, he would start receiving verbal and written warnings, and his job could be in jeopardy. Alan had seen this occur with other employees in the past, and he did not want it to happen to him.

In an effort to curb these interpersonal processes, Alan considered: What would it look like to relate to others in a manner that reflected their value as people, and his value as well? When Larry spoke with Alan about his work projects, Alan worked to hold his tongue and not argue with him. Instead, Alan actively tried to take in Larry's perspective about how these projects were going, along with what Alan could do to improve his efficiency and quality control. Recognizing that all of his avoidance was quite disempowering to *him*, Alan worked to be more consistent at his job, regardless of how he happened to be feeling in the moment. As he begrudgingly responded to colleagues' e-mails, he saw himself as showing them some basic level of respect and care, even while he struggled to fully trust them. In these ways, Alan cultivated a more flexible interpersonal approach that was simultaneously validating of his colleagues, Larry, *and* himself as a person.

Alan gradually noticed a shift in his emotional experience in the workplace. He felt less inadequate there, and less apprehensive that everyone was looking down on him. His resentment toward Larry subsided, and he wondered if perhaps he had been giving Larry too hard of a time. Sure, Larry could be cold and condescending, but he had also been quite understanding of Alan's difficulties this year, in a way that many bosses would not have been. For the first time in a long time, Alan started enjoying his coding work again, experiencing a newfound sense of confidence in his own strengths and abilities. While he still kept largely to himself, he felt more at peace with that, as if he had attained some new, solitary equilibrium.

Feeling more secure in himself at work, Alan realized how much he had been relying on Maggie to regulate his emotions throughout all of this, and really since they began dating way back in college. What was *that* about? Perhaps it was time to work on this as well. . . .

Chapter Review 8.1
What is Your Attachment Style?

Attachment Theory

- Attachment theory is a school of thought in psychology that suggests that infants need to develop an emotionally attuned relationship with at least one primary caregiver for their successful development.

- When caregivers are consistently available and responsive to the child, the child feels secure and confident in the caregivers' accessibility.

- When caregivers are more aggressive, rejecting, or emotionally neglectful, the child feels insecure about the caregivers' availability and responsiveness.

- These processes are internalized by the child in the form of **attachment styles**—a person's characteristic manner of experiencing and regulating closeness in their relationships, in childhood and throughout development.

Attachment and Mentalization

- Borderline personality disorder (BPD) is significantly associated with insecure attachment.

- If you feel insecure and rejected in your relationships, you are more likely to experience problems with mentalizing yourself and other people.

- Mentalization-based treatment (MBT) underscores several key points about attachment styles:

  - Attachment styles encompass *both* internal processes (e.g., thoughts, emotions, desires) and behaviors.

  - Many people exhibit different attachment styles in different relational contexts: in specific types of relationships (e.g., friendships, family relationships, intimate partnerships), with particular individuals, and when interacting with people who have specific qualities or characteristics.

  - Attachment strategies can vary based on *what happens* in your relationships—that is, whether or not people treat you in a positive, negative, or "neutral" manner.

  - MBT focuses on *how* you relate to other people in your current life, rather than "why" you developed your attachment style based on your history.

[continued on next page]

Two Different Theories of Attachment Styles

- The most fundamental types of insecure attachment are attachment anxiety and attachment avoidance.

  - **Attachment anxiety** involves seeing yourself in a negative light, fears of rejection and abandonment, coping with distress by moving closer to other people, and feeling angry or upset when others are not responsive to you.

  - **Attachment avoidance** entails seeing others in a negative light, desire to avoid other people, reticence around expressing your feelings, and discomfort surrounding "asking for help" and relying on others.

- Another theory of attachment centers on the different types of *value* that you ascribe to yourself and other people.

  - **Secure attachment:** You have a sense of your own inherent worth and self-esteem *[positive view of Self]*, and you see other people as generally accepting and responsive to you *[positive view of Other]*.

  - **Preoccupied attachment:** You struggle with low self-esteem *[negative view of Self]*, only feeling good about yourself when you receive validation from others, whom you see as "better" than you *[positive view of Other]*.

  - **Fearful attachment:** You see yourself as deficient and unlovable *[negative view of Self]*, and you also expect that other people are going to see you the same way *[negative view of Other]*.

  - **Dismissive attachment:** You have a largely stable sense of self-esteem *[positive view of Self]*, but you see others as problematic, leading to self-reliance, invulnerability, superiority, and arrogance *[negative view of Other]*.

Chapter Review 8.2
Mentalizing Practice Points: Evolving Your Attachment Style

Identify Maladaptive Attachment-related Behaviors

Consider actions, interpersonal tendencies, or relational patterns that you want to change.

These behaviors could negatively affect how you feel, how other people feel, your ability to function effectively in your relationships, and your capacity to achieve the kinds of relationships that you want.

Stay on the Lookout for Attachment-related Impulses

- Outside the heat of the moment, reflect on your mental states leading up to your attachment-related problem behaviors.

  - "What do I feel in my body before I engage in the behavior? What physical sensations do I experience?"

  - "Are there any thoughts, ideas, or images that go through my mind, when I am really wanting to do this thing?"

  - "What emotions do I experience before taking the action? How do I feel about myself?"

  - "What does the impulse *itself* feel like? Can I put words on it in any way?"

- When you notice these feelings arise, privately articulate the impulse: "I am experiencing the desire to _____."

Mentalize your Attachment-related Motives

- "What do I want to happen by engaging in this behavior?"

- "What do I wish to feel by taking this action? Are there emotions from which I am trying to distance myself?"

- "If I take this action, how am I hoping to feel about myself? Are there benefits I am seeking, at the level of my self-worth and self-esteem?"

- "Could there be any avoidance at play for me here? Am I trying to prevent negative events from happening? Am I attempting to avoid certain feelings in myself, or to stop other people from seeing me in a particular way?"

- If the behavior directly involves an interpersonal interaction:

  - "If I take this action, how do I want the other person to feel? How do I want them to feel about *me*? How do I want them to view me?"

  - "If I engage in this behavior, what do I want the other person to do? How am I hoping they will respond to me, or engage with me?"

[continued on next page]

Reflect on the Behavior's Negative Consequences

- "Are there any downsides to taking this action? What is the worst case scenario if I move forward with this?"

- "Could doing this lead to any negative consequences in me? How might this affect my emotions, mood, and self-esteem?"

- "Could taking this action negatively affect other people at all: their emotions, desires, and feelings about themselves?"

- "If I engage in this behavior, could that ever make me want to engage in *other* problematic behaviors, which may cause more trouble for me or other people?"

Consider Alternative Attachment-related Behaviors

- "In this situation, how could I conduct myself with a greater sense of integrity and self-respect? What would allow me to maintain my dignity—to affirm my inherent worth as a person?"

- "What actions could I take that are more consistent with other people's worth and value? How could I treat them with respect and care, in the manner they most deserve?"

- "Are there any behaviors that could *simultaneously* reflect my own value and the value of other people? What would it look like for me to engage with others in that way? What would that be like for me, and for other people?"

9

How to Recognize
"What" People Are Feeling

Martha struggled with a long history of depression and suicidal thinking. While she had achieved some success in her career as a cardiac nurse, over the past decade, she had found it difficult to hold down a job for longer than one year. She would quickly impress her colleagues with her clinical skills and warm manner with patients, but inevitably the same pattern would repeat itself: falling behind in paperwork, feeling deeply insecure in her interactions with co-workers, arriving hours late to shifts, feeling more insecure and ashamed, and finally failing to show up to work altogether, at which point she would either quit or get fired. She was sure that her colleagues were judging her for her inconsistency; she would rather lose these jobs than experience their negative views of her.

Now in her 40s, Martha lived a life of profound isolation. Her only living family member was an older sister Sarah, whom she saw as her antithesis—married with two young boys, emotionally stable, and professionally successful. Martha, on the other hand, had not dated anyone in over a decade, and she spent most of her time alone in her apartment—watching TV, eating junk food, languishing in bed, making endless lists, and moving piles of papers from one surface to another. Feeling abandoned by the world, Martha would start to fantasize about ways to take her life, which gave her a temporary feeling of relief that there might be some escape from this maddening cycle of meaninglessness.

Concerned about her suicidality, Martha decided to seek out an individual therapist who provided mentalization-based treatment (MBT). Martha had never received therapy before, and she was not expecting all of this talk about *feelings*. The therapist would doggedly inquire about Martha's emotions, desires, and feelings about herself. "What emotions were you experiencing at that moment?" "Do you have a sense of how you are wanting your sister to engage with you?" "How does that make you feel about yourself—to not be working anymore?" Martha was surprised that she actually did not know the answers to these questions. She rarely stopped to consider what she was feeling, as she was so focused on more "visible" factors in her life, whether those be objects or activities in her apartment, or (when she was working) all of the concrete tasks that overwhelmed her.

As the therapy progressed, Martha shared more about her challenges in her relationship with her sister Sarah. While Sarah would reach out to Martha by phone to check in on her, she rarely initiated in-person get-togethers. Martha would often learn after the fact that Sarah and her children had done some activity to which they could have easily invited Martha. Martha conveyed: "She sees me as a burden; she's completely overwhelmed by me. She just wants to live her life—to go to work, take care of her kids, and not have to deal with me and my issues." Mentalizing Sarah in this way, Martha felt even more isolated and alone. If her sister—the person in the world to whom she was closest—did not even care about her, what was the point of trying to get better?

Mentalization. Robert P. Drozek, Oxford University Press. © Oxford University Press 2025.
DOI: 10.1093/oso/9780198916857.003.0009

DIFFICULTIES RECOGNIZING YOUR OWN MENTAL STATES

As we discussed in Chapter 3, a foundational component of mentalizing is reflecting on mental content—that is, observing and identifying specific mental states (e.g., thoughts, beliefs, emotions, needs, desires, self-states, and attitudes) in yourself and other people. This is the "what" form of mentalization, also referred to as *content-mentalizing* (Drozek et al., 2023; Drozek & Henry, 2021). If you have borderline personality disorder (BPD), you might find it difficult to mentalize in these ways, especially when facing one of your triggers (Chapter 7), or when experiencing any intense emotion. Examples of problems content-mentalizing your own emotions include:

- confusion about what you are feeling;
- drawing inaccurate conclusions about your own internal processes;
- tendency to "miss" or ignore particular subjective states in yourself;
- difficulty identifying and "putting words on" certain mental states in yourself; and
- "biases" toward identifying some feelings in yourself, while neglecting others.

Given its importance in BPD, this last difficulty in mentalizing deserves special attention. When confronted with outside factors that you see as "wrong" or "unjust," you may find yourself quickly jumping to an experience of anger, where you focus extensively on other people's problematic qualities or actions. In such moments, you are most likely noticing emotions of anger in yourself, as well as other anger-related feeling states: frustration, agitation, resentment, rage, a desire to "get back at" the person, a wish to enumerate all the ways they have harmed you, and so on.

However, it could be more challenging to identify the "softer" or more vulnerable feeling states in yourself: sadness, insecurity, shame, fear of abandonment, and desires for attention or care. You might cognitively know that such feelings are present in you, but at an experiential level, they exist just outside your field of peripheral vision. This is an example of what we call a *bias* in content-mentalizing: You easily recognize certain mental states in yourself, but other mental states are less "on your radar."

Problems in content-mentalizing can lead to significant challenges in BPD. If you struggle to recognize your feelings, you lack a full sense of agency in relation to them. You can be blindsided by your emotions—they control you rather than you controlling them. This theory is supported by extensive research linking difficulties identifying emotions with BPD symptoms (Derks et al., 2017), including emotional instability and self-injurious behavior (Edwards et al., 2021; Sleuwaegen et al., 2017).

Along similar lines, when you are unable to identify your own feelings, you lack a core element in a coherent sense of self. You can feel confused, empty, aimless, and easily overwhelmed. You are like a house without a foundation: At any moment, the weather might change, and the whole structure could topple over. These deficits explain the identity diffusion associated with BPD, reviewed in Chapter 1. Without a clear understanding of your own emotions and desires, you can be significantly influenced by *other people's* emotions and desires. This places you at risk for unstable relationships, mistreatment, and exploitation by others.

These problems with mentalizing can also impact your sense of direction in life. If you do not know what matters to you, then you cannot pursue those things. This gives rise to a sense of stuckness and paralysis, where you continuously feel like you are not reaching your full potential as a person. It is like you are using a roadmap that is missing an entire section, so you cannot get where you need to go. As it turns out, that missing section is YOU!

In addition, when you struggle with content-mentalizing, your actions fail to reflect the full spectrum of your internal experiences. For example, if you are not attuned to how much you crave relationships, you may be more cold, distant, and aloof when you are interacting with other people. If you ignore your own values and ethics, you might mistreat other people, or take actions that undermine your own dignity and self-respect. If you are only in touch with your anger in a situation, then you will naturally *show and express* that anger to others, rather than all of the other feelings unfolding inside of you (e.g., sadness, hurt, insecurity). People can thus feel criticized and attacked by you, leading to upset feelings, conflict, and broken relationships. In contrast, when you are mentalizing these "softer" feelings in yourself, you will come across as more open, approachable, and emotionally engaged. People will want to move closer to you in these moments, or at least not to pull away from you. Most of us would rather pet a sweet puppy than an aggressive pit bull![1]

When you are identifying your difficulties mentalizing yourself in MBT, it is helpful to keep a handful of things in mind. First, MBT tends to prioritize your problems mentalizing specifically *affective* content—that is, emotions, desires, and feelings about yourself. To refresh your memory, see here for some definitions of these terms from Chapter 3.

- **Emotion:** a feeling, sentiment, or mood, usually carrying some positive or negative valence. Examples include sadness, anxiety, anger, happiness, and hurt.
- **Desire:** a wish or impulse that some event will happen, or that some other situation will *not* happen. Examples include the desire to feel a certain way; a longing for other people to feel a certain way (e.g., in themselves, about you); the wish to take a specific action (e.g., using substances, asking someone out, going to the gym); or the urge for some visible circumstance to transpire in the world (e.g., getting a promotion, receiving a good grade on a test, a loved one recovering from a medical illness).
- **Self-state:** a feeling about oneself—who one is as a person, usually concerning one's own value and worth. Examples include shame, embarrassment, pride, and self-doubt.

These affective processes are more "in your gut," rather than "in your head"—processes like thoughts, beliefs, attitudes, and values. As discussed in Chapter 4, MBT suggests that the ability to mentalize emotions serves as the foundation for the core sense of mental selfhood. By strengthening your ability to mentalize these "deeper" parts of yourself, MBT helps you to lay the groundwork for an embodied, coherent sense of self.

Furthermore, when describing your particular mentalizing vulnerabilities, consider those mental states that (a) are probably present in you to some degree, but (b) you struggle to recognize when they are there. For example, you suspect that you probably want to say things to hurt your romantic partner, but you also really judge yourself for that, so it is difficult for you to experientially "locate" these desires in yourself. However, if the mental states in question are probably *not* present in you at all, we would not say that you are struggling to mentalize them. For instance, you would not list "happiness and contentment" on your list of neglected emotions if you simply do not tend to feel happy and content much of the time. So specify the emotions that are difficult to *see*, not difficult to *generate*.

Finally, actually spell out the specific feelings that are more challenging for you to identify in yourself—that is, particular emotions, desires, and feelings about yourself. What do you tend to miss, to pass over? See here for some examples.

- *Emotions:* "I struggle to recognize any 'anger'-related feelings in myself: frustration, resentment, and annoyance. I often don't recognize that I am feeling that way until I hit a breaking point and say something aggressive." Or: "When people mistreat me, I often immediately get angry at them, but I 'skip over' other emotions in myself that I find more painful, like hurt and sadness."

[1] No offense to any pit bull owners out there! I am playing on stereotypes to land the metaphor.

- *Desires:* "I can sometimes 'miss' that I am desiring care, attention, and validation from other people, especially romantic partners. I don't think that I deserve those things, so I find it hard to acknowledge that I want them."
- *Self-states*: "In social situations, I often ignore my feelings of insecurity, embarrassment, and shame. At the time, I always say 'I'm fine,' but after the fact, I realize that I have been comparing myself to other people, and feeling defective and unworthy in relation to them."

Mentalizing Warm-up

With these problems in mentalizing in mind, consider Martha's story at the start of the chapter, on page 151. How does Martha struggle with noticing and identifying her own emotions, desires, and self-states? How might these difficulties negatively impact Martha in her life?

We cannot try to find a thing unless we first know that it is missing. By recognizing the parts of yourself that might be "harder to see," you can keep an eye out for these neglected emotions, wishes, and feelings about yourself. It is like you are filling in that missing part of your roadmap. Now you can start to *explore* that uncharted terrain as you move throughout your life. Worksheet 9.1 helps you to identify your unique challenges with content-mentalizing.

Worksheet 9.1
Challenges Mentalizing "What" You are Feeling

(1) People with BPD experience various types of challenges with mentalizing their own internal states. Circle any of these challenges that you have encountered in your life.

Tendency to "miss" or ignore particular subjective states in yourself

Drawing inaccurate conclusions about your own internal processes

Difficulty identifying and "putting words on" certain mental states in yourself

Bias toward noticing some feelings in yourself, while neglecting others

Confusion about what you are feeling

(2) What do these mentalizing problems look like for you? Have they caused any disruptions in your mood, self-esteem, relationships, or functionality? Provide at least three examples.

Difficulties Reflecting on Your Emotions

(3) See below for a list of emotions that many people experience. Draw a square around any emotions that you are easily able to notice in yourself, when you are experiencing them. Then draw an "X" through any emotions that you find more challenging to identify in yourself, if you happen to be feeling them. You do not have to mark all of the emotions listed.

Anger	Fear	Sadness	Happiness
Love or care	Disgust	Jealousy	Surprise
Dread	Hurt	Relief	Helplessness
Amusement	Boredom	Rage	Satisfaction
Hope	Grief	Trust	Horror, terror
Loneliness	Impatience	Frustration	Guilt, remorse
Envy	Anxiety, worry	Satisfaction	Disappointment

[continued on next page]

Hatred, contempt	Joy	Depression	Tension, stress
Panic	Awe, wonder	Contentment	Excitement
Calm, relaxation	Overwhelmment	Gratitude	Pity
Rejection, abandonment	Pleasure, enjoyment	Hopelessness, despair	Annoyance, irritation
Other emotion:	Other emotion:	Other emotion:	Other emotion:

(4) Now look back at the emotions above with X's through them. Are there any contexts (e.g., specific events, interactions, or interpersonal situations) where you find it easier to recognize these emotions? Are there any contexts where you find it more difficult to notice them?

Difficulties Reflecting on Your Desires

(5) List any desires you find more challenging to identify in yourself, if you happen to be feeling them. These could include the desire to feel a certain way, a yearning for other people to feel a specific way (e.g., in themselves, about you), the wish to take a particular action, or the urge for some event to happen.

(6) Are there any contexts (e.g., specific events, interactions, or interpersonal situations) where you find it easier to recognize these desires? Are there any contexts where you find it harder to notice these desires?

[continued on next page]

Difficulties Reflecting on Your Feelings about Yourself

(7) See below for a list of self-states, or "feelings about oneself," that many people experience. Draw a square around any self-states that you are easily able to notice in yourself, when you are experiencing them. Then draw an "X" through any self-states that you find more challenging to identify in yourself, if you happen to be feeling them. You do not have to mark all of the feelings listed.

Embarrassment	Shame	Pride	Worthlessness
Self-confidence	Humiliation	Insecurity	Self-pity
Self-love	Inadequacy	Self-doubt	Self-blame
Self-loathing, self-hatred	Empowerment, triumph	Self-consciousness	Self-satisfaction
Other self-state:	Other self-state:	Other self-state:	Other self-state:

(8) Now look back at the self-states above with X's through them. Are there any contexts (e.g., specific events, interactions, or interpersonal situations) where you find it easier to recognize these feelings about yourself? Are there any contexts where you find it more difficult to notice these feelings?

DIFFICULTIES READING OTHER PEOPLE'S MENTAL STATES

Content-mentalizing also involves "reading" and recognizing mental states in other people. In BPD, problems with mentalizing others include:

- difficulty "reading" or understanding mental states in others;
- drawing inaccurate conclusions about others' internal processes;
- tendency to "miss" or ignore specific subjective states in other people;
- difficulty identifying and "putting words on" certain mental states in others; and
- biases toward identifying particular feelings in other people, while neglecting others.

Let's consider the most common examples of these challenges in BPD. You might be exceptionally attuned to other people's potentially negative feelings about you (e.g., judgments, criticisms, anger), assuming that is how people are *really* feeling about you. You might "miss" others' positive or neutral feelings toward you, thus feeling more insecure and anxious in your interactions with them.

On the other hand, you could focus mostly on people's *positive* feelings toward you—the things they have said or done that indicate their interest, investment, and care for you. This can arise when you are highly dependent on a particular person, or if you are craving attention and care from someone. However, you might be less cognizant of others' mental states indicating their more challenging feelings toward you, including anger, impatience, apathy, and indifference. You can thus assume that other people care more about you than they actually do, which places you at risk for neglect and mistreatment in your relationships. You focus on the good, ignore the bad, and end up settling for less than you deserve.

You could also be hyper-focused on how other people feel about *you*, paying less attention to their other mental states. Especially when you are struggling, you might be less attuned to people's feelings that have nothing to do with you, such as their emotions or desires about other situations in their lives, or their feelings about themselves. This can manifest itself in difficulties with self-focus and self-centeredness, where you experience the world primarily in light of *your* feelings and desires, rather than in terms of other people's needs and wants. These tendencies can generate distance and conflict in relationships, especially if people feel like you are not sufficiently "taking them in" and considering their independent viewpoints.

In addition, you might have the tendency to take things personally in your interactions with others—that is, to assume that other people's actions and comments are "about" you in some way. For instance, your friend has been texting you a lot less frequently lately, and you worry that she is upset with you, and trying to distance herself from you. However, you fail to consider all of the other mental states that might explain her decreased communication: her excitement about starting a new relationship, her anxiety and preoccupation about applying to graduate school, and her distress about recent conflicts in her family.

Along similar lines, you could fail to consider other people's motives and personality traits that might be leading them to treat you in the way that they do. You thus end up "blaming yourself" for other people's psychological vulnerabilities. For example, you might be quite attuned to your partner's dissatisfaction about how you load the dishwasher, feeling guilt and shame about your approach: "It is true that I am totally disorganized and chaotic. Why can't I just do it their way?" But you could be less attentive to the ways in which your partner's displeasure likely reflects their own rigidity, perfectionism, and desire for control—traits which they are likely to display in other areas of their life as well.

When identifying your problems mentalizing other people, MBT recommends that you utilize the same principles that we discussed for describing your challenges with self-mentalizing:

- Prioritize your problems mentalizing specifically affective content in other people—that is, your difficulties identifying other people's emotions, desires, and feelings about themselves.
- Consider those mental states that (a) are probably present in the other person to some degree, but (b) you struggle to recognize when they are there.
- Spell out and "put words on" the specific mental states are more challenging for you to identify in other people: sadness, desires for attention, insecurities, emotions about life circumstances that are unrelated to you, and so on.

Mentalizing Warm-up

Now that you understand the various problems mentalizing others, revisit Martha's story at the start of the chapter, on page 151. How might Martha struggle with "reading" and identifying other people's emotions, desires, and self-states? In what ways could these difficulties affect Martha's mood, self-esteem, relationships, and functionality?

With these examples in mind, start reviewing Worksheet 9.2, which explores your difficulties identifying other people's mental states.

Worksheet 9.2
Challenges Mentalizing "What" Other People are Feeling

(1) People with BPD experience various types of challenges with mentalizing what others are feeling. Circle any of these challenges that you have encountered in your interactions with others.

Tendency to "miss" or ignore specific subjective states in other people

Drawing inaccurate conclusions about others' internal processes

Difficulty identifying and "putting words on" particular mental states in others

Bias toward noticing some feelings in other people, while neglecting others

Trouble "reading" or understanding mental states in others

(2) What do these mentalizing problems look like in your life? Have they caused any disruptions in your mood, self-esteem, relationships, or functionality? Provide at least three examples.

Difficulties Reflecting on Other People's Emotions

(3) See below for a list of emotions that many people experience. Draw a square around any emotions that you are easily able to notice in other people. Then draw an "X" through any emotions that you find more challenging to identify in others. You do not have to mark all of the emotions listed.

Anger	Fear	Sadness	Happiness
Love or care	Disgust	Jealousy	Surprise
Dread	Hurt	Relief	Helplessness
Amusement	Boredom	Rage	Satisfaction
Hope	Grief	Trust	Horror, terror
Loneliness	Impatience	Frustration	Guilt, remorse
Envy	Anxiety, worry	Satisfaction	Disappointment

[continued on next page]

Hatred, contempt	Joy	Depression	Tension, stress
Panic	Awe, wonder	Contentment	Excitement
Calm, relaxation	Overwhelmment	Gratitude	Pity
Rejection, abandonment	Pleasure, enjoyment	Hopelessness, despair	Annoyance, irritation
Other emotion:	Other emotion:	Other emotion:	Other emotion:

(4) Now look back at the emotions above with X's through them. Are there any contexts (e.g., specific events, interactions, or interpersonal situations) where you find it easier to recognize these emotions in others? Are there any contexts where you find it more difficult to notice them?

Difficulties Reflecting on Other People's Desires

(5) List any desires you find more challenging to identify in other people. These could include their desires to take some action, to feel a certain way, for others to feel some way, or for specific events to happen.

(6) Are there any contexts (e.g., specific events, interactions, or interpersonal situations) where you find it easier to recognize these desires in other people? Are there any contexts where you find it harder to notice these desires?

[continued on next page]

Difficulties Reflecting on Other People's Feelings about Themselves

(7) See below for a list of self-states, or "feelings about oneself," that many people experience. Draw a square around any self-states that you are easily able to notice in other people. Then draw an "X" through any self-states that you find more challenging to notice in others. You do not have to mark all of the feelings listed.

Embarrassment	Shame	Pride	Worthlessness
Self-confidence	Humiliation	Insecurity	Self-pity
Self-love	Inadequacy	Self-doubt	Self-blame
Self-loathing, self-hatred	Empowerment, triumph	Self-consciousness	Self-satisfaction
Other self-state:	Other self-state:	Other self-state:	Other self-state:

(8) Now look back at the self-states above with X's through them. Are there any contexts (e.g., specific events, interactions, or interpersonal situations) where you find it easier to recognize these feelings in other people? Are there any contexts where you find it more difficult to notice these feelings?

MENTALIZING PRACTICE POINTS: RECOGNIZING WHAT YOU AND OTHERS ARE FEELING

In MBT, you will learn to identify and recognize a broader array of mental states in yourself: your beliefs, emotions, desires, values, and feelings about yourself. In this way, you gain an increased ability to regulate your emotions, and you develop a more secure, emotionally grounded sense of who you are as a person. This helps you to feel more confident and safe in your relationships, and to conduct yourself in a manner that reflects *all* of who you are, rather than just what you happen to be feeling in the moment. Research suggests that the ability to mentalize yourself is linked with significant psychological benefits: a greater sense of personal well-being (Greenberg et al., 2017; Jurist, 2018); increased ability to regulate your emotions (Fitzpatrick et al., 2019); and increased self-esteem and motivation to pursue life goals (Ballespi et al., 2021).

At the same time, you will work to understand and appreciate other people's internal experiences: who *they* are as people, what drives them, and what is important to them. Interestingly, the ability to mentalize others has tremendous benefits for *you*, with one study linking this ability with increased happiness and functionality (Ballespi et al., 2021). Taken together, these two types of mentalizing—mentalizing yourself and mentalizing others—forms the basis for stable connectedness with other people. You are able to "hold on to" a core sense of yourself as a unique individual engaged with other unique individuals, all experiencing a wide range of emotions and desires in relation to each other.

Let's review MBT's primary strategies for mentalizing yourself and other people.

Map out your mentalizing blind spots. Instructing someone to "find a feeling" that they cannot easily identify may sound like an impossible proposition, akin to saying, "Go and see that invisible thing." And yet there is a first step in this process—namely, charting out the mental states that you find harder to "see" in yourself and other people. This is called "mapping out your mentalizing blind spots." You have already begun to do this with Worksheets 9.1 and 9.2. The next step is to whittle things down a bit, to make this practical and usable in your everyday life. Turn back to these worksheets, and take a look at all the emotions, desires, and self-states that you struggle to recognize in yourself and others. Which of these "blind spots" affect your life most negatively? Which ones cause the most trouble in your mood, self-esteem, relationships, and functionality? Or considered from a different perspective: If these blind spots were resolved, which ones would have the most positive impact on how you feel, and how you live? Pick the "heaviest hitters" in each category (e.g., emotions, desires, feelings about yourself), which you most want to address in treatment. See here for an example.

Mentalizing Blind Spots Toolkit	
With Yourself	With Other People
Emotions: Sadness or hurt (especially when I feel angry)	*Emotions:* Their positive feelings toward me; anxiety and worry about things in their life not related to me
Desires: Desires for attention and admiration from other people	*Desires:* Desires for power or control
Self-states: Insecurity, shame	*Self-states:* Inadequacy, self-doubt

Now try doing this for yourself, on the Mentalizing Blind Spots Toolkit below. If you think it would be helpful, feel free to discuss this with your therapist, loved one, or close friends, to get their feedback about which mental states you tend to "miss" in yourself and other people.

Mentalizing Blind Spots Toolkit	
With Yourself	With Other People
Emotions:	*Emotions:*
Desires:	*Desires:*
Self-states:	*Self-states:*

Stay on the lookout for less-mentalized feelings. All else being equal, you naturally notice the things that are already in your direct field of vision. In order to start noticing things in your *peripheral* vision, you need to remember to turn your head from side to side—to intentionally look around and search for what you might be missing. So now that you have mapped out the mental states you struggle to recognize in yourself and others, your work is to start to *look* for them. This can be done in several ways. Take a picture of the Mentalizing Blind Spots Toolkit on your smartphone, or (if you are old like I am) write them down on an index card, and carry it around with you in your back pocket. As you move throughout your day, take out the Toolkit, and ask yourself the question: Can you notice any of these feelings in yourself at this moment? If you are interacting with someone else, do you see any signs of these feelings unfolding in the other person?

If you think it would be helpful, set a "mentalizing reminder" or alarm on your phone, smartwatch, or Alexa—two times per day, four times per day, or even more. When the alarm goes off, take that as a cue to mentalize these less-mentalized feelings.

In addition, at the start of your day, pick a particular mental state to "track" for the next twenty-four hours. For example, if you struggle to notice anger and resentment in yourself, or if you find it challenging to recognize insecurity in others, decide to "stay on the lookout" for these internal processes, one day at a time. Do this with a different mental state each day, until you have worked your way through all of the feelings listed on your Mentalizing Blind Spots Toolkit. Once you are done, do it again! Over time, by doggedly turning your attention to these less-mentalized feelings, you will increasingly recognize and identify a broader range of emotions in yourself and other people.

Mentalize the "what" in yourself and others. You can also expand this process beyond these less-mentalized emotions, instead considering *all* of the potential feelings unfolding between yourself and other people. See here for the Content-mentalizing Toolkit, which summarizes the core mentalizing questions about "what" you and other people are feeling.

Content-mentalizing Toolkit: Considering "What" People are Feeling	
Yourself	Other People
EMOTIONS: "What emotions am I experiencing right now?"	*EMOTIONS:* "What emotions does it seem like this other person is feeling?
DESIRES: "What am I wanting and desiring?"	*DESIRES:* "What could the other person be wanting?"
SELF-STATES: "How am I feeling about myself? What am I experiencing, at the level of self-worth and self-esteem?"	*SELF-STATES:* "How might the other person be feeling about themself? What could they be experiencing, at the level of self-worth and self-esteem?"

In asking yourself these questions, the purpose is not to "get it right." When it comes to mentalizing, it is very difficult (if not impossible) to fully "know" what other people are feeling, or even what you are truly feeling. However, by slowing things down and trying to better understand yourself and others, you gradually notice emotions and desires that had never been on your radar, or that were only vague and blurry in your field of emotional vision.

As you work on strengthening your mentalizing in these ways, MBT offers a handful of suggestions, summarized below.

Pay attention to nuance in emotional experience. When you are mentalizing yourself and other people, rather than lump all of the feelings together into one big heap, start to take these feelings *off* of the heap, so that you can see them all laid out next to each other, each with its own unique shape, texture, qualities, and bodily location. In MBT, we are always going for increased complexity, specificity, and differentiation in internal experience. So rather than just use a single word to describe someone's feelings (e.g., "sad," "guilty," "jealous," "angry"), do your best to articulate what that feeling is *about* for the person. For example, rather than just saying, "I bet she's anxious," elaborate on the emotion a bit: "I get the sense she is anxious about how things are going at work. She just got that promotion, so she probably feels a lot of pressure to do a good job. She can also feel insecure about her intelligence and abilities, so she might be worried that she isn't good enough to succeed there."

Similarly, when you are mentalizing multiple feeling states, work to pay attention to the *differences* between the emotions in question. For example, you might reflect, "I feel angry that she treated me that way, but also maybe a little sad, since it seems like she doesn't care about me as much as I care about her. I don't like feeling this way, and I want to do something to get back at her, so that maybe I will feel better. I also feel a bit embarrassed about what has happened between us, but that irritates me even more—that she has the power to make me feel bad about myself in that way."

"Take inventory" of emotions in yourself and others. Once you have a hunch about what you or others are feeling, it is often helpful to explicitly *label* those internal states—to define

them in a more explicit way. "I am experiencing a sense of shame and embarrassment—like I sounded so stupid during that presentation, and people might be judging me for it." "I suspect that my mother might be feeling some anxiety. She could be worried about my safety, and that we could have another conflict if we keep talking about this."

This form of "taking inventory" of emotions is a therapeutic technique that has been extensively studied and developed within acceptance and commitment therapy (ACT), an evidence-based psychotherapy for depression, anxiety, and chronic pain (Harris, 2022; Hayes, 2020). By "putting words on" what you and others are feeling, you affirm the difference between the *emotion* and the *person*. These feelings are rattling around inside of you, but they are not YOU, so they do not have to define and control you. They are a *part* of what other people might be experiencing, but they are not the whole person. This helps you to feel less overwhelmed by emotions—to feel a greater sense of agency and self-control in relation to them.

"Go solo" with your mentalizing. With BPD, it is often more challenging to mentalize when you are in the midst of an interpersonal interaction. You might feel uncomfortable, overwhelmed, or anxious, and that can make it harder to think about what is going on inside of yourself and other people. So when you are trying to understand what people are feeling, give yourself permission to take some time to yourself, and devote yourself to some focused, intensive mentalizing. Try going for a walk in nature, so that you can mentalize some situation that is bothering you in a peaceful and tranquil environment, without any outside distractions.

Or stay home, turn the lights down low, and spend some time journaling about your own emotions and desires, or what your loved ones could be going through. To better recognize your own feelings, feel free to close your eyes, so that it is just you and your emotions, unencumbered by the outside world. What feelings are the most prominent, the stars of the show? What do you notice bubbling up inside you, just rumbling beneath the surface? Once you have given yourself sufficient space to mentalize on your own, you are ready to reengage with your life, armed with a clearer understanding of what you and other people might be feeling.

"Go public" with your mentalizing. When you are really confused about what you or someone else might be feeling, another option is to try to work this out *with* other people. It is often tempting to seek out feedback from someone you are quite confident will "take your side" and see things your way. You know who I'm talking about: that person who, whenever you describe an interpersonal conflict you have had with someone, usually responds with, "How could they do that to you? They are being a complete asshole. You don't need them anyway." While it can be nice to get this sort of support sometimes, this is not really *mentalizing*. Mentalizing is about seeing things from *multiple* perspectives, rather than hammering home a single viewpoint. In contrast, try soliciting feedback from someone you see as thoughtful, balanced, unbiased, and flexible—someone who also seems to have their own life in order, and who is largely stable in their mood and relationships. This could be a loved one, close friend, therapist, fellow member of a support group or 12-step group, or if you belong to a religious community, a trusted person from your faith.

Share about the situation in as objective a manner as possible, not delivering the information in a way that slants things toward your existing perspective. And then seek out feedback about the situation: What could you be feeling in the scenario, and what might the other person be experiencing? For some helpful prompts, feel free to utilize the questions in the Content-mentalizing Toolkit above. The purpose here is not to solicit advice, or to arrive at some definitive "solution" to the problem. It is just to utilize another, trusted mind to enable you to attain a broader perspective on what you or other people could be going through.

Acknowledge confusion and ambiguity around mental states. Feelings are often very, very confusing. They can be messy, ill-defined, chaotic, and constantly shifting, such that it is difficult to recognize what you are feeling, or what is happening inside of other people. Accordingly, you might feel discouraged when you try to mentalize, and you struggle to identify the mental states in question. However, remember that mentalizing is not about "knowing" what people are feeling; it is simply about TRYING to understand yourself and others. So when you feel confused about what is happening inside of people, start by naming and identifying that confusion. Spell out whatever you *do* understand about the experience, along with the parts of the experience that are unclear to you.

"I know that I am not feeling good right now, but I cannot figure out what the feeling is. I am uncomfortable in my body, like I want to DO something in order to make myself feel better. But I don't even understand what I want to do!" Or: "My boyfriend seems a bit withdrawn and preoccupied today, but I cannot really tell what he is feeling. Is he upset with me, or is he just worried about something else going on in his life? I know that his work has been quite stressful lately, but usually that would not bleed into how he is at home. It is hard to sort this out!"

Once you have done your best to articulate these things, take a break and pat yourself on the back. Paradoxically, by articulating your own confusion and uncertainty about feeling states, you have begun mentalizing! Now just try to go about your business, weaving in other strategies in this book as things unfold. Live your life, and do not pressure yourself. You cannot force yourself to understand something that is automatically perplexing to you. However, by acknowledging what you do NOT understand in yourself and others, you cultivate a mentalizing attitude of openness, receptivity, and discovery. Over time, you will naturally arrive at new hypotheses and intuitions about what might be happening inside of yourself and other people, without having to harangue or browbeat yourself.

Work your way from the "outside" to the "inside." As discussed in Chapter 3, we cannot "see" mental states in the same way that we can see people, places, and objects. That said, we are able to infer the presence of particular mental states based on what *can* be experienced in the outside world: actions, physical characteristics, outward appearance, bodily experiences, the external environment, visible circumstances and events, and non-verbal cues like facial expressions, eye contact, bodily posture and movements, vocal tone, and voice volume. So another way to sort out what people might be feeling is to use these external markers as "clues" that indicate internal processes like emotions, desires, and self-states.

Start by making a list of visible factors that potentially "point" to what you or another person might be feeling. Once those external factors are listed in front of you in black and white, consider the top three feelings that could be present in the person, possibly driving and explaining the external factors in question. See here for an example of this approach, using the Mentalizing from the Outside In Toolkit.

Mentalizing from the Outside In Toolkit	
Working to Mentalize (*circle one*)	
Yourself　　　OR　　　Another Person: Leila	
External Factor	**Potential Mental State**
She did not respond to my text for 4 hours	1. She could be upset with me (not sure why)
She is giving that big presentation today	
She hugged me and said, "I love you" before she left this morning	2. She could be telling the truth— she loves me and wants to be with me.
She often does not look at her phone when she is at work	3. She might be anxious and preoccupied about the presentation. Her promotion is on the line.
She has seemed more distracted lately—not been as physically affectionate	

In this example, the patient focused on his girlfriend Leila, who had not been responding to his texts. He listed a range of external factors, including the triggering event itself (i.e., Leila not texting him back for four hours), important contextual factors in Leila's life (i.e., having to make a big presentation at work), Leila's broad behavioral pattern in this area (i.e., not checking her phone when she is at work), and potentially relevant recent interactions in their relationship (e.g., Leila's decreased physical affection, Leila hugging him and saying "I love you" that morning). In light of these "outside" things, the patient reflected on the possibility that his girlfriend might genuinely love him and be committed to him, that she could be upset with him for some reason (thus explaining her non-responsiveness and decreased affection), as well as the less-personalized hypothesis that she could simply be anxious and preoccupied about the presentation—a mental state that would simultaneously explain Leila not responding to his texts, her recent distractedness, and her reduced physical affection lately.

Now let's review an example of this approach focused on a different patient, who was trying to better understand her own feeling states.

Mentalizing from the Outside In Toolkit	
Working to Mentalize (*circle one*) ⟨Yourself⟩ OR Another Person:	
External Factor	**Potential Mental State**
I am feeling a tightness in my chest, like I want to jump out of my skin	1. I could be feeling hurt and rejected by my co-workers—I thought they were my friends.
I have been snapping at people lately, especially my mom	
This seems to have started when I did not get invited to that party at work	2. I want to withdraw from them, to show them how they hurt me
I've been smoking more pot, every night after my parents go to bed	3. I have a desire to avoid these feelings: by staying away from people, smoking pot, and criticizing my mom.
I have not been talking with people as much at work. Been keeping to myself	

Here, the patient surveyed a range of external factors that seemed potentially relevant to her emotions: her physical experience of the emotion; her recent behaviors (e.g., snapping at her mom, increased cannabis use, withdrawal from co-workers); and an event that correlated with the start of these feelings—namely, her learning that she was not invited to a party with her co-workers. Given these external factors, the patient identified several different internal states that could have been in play for her, including feeling hurt and rejected by her co-workers for not inviting her to the party, a desire to withdraw from them in order to communicate her distress, and a wish to avoid the pain she had been experiencing surrounding this scenario.

While the above two examples are quite different from each other, they illustrate a core strategy that you can utilize when you are working to mentalize yourself and other people: First work to get grounded in the basic "facts" of the situation, and then use these facts to illuminate potential internal processes that could be unfolding inside of the person in question. Now give this technique a shot on your own, using the blank toolkit below.

Mentalizing from the Outside In Toolkit	
Working to Mentalize *(circle one)* Yourself　　OR　　Another Person:	
External Factor	Potential Mental State
_____ _____ _____	1. 2. 3.

Try to avoid judging, evaluating, or explaining the feelings. Throughout this chapter, we have considered mentalizing techniques for identifying what you and other people might be feeling. However, for many people with BPD, there is a fine line between mentalizing and *evaluating.* Mentalizing always involves curious, open-minded, flexible, and empathic reflection on mental states. However, when reflecting on mental states, you might naturally fall into a more evaluative or judgmental stance toward yourself and other people.

This could variously involve:

- *Judging, criticizing, or dismissing your emotions.* "This is so stupid. I have no reason to be upset. Why I am making such a big deal about this?" You can then end up feeling bad about yourself for feeling a certain way, which can perpetuate a sense of shame, self-hatred, and worthlessness. This approach can also interfere with mentalizing the emotions themselves. If you are judging a particular emotion, then it will be more difficult to "see" the internal state in question, since (in your view) it should not be there in the first place!
- *Evaluating your feelings as "good" or "bad," "healthy" or "unhealthy," "positive" or "negative."* This automatically sets up a bias in emotional

experiencing, where you try to generate and promote specific feelings in yourself (e.g., happiness, contentment, confidence), and to stay away from others that you deem to be unacceptable (e.g., anxiety, sadness, shame, anger). You might then try to distract yourself from your emotions, or to avoid or suppress certain parts of yourself. While this approach might reduce painful feelings in the short term, research suggests that it paradoxically *intensifies* the very emotions you are trying to extinguish in yourself, for people with BPD and also among individuals with mood and anxiety disorders (Akbara et al., 2022; Bud et al., 2023).

- *Trying to explain or analyze your feelings.* You also might take a more intellectual or abstract approach to your emotions: trying to figure out "why" you are feeling a certain way; considering what your feelings say about you and your broader patterns in relationships; relating your emotional experiences to theories and concepts from popular psychology (e.g., trauma bonding, codependency, people-pleasing, being an "empath"); wondering about how your emotions and mood relate to your personal background (e.g., how you were raised, your relationships with your parents, history of traumatic experiences); or even pondering the connection between your emotions and broader societal and cultural issues. While these forms of reflection can sometimes be helpful, they tend to "skip over" the heart of content-mentalizing: recognizing and identifying your emotions themselves, in all of their nuance and complexity. These intellectualized tendencies can inadvertently distance you from your feelings, contributing to difficulties with emptiness, emotional dysregulation, and unstable sense of self.

- *Judging or criticizing how other people are feeling.* Especially when you are upset with people, you might fall into judging *their* emotions and desires. "My mom should not be angry with me and giving me so much trouble. I have not done anything wrong!" "My therapist is completely over-reacting here. I am totally fine, and there is no reason to worry about me." "It's not healthy: She just wants to be with him 24 hours a day, even though they just started going out. She is completely codependent." When taking this stance toward others, you are focusing on how they "should" be feeling, rather than what they actually *are* feeling. You are then less likely to try to see things from their perspective, and more likely to be dismissive of other people. This can lead to misunderstandings, interpersonal conflicts, and emotional distance in your relationships.

For all of these reasons, when you are working to mentalize yourself and other people, MBT recommends that you do your best to not judge the feelings under consideration. Similarly, try to not judge yourself or others for feeling a certain way. Dialectical behavior therapy has famously made a similar point with the "Mindfulness of Current Emotion" skill, which states: "Do not judge your emotion. Practice willingness. Radically accept your emotion" (Linehan, 2015a, p. 264).

Of course, this is all easier said than done. When mentalizing, if you find yourself starting to judge yourself or other people, work to reorient to the mental state in question. For example, if are drawn to criticize yourself for feeling angry with someone, just gently return to noticing and considering the anger itself. If your mind keeps returning to the judgment, it can be helpful to then just articulate the judgment, explicitly in terms of mental states.

- "I am judging myself for feeling _____."
- "I am assuming that I should not be wanting _____."
- "I believe that this other person should not feel _____."

Interestingly, by framing your judgments of yourself and other people as *mental states* (e.g., assumptions, beliefs), you have placed them into the basket of all of the other feelings you are trying to mentalize! "I am feeling angry, and I am also judging myself for feeling angry. I want to feel more positive emotions toward this person, since I am worried that they will reject me if they see how upset I am toward them."

The benefit of this approach is that you do not need to expunge all of your judgments from yourself, in order to productively utilize the principles of MBT. Just let them be there, and continue your efforts to mentalize yourself and other people. At this stage of the process, do not try to "argue with" these judgments, or to change them into something more positive— this would just be more criticism of the feelings! In Chapter 12, "Addressing Problems with Certainty and Rigidity," we will consider how to generate greater flexibility in your negative views of yourself and others, as they continue to crop up in your life.

Mentalizing Cool-down

Now that you have learned about MBT's techniques for recognizing what you and others are feeling, return to Martha's story at the start of the chapter, on page 151. How might Martha work to implement these strategies in her own life, especially with her difficulties with mood, work, and relationships?

RETURNING TO MARTHA

In the earliest phase of MBT, Martha and her therapist decided to prioritize her challenges understanding emotions in herself and other people, especially her significant confusion about what she was feeling, and her "bias" toward focusing on other people's negative views of her. To that end, Martha and her therapist started exploring Martha's "mentalizing blind spots." When mentalizing other people, Martha often automatically assumed that others were judging her, as indicated by her conviction that her co-workers were looking down on her for her inconsistency, and her certainty that her sister Sarah was seeing her as a burden. Focusing only on those "judgment"-related mental states, Martha would understandably *feel* more rejected by the other person, which led her to withdraw and avoid those relationships. In those moments, Martha was far less likely to notice mental states in others that did *not* directly involve her and her deficiencies. For example, she often overlooked her colleagues' potential feelings of concern for her, as well as Sarah's love for her and desire to spend time with her.

In herself, while Martha was especially attuned to her feelings of rejection and sadness, she did not naturally notice her loneliness, her desire to spend time with other people, and her wish to feel important to others, especially Sarah and her children. In fact, Martha only realized these feelings were there *after* she felt rejected by others! With all these ideas in mind, Martha worked to "stay on the lookout" for these emotions as she puttered around her apartment throughout the day. When she texted with her sister Sarah, she started considering the possibility that Sarah *did* really care about her, despite how rejected and abandoned Martha felt by her at times.

Utilizing the "Mentalizing from the Outside In Toolkit," Martha listed the various external facets of Sarah's experience, including the fact that Sarah would call to check in on her every other day; Sarah's various parenting responsibilities and obligations; Sarah NOT inviting Martha to larger family outings; as well as Sarah's specific language that she used in texts and phone calls: "I miss you, Martha." "You know how much I love you, don't you?" "You're my only sister. You're not going to get rid of me that easily!" What could Sarah be feeling, which might account for some of these things? It was possible that Sarah actually did miss her and want to spend time with her, as she was claiming. It was also possible that Sarah felt overwhelmed by her and did not want to have to deal with her. No matter what, Martha knew that Sarah loved her. When Martha was feeling hurt by Sarah, she could sometimes forget that, but when she started thinking about all of the things Sarah did and said affirming her care for Martha, it was impossible to deny.

Considering things in this way, Martha started feeling warmer toward Sarah, and more in touch with her own desires to strengthen their relationship. Employing the Content-mentalizing Toolkit, Martha began to intentionally consider her various feelings surrounding her relationship with her sister. "What emotions am I feeling toward Sarah?" "What do I want from her?" "How do I feel about myself in this relationship?" As she reflected on these feelings, Martha worked to explicitly articulate the complex array of internal processes that were coming up for her, "taking inventory" of them in a nuanced way. Martha tried journaling about these feelings ("going solo" with mentalizing), also talking about them directly in therapy ("going public" with mentalizing). See here for some of Martha's reflections, including some brackets I am adding to categorize the different sorts of feelings she mentalized in herself.

"I am still feeling angry and resentful at Sarah, since I feel like she should have been including me in these family outings *[emotion]*. I also feel hurt by her, and worried that she does not really want to spend time with me *[additional, more vulnerable emotions]*. I want her to *want* to spend time with me—for our relationship to be as important to her as it is to me *[desire for the other person to feel a certain way]*. I am embarrassed to admit this *[feeling "about" a feeling]*, but I also feel sort of jealous of Sarah *[emotion]*. She has so much going on in her life—and so many *people* in her life!—that I don't have, and I want that for myself, too *[desire for something in the world]*. This makes me feel inferior to her sometimes *[self-state, AKA a "feeling about the self"]*. I mean, I love her more than anyone else in the world *[emotion]*, but sometimes I feel like I am not good enough to be close to her *[additional description of the self-state]*. This makes it hurt even more when she doesn't want to spend time with me—it's like she's confirming the way that I already feel about myself *[complex emotion]*."

As she engaged in these forms of reflection, Martha began to feel more grounded in herself—less aimless, disoriented, and confused. She still did not feel *good*, but there was something comforting and relieving about knowing what was happening inside of her. Then one day when Martha was talking with her sister, without planning it, Martha playfully blurted out, "Why don't we hang out together anymore?" Sarah shared that she has been worried about inviting Martha to things. Martha had missed so many family events over the years, openly admitting how anxious and overwhelmed she felt being around people. Sarah did not want to do anything to pressure Martha, which she worried could make Martha feel more depressed and suicidal.

This all floored Martha. She had never considered that Sarah was actually trying to *help* her by limiting these invitations. Feeling much less rejected by Sarah, Martha started to reach out to Sarah herself, expressing her interest in spending time with Sarah and her family. The timing was right, as Sarah's nanny had recently given her notice, and they were desperately searching for help with childcare. Martha started taking care of her nephews several days a week, also going over for family dinners and movie nights on the weekends. Martha experienced a significant sense of purpose and meaning from these activities. For the first time in a long time, she felt like people *needed* her, which made her feel like she might actually have a reason to be around. Her mood improved, and she noticed an increased sense of motivation in her life more broadly, even on the days when she was not helping with the boys. Martha ended up applying for a per diem position as a nurse at her old hospital. To her surprise, her old boss was grateful to have her, and she began picking up relief shifts when she could, which gave her flexibility to continue taking care of her nephews.

Martha's progress has continued for years now. Looking back on this period in her life, she continues to be struck by the dramatic shift in her experience over a relatively brief period of time, after years and years of suffering. These improvements underscore an essential point in the treatment of BPD: By intentionally working to broaden and deepen your understanding of feeling states in yourself and other people, you can move forward in areas of your life where historically you have been stuck.

Chapter Review 9.1
Challenges Understanding "What" People are Feeling

Problems with Content-mentalizing in Borderline Personality Disorder

- Content-mentalizing involves observing and identifying specific mental states (e.g., thoughts, beliefs, emotions, needs, desires, self-states, and attitudes) in yourself and other people.

- People with borderline personality disorder (BPD) can experience significant problems with content-mentalizing, especially (a) when facing one of their triggers, or (b) when experiencing any intense emotion.

- To identify your problems in content-mentalizing, mentalization-based treatment (MBT) suggests that you utilize the following principles.

  - Prioritize your difficulties mentalizing specifically affective content—that is, emotions, desires, and feelings about self.

  - Consider those mental states that (a) are probably present to some degree, but (b) you struggle to recognize when they are there.

  - Spell out the specific mental states that are more challenging for you to identify: sadness, insecurity, desires for attention, anger, and so on.

Difficulties Identifying Your Own Mental States

- With yourself, problems with content-mentalizing include:

  - confusion about what you are feeling;

  - drawing inaccurate conclusions about your own internal processes;

  - tendency to "miss" or ignore particular subjective states in yourself;

  - difficulty identifying and "putting words on" certain mental states in yourself; and

  - "biases" toward identifying some feelings in yourself, while neglecting others.

- These difficulties mentalizing yourself can lead to significant challenges in BPD:

  - *Emotional instability and dysregulation:* Your emotions control you, rather than you controlling them.

  - *Unstable sense of self:* You can feel confused, empty, aimless, and easily overwhelmed.

  - *Unstable relationships:* You might be easily influenced by other people's emotions and desires, placing you at risk for mistreatment.

  - *Stuckness and paralysis in life:* If you do not know what matters to you, then you cannot pursue those things.

  - *Your actions fail to reflect your feelings:* If you are not recognizing all of your emotions, you will not ACT on those neglected emotions, and people will be less likely to see those emotions in you. For example, if you are in touch with your anger but not your sadness in a situation, you will probably behave more aggressively, and people might not pick up on your feelings of sadness.

[continued on next page]

Difficulties Reading Other People's Mental States

- Problems with content-mentalizing of other people include:
  - difficulty "reading" or understanding mental states in others;
  - drawing inaccurate conclusions about others' internal processes;
  - tendency to "miss" or ignore specific subjective states in other people;
  - difficulty identifying and "putting words on" certain mental states in others; and
  - biases toward identifying particular feelings in other people, while neglecting others.
- Common examples of these challenges in BPD include:
  - You may be exceptionally attuned to other people's negative feelings about you and "miss" others' positive or neutral feelings toward you.
  - You could focus mostly on people's *positive* feelings toward you, while being less cognizant of others' more challenging emotions toward you (e.g., anger, apathy, decreased emotional investment).
  - You might be hyper-focused on how others feel about *you*, paying less attention to their mental states not directly related to you: their emotions or desires about other situations in their lives, or their feelings about themselves.
  - You could take things personally, assuming that other people's actions and comments are "about" you in some way.
  - You may reflexively "blame yourself" for problems in relationships, failing to consider others' mental states in and about *them* (e.g., personality traits, psychological vulnerabilities, feelings about other situations in their lives) that might be leading them to treat you in the way that they do.

Chapter Review 9.2
Mentalizing Practice Points: Recognizing What You and Others are Feeling

Mentalize the "What" in Yourself and Other People

Consider all of the potential feelings unfolding inside yourself and others.

Content-mentalizing Toolkit: Considering "What" People are Feeling	
Yourself	Other People
EMOTIONS: "What emotions am I experiencing right now?"	*EMOTIONS:* "What emotions does it seem like this other person is feeling?"
DESIRES: "What am I wanting and desiring?"	*DESIRES:* "What could the other person be wanting?"
SELF-STATES: "How am I feeling about myself? What am I experiencing, at the level of self-worth and self-esteem?"	*SELF-STATES:* "How might the other person be feeling about themself? What could they be experiencing, at the level of self-worth and self-esteem?"

Pay Attention to Nuance in Emotional Experience

Articulate what the emotion is "about" for the person: "I get the sense she is anxious about how things are going at work. She just got that promotion, so she probably feels a lot of pressure to do a good job."

When mentalizing multiple feeling states, consider the *differences* between the feelings in question. "I feel angry that she treated me that way, but also maybe a little sad, since it seems like she doesn't care about me as much as I care about her."

[continued on next page]

"Take Inventory" of Emotions in Yourself and Others

Once you have a hunch of what you or others are feeling, explicitly *label* those internal states, defining them in a more explicit way.

- "I am experiencing a sense of shame and embarrassment—like I sounded so stupid during that presentation, and people might be judging me for it."

- "I suspect that my mother might be feeling some anxiety. She could be worried about my safety, and that we could have another conflict if we keep talking about this."

"Go Solo" With Your Mentalizing

When you are trying to understand what people are feeling, give yourself permission to take some time to yourself, and devote yourself to some focused, intensive mentalizing.

- Try going for a walk in nature, so that you can mentalize some situation that is bothering you in a peaceful and tranquil environment.

- Stay home, turn the lights down low, and spend some time journaling about your own emotions and desires, or what your loved ones could be going through.

- To better recognize your own feelings, feel free to close your eyes, so there is just you and your emotions, unencumbered by the outside world. What do you notice unfolding inside of you?

"Go Public" With Your Mentalizing

Seek out feedback from someone you see as thoughtful, balanced, unbiased, and flexible. This could be a loved one, close friend, therapist, fellow member of a support group, or a trusted person from your faith.

Share about the situation in as objective a manner as possible, not delivering the information in a way that slants things toward your existing perspective.

Then seek out feedback about the situation: What could you be feeling in the scenario, and what might the other person be feeling?

[continued on next page]

Acknowledge Confusion and Ambiguity Around Mental States

When you feel confused about what is happening inside of people, start by naming and identifying that confusion.

Spell out whatever you *do* understand about the experience, along with the parts of the experience that are unclear to you.

- "I know that I am not feeling good right now, but I cannot figure out what the feeling is. I am uncomfortable in my body, like I want to DO something in order to make myself feel better. But I don't even understand what I want to do!"

Once you have done your best to articulate these things, just try to go about your business. Do not pressure yourself. Over time, you will naturally arrive at new hypotheses and intuitions about what might be happening inside of yourself and other people.

Chapter Review 9.3
Mentalizing Practice Points: Additional Strategies for Content-mentalizing

Map Out Your Mentalizing Blind Spots

Consider the emotions, desires, and self-states that you struggle to recognize in yourself and others. Which of these "blind spots" affect your life most negatively? Try filling out the following table.

Mentalizing Blind Spots Toolkit	
With Yourself	With Other People
Emotions:	*Emotions:*
Desires:	*Desires:*
Self-states:	*Self-states:*

Stay on the Lookout for Less-mentalized Feelings

- Take a picture of the Mentalizing Blind Spots Toolkit on your phone, or write down your blind spots on an index card. As you move throughout your day, take out the toolkit and ask yourself:
  - "Can I notice any of these feelings in myself at this moment?"
  - "Do I see any signs of these feelings unfolding in other people?"
- Set a "mentalizing reminder" or alarm several times per day on your phone, smartwatch, or Alexa. When the alarm goes off, take that as a cue to mentalize these less-mentalized feelings.
- At the start of your day, pick a particular mental state to "track" for the next 24 hours. "Stay on the lookout" for these internal processes, one day at a time.

[continued on next page]

Work Your Way from the "Outside" to the "Inside"

Start by making a list of visible factors that "point" to what you or another person could be feeling. Then consider the top three feelings that could be present in the person, potentially driving and explaining the external factors in question.

Mentalizing from the Outside In Toolkit	
Working to Mentalize *(circle one)* Yourself OR Another Person:	
External Factor	Potential Mental State
	1. 2. 3.

[continued on next page]

Try to Avoid Judging or Evaluating the Feelings

- When you are mentalizing what you or another person is feeling:
    - DON'T judge, criticize, or dismiss the feelings.
    - DON'T evaluate the feelings as "good" or "bad," "healthy" or "unhealthy," "positive" or "negative."
    - DON'T explain or analyze the feelings.
- If you find yourself starting to judge yourself or other people, work to reorient to the mental state in question.
- If your mind keeps returning to the judgment, just articulate the judgment, explicitly in terms of mental states.
    - "I am judging myself for feeling _____."
    - "I am assuming that I should not be wanting _____."
    - "I believe that this other person should not feel _____."
- Just let your judgments be there, and continue your efforts to mentalize yourself and other people. For now, do not try to "argue with" these judgments, or to change them into something more positive.

10

How to Consider "Why" People Are Feeling Something

William struggled with a long history of self-loathing, social isolation, and alcohol abuse. Highly intelligent but socially awkward, he had always felt fundamentally "different" from other people, and he found it challenging to make friends. An Air Force veteran and captain in the fire department, William prioritized his work above everything else, attaining significant professional success by an early age. His romantic relationships were brief and intense: He would meet some woman at a bar, they would have sex, and then suddenly they were in a relationship together! This would not last long, as inevitably William would meet some new woman at a bar, becoming intimate with her and disrupting his current relationship. When William was unable to distract himself with work and promiscuity, he endured intense feelings of emptiness and self-hatred, hitting himself in the head in order to punish himself for his insufficiency.

This all changed when he met Catherine, a successful lawyer at a large law firm. On paper, they were an unlikely pair, but they connected around their shared ambitiousness, hardheadedness, love of politics, and tendencies toward argumentation and intellectualization. They fell quickly and passionately in love, and they were married within months.

The honeymoon did not last long, as William's alcohol use was steadily increasing, leading to absences, interpersonal conflicts, and inconsistency at work. His supervisees began to complain about him, and the fire chief confronted William about his deteriorating performance. Humiliated and rejected, William decided to take his own life, shooting himself in the stomach with one of his many firearms. The doctors were able to save him, but he suffered severe nerve damage, leaving him disabled with a permanent limp. He was forced to retire on a medical disability.

William presented to treatment several years later, in the context of continued alcohol use, depression, and arguments with Catherine. Without a job to anchor him, and with virtually no other people in his life, William felt like his entire world centered around Catherine. While they had brief periods of connectedness and stability, they bickered almost constantly, especially when William felt like Catherine was criticizing him (e.g., about his driving, alcohol use, hardheadedness, or manner of completing some household task). William was highly defensive in these moments, immediately telling Catherine how she was wrong in her manner of viewing the situation. This escalated into full-on arguments, resulting in yelling, name-calling, and estrangement in the relationship. When William's anger subsided, he felt increasingly desperate and hopeless: crying, drinking more alcohol, and hitting himself in the head. This pattern continued until William and Catherine were able to make up, when William could finally feel stable and connected again.

At the start of mentalization-based treatment (MBT), William identified his goals as decreasing his depression and improving his relationship with Catherine. The therapist tried to explore William's experience of his depression, as well as its precipitants. William responded, "I have no idea why I'm depressed. This is the way I've been my whole life."

Mentalization. Robert P. Drozek, Oxford University Press. © Oxford University Press 2025.
DOI: 10.1093/oso/9780198916857.003.0010

When the therapist asked if there could be any connection between his depression and various objective circumstances in his life (e.g., arguments with Catherine, lack of employment, social isolation), William was emphatic that there was no relationship between these things. "I have been depressed even before I lost my job, and even when Catherine and I are not fighting. This is just how I am."

In sharing about his arguments with Catherine, William focused extensively on *her* behavior in the relationship: what he saw as her controlling tendencies, her tendency to criticize and dismiss him, and her inability to take responsibility for her own contributions to their conflicts. Whenever the therapist encouraged William to consider his own part in these dynamics, he naturally gravitated back to Catherine and what she was doing wrong. "I am largely a very passive, peaceful person. If she were not so critical of me, I would not have to defend myself. All her colleagues say the same thing about her—it has to be her way, all the time." The therapist invited William to reflect on Catherine's *emotions* involved in their arguments, and William responded, "She's just mad at me for drinking. She can't get me to stop drinking, so she criticizes me about everything else."

When the therapist tried to explore William's emotions surrounding these arguments, William displayed a similar form of concreteness. He acknowledged only that he felt "annoyed" and "frustrated" with her, but he was unable to locate any other emotions in himself surrounding these conflicts. "Of course I hate myself for a lot of reasons: for trying to kill myself, for destroying my career, for drinking as much as I do. But I don't really feel bad about myself in these arguments with Catherine. She's the one who is being unreasonable, not me."

William thus found himself largely dominated by factors beyond his control (e.g., Catherine, his emotions, his own behavioral tendencies), without any clear foothold to implement any change in his life.

DIFFICULTIES IDENTIFYING "WHY" YOU ARE FEELING SOMETHING

As we reviewed in Chapter 3, context-mentalizing involves reflecting on the relationship between some feeling state and the broader "context" of the feeling itself, namely situations, behaviors, and other psychological processes. This can involve considering "why" a person might be feeling a certain way—that is, how some situation, behavior, or other internal state (e.g., belief, desire, emotion, value) is affecting the person's emotions. It also can involve reflecting on how the emotion influences other aspects of experience: what actions the person takes, other things the person might feel, and how these behaviors and feelings then impact other people. From this perspective, context-mentalizing encompasses the "why?" as well as the "what's next?" in emotional experience.

For example, you notice that you have been feeling more anxious *[emotion]* ever since you learned that your partner has been thinking about changing jobs *[situation]*, and you become curious: "What is making me feel so concerned about this?" Perhaps you are worried that your partner would be unhappy at the new job, that the job might not pay as much, or that the work could be more demanding, thus interfering with how much time you spend together. Or you might reflect on how these feelings of anxiety could be affecting you in other ways. Perhaps the anxiety is making you feel more irritable and frustrated *[another emotion]*, leading you to be more critical and impatient with your partner *[behaviors]*.

All of these forms of reflection are examples of what MBT calls *context-mentalizing*, where you consider the association between mental states and other aspects of experience: situations, behaviors, and other psychological processes. If you have borderline personality disorder (BPD), you might experience certain problems with mentalizing the broader context of your emotions. Examples of problems in context-mentalizing in yourself include:

- *Feeling unsure about "why" you are feeling a certain way.* You might feel like your emotions just *happen* to you, with no rhyme or reason. This can be stressful and overwhelming: You feel like a stranger to yourself, and you are unable to predict when some new emotion is going to hit you and knock you over.
- *Difficulty identifying situational/environmental factors that might be influencing your mood and emotions.* You know that you are feeling a certain way (e.g., irritable, worried, happy), but you "miss" the role that outside circumstances (e.g., interactions with others, recent events) are playing in generating that emotion. This can make you feel more isolated and separate from others, since you fail to appreciate the significance of specific relational experiences in how you are feeling, and how you are feeling about yourself. This problem in mentalizing can hinder your ability to effectively relate to other people. If you are not fully attuned to how your environment is affecting you, you will be less likely to take actions to address your interpersonal problems, or to ensure that your needs get met in your relationships.
- *Trouble recognizing how other psychological factors (e.g., specific thoughts or emotions) might be influencing your mental states.* Moods and emotions are not simply instigated by what is going on around you; they are also impacted by what is going on *inside* of you. For example, you feel angry at your best friend for blowing you off the other day, but this anger could also be affected by you feeling hurt by your friend, as well as recent loneliness you have been experiencing. In BPD, however, you might not consider the various other internal processes (e.g., thoughts, emotions, desires, self-states, values) that could be influencing how you are feeling in any given moment. This can make it more difficult for you to resolve your emotional difficulties, since you are not fully understanding and addressing the range of emotions that are causing you to feel upset.
- *Challenges discerning how your emotions impact your behaviors.* Sometimes you could take a certain action, but you fail to mentalize the internal processes triggering that behavior. For example, you have been experiencing an increased desire to self-injure recently, but you do not consider the various feeling states (e.g., hurt or rejection by a romantic partner, insecurity at work or school, anger in family relationships) that could be fueling those impulses. Or you have been struggling to complete your school assignments, and you do not reflect on the internal processes (e.g., fear of failure, desire to binge on alcohol, feelings of insecurity and shame) that might be contributing to these difficulties. Accordingly, your behavioral challenges just continue, since you are not tackling the emotional difficulties that are setting them in motion.
- *Difficulties understanding how your behaviors impact your mood, emotions, and desires.* You also might know that you are feeling a certain way (e.g., depressed, anxious, angry), but you fail to consider actions you are taking that could be playing a significant role in generating these feelings in the first place. For example, you do not appreciate the impact that your promiscuity could be having on your feelings of shame, that your substance use might be having on your poor motivation, or that your avoidance and isolation may be having on your ongoing feelings of anxiety. So you know that you want to "feel better," but you lack the essential information about how to MAKE yourself feel better, which often involves an attentiveness to implementing effective behavioral changes.

- *Tendency to focus on your discrete behaviors, and to "miss"/fail to recognize your broader patterns in relationships.* When you are suffering, it is easy to get tunnel vision—that is, to focus on the situation right in front of you that is causing you pain (e.g., what you are doing, what other people are doing and saying), rather than taking a step back and asking, "How does this scenario relate to my challenges in life more generally?" or "What role might I be playing in this dynamic?" Without this form of mentalizing in play, you are more likely to blame other people for your instability, to keep repeating the same interpersonal patterns, and to feel like a perpetual victim in your own life. In addition to leading to interpersonal disruptions with others, this approach can generate feelings of anger, hopelessness, and powerlessness in your relationships.
- *A "passive," non-proactive stance toward your own problems and behaviors.* When you are struggling in your life (e.g., with depression, negative feelings about yourself, maladaptive behaviors, interpersonal conflicts), you might naturally adopt a stance of passivity toward your own difficulties: feeling like there is nothing you can do about the issue, assuming that other people (e.g., romantic partners, parents, therapists) need to fix the problem for you, or just saying "fuck it" and going along with whatever is happening at the time. In these moments, you are less likely to actively wrestle with questions like "What can I do to address this problem?" or "How do I move myself forward in this area?" You thus end up overlooking the behaviors and interpersonal approaches that *are* under your control, which could help you experience a greater sense of agency, fulfillment, and well-being in your life.

Mentalizing Warm-up

With these problems in mentalizing in mind, return to William's story at the start of the chapter, on page 181. How could William struggle to reflect on the relationship between his feelings and additional aspects of his experience: external circumstances, his behaviors, and other psychological processes in himself?

Can you identify with any of these problems in mentalizing yourself? Try completing the following worksheet, which walks you through the different ways you might find it challenging to reflect on the "why" of your own experience.

Worksheet 10.1
Difficulties Mentalizing "Why" You Are Feeling Something

(1) Do you ever feel a certain way (e.g., irritable, worried, happy), but you do not understand "why" you are experiencing that emotion? Describe any examples of this, as well as the impact this has had on you.

(2) If you have borderline personality disorder (BPD), you might sometimes find it difficult to recognize the impact of external circumstances (e.g., interpersonal interactions, valued interactions NOT happening, impersonal events) on your moods and emotions. Recount any examples of this, as well as how they have affected you.

(3) You also might struggle to acknowledge other psychological factors (e.g., specific thoughts or emotions) that influence how you feel. For example, you could feel angry, but you "miss" your feelings of hurt or insecurity that could be making you angry. List instances where you have failed to notice that additional internal processes could be affecting your mood and emotions.

[continued on next page]

(4) You could find yourself drawn to take certain actions (e.g., criticizing someone, avoiding a situation, hurting yourself, addictive behaviors), without fully reflecting on your internal states (e.g., emotions, desires, feelings about yourself) potentially fueling these impulses. Detail at least three examples where you have engaged in maladaptive behaviors, while neglecting to consider relevant feelings leading you to take these actions.

(5) You may also overlook your behaviors that could be impacting your mood, emotions, and desires. Identify at least three actions you take that (a) likely affect your mood or emotional stability in a negative way, but (b) you fail to recognize their harmful impact on you.

(6) With BPD, you might find yourself blaming other people for your challenges in relationships, feeling perpetually mistreated by the people in your life. Outline at least three examples where you have found it challenging to discern your own broader patterns in relationships—that is, what YOU tend to do that causes difficulty for you and other people.

(7) You might sometimes adopt a "passive," non-proactive stance toward your own problems and behaviors: feeling like there is nothing you can do about the issue, and failing to ask yourself, "What can I do to address this problem?" Describe at least three scenarios where you struggle to maintain a sense of agency and autonomy in relation to your difficulties.

DIFFICULTIES UNDERSTANDING "WHY" ANOTHER PERSON IS FEELING SOMETHING

You also might struggle to context-mentalize other people—that is, to reflect on the potential connection between their emotions and other aspects of their experience: external events and situations, their behaviors, and other psychological processes in them (e.g., emotions, desires, feelings about themselves). See here for some examples of problems with mentalizing the broader context of other people's experiences:

- *Difficulty identifying situational/environmental factors that might be influencing other people's mood and emotions.* You notice that people are feeling a certain way (e.g., happy, anxious, irritated), but you fail to consider the objective situations in their lives that might be contributing to that feeling state. These circumstances could involve work, family, romantic relationships, friendships, or more "concrete" factors (e.g., finances, living situation, medical issues). If you are not recognizing the impact of these domains on other people's experience, it will be more challenging to understand and empathize with others—to really "see" what is happening in their life, and what they are going through. You also could be more likely to "take things personally" in your interactions with other individuals—to assume that others' feelings are related to you, rather than connected to important situations in their lives that have little or nothing to do with you.

- *Trouble recognizing additional psychological factors that might be influencing other people's feelings.* You may observe a particular emotion in other individuals (e.g., anger, excitement, shame), but you could "miss" the role of other mental states in influencing these emotions. For example, you can tell that your grandmother is frustrated with you because you forgot to call her back when she reached out to you the other day. In the heat of the moment, you might think less about your grandmother's feelings of hurt, loneliness, and a desire to connect with other people—all feelings that are likely contributing to her anger toward you. When you fail to mentalize the impact of these additional emotions on people's experience, you are left only with your "first impression" of what someone seems to be feeling. The person seems mad, so they are mad. The person seems happy, so of course everything is fine. What you see is what you get. You can thus end up making snap judgments of other individuals, leading to difficulties with reactivity, naivete, and even paranoia in your relationships.

- *Challenges understanding the connection between others' mental states and their behaviors.* You could fail to consider how other people's feelings affect their behaviors, or how their behaviors impact their emotions. For example, you know that your sibling always tries to "one-up" you in conversations. This really frustrates you, but you do not stop to consider your sibling's emotions potentially driving this behavior, including insecurity, jealousy, or hurt about how your parents have treated them over the years. Or you see that your partner has been more emotionally disconnected lately. You worry that they are pulling away from you, but you think less about their various actions (e.g., extensive video game usage, doomscrolling, increased marijuana use) that could be making them feel numb and empty. Without a clear understanding of other people's feelings and behaviors, you feel more confused and overwhelmed in your relationships, finding it challenging to figure out how to effectively relate to other people.

- *Problems recognizing how **YOU** are often the context of other people's mental states.* If you have BPD, you likely often feel hurt and upset by how other people are treating you: Others can come across as cold, uncaring, withdrawn, rejecting, or aggressive, as the case may be. However, you could "miss" the fact that these tendencies are sometimes *reactions and responses* to how you are engaging with the person in question. For example, the individual you were messaging on a dating app gradually stops responding to you. Of course you feel rejected by this, but you do not consider that they could be feeling less interested in you not because of how you look, but because of aspects of how you were communicating with them: sharing about your psychiatric issues, sending them multiple messages in quick succession, or not asking them questions about themself. When you fail to mentalize the impact you are having on other people, you can end up feeling perpetually victimized and mistreated in your interactions with others. This can lead to feelings of anger, hopelessness, and worthlessness, while also stopping you from recognizing the changes you could make to improve the quality of your relationships.

Mentalizing Warm-up

With these ideas in mind, return to William's story at the start of the chapter, on page 181. How does William struggle to consider the connection between other people's emotions and additional aspects of their experience: other feeling states in them, their behaviors, and external circumstances, including William's own manner of relating to the person in question?

Can you identify with any of these problems in mentalizing other people? Take a crack at Worksheet 10.2, which explores the ways you find it challenging to reflect on "why" people are feeling something.

Worksheet 10.2
Difficulties Mentalizing "Why" Another Person
Is Feeling Something

(1) If you have borderline personality disorder (BPD), you might sometimes find it difficult to recognize the impact of external circumstances (e.g., interpersonal interactions, valued interactions NOT happening, impersonal events) on other individuals' moods and emotions. Recount any examples of this, as well as how this has affected you and your relationships.

(2) You may have trouble recognizing other psychological factors influencing other people's feelings. For example, you notice that someone feels angry with you, but you think less about their feelings of anxiety and shame that could be fueling their anger. List instances where you have failed to notice that additional internal processes could be affecting another person's moods and emotions.

(4) You also could fail to examine how other people's emotions affect their behaviors. For instance, your sibling tries to one-up you in conversations, but you do not naturally consider their feelings of insecurity, jealousy, and hurt that could be leading them to take this action. Describe any scenarios where you skip over the emotions that could be influencing another person's actions.

[continued on next page]

(5) You might sometimes overlook the behaviors that could be impacting other people's mood, emotions, and desires. For example, your partner has been emotionally disconnected lately, but you don't reflect on their various actions (e.g., extensive video game usage, doomscrolling, increased marijuana use) that could be making them feel numb and empty. List any examples where you "miss" the actions that could be affecting another person's emotional states.

(6) With BPD, you might struggle to recognize the impact that you have on other people. You "see" that another person is feeling a certain way toward you (e.g., frustrated, uncomfortable, anxious, disinterested), but you fail to appreciate that these feelings are sometimes *reactions and responses* to how you are engaging with the person. Discuss at least three examples where (a) someone was feeling a difficult emotion toward you, but (b) you found it challenging to understand that YOU were playing a role in generating that emotion in the person.

MENTALIZING PRACTICE POINTS: RECOGNIZING "WHY" YOU AND OTHERS ARE FEELING A CERTAIN WAY

In Chapter 9, you learned MBT's strategies for identifying "what" you and other people are feeling. Once you have put words on that ("I am feeling a sense of sadness," "He seems to be feeling angry"), what do you do next? MBT recommends that you work to *broaden the context* of these mental states—that is, to consider the factors happening "around" the feeling state, and how they might be impacting the feeling itself. As mentioned earlier, this is called "context-mentalizing."

By and large, context-mentalizing strategies invite you to "step back" from the immediacy of your experiences, and to occupy a vantage point where you can consider

(a) Some emotion in yourself or other people;

(b) Some additional element, such as an event, behavior, or other mental state; and

(c) How these two things interact and connect with each other.

As you gain the ability to reflect in these ways, you experience a greater sense of agency and autonomy in your life. By reflecting on what is impacting how you feel, you understand yourself better, and you feel like you have greater control over your emotions and reactions. Similarly, as you become more curious about what is leading other people to feel a certain way, people start to make sense to you, and they become less threatening. You feel more stable in yourself, and more able to respond effectively in your relationships.

Now let's review MBT's techniques for considering "why" you and other people are feeling certain emotions.

"Stop and rewind" the emotional experience. In Chapter 7, we reviewed MBT's "stop and rewind" technique for identifying triggers, where you rewind the movie of your life to the moment just BEFORE you start to feel upset, excited, or worked up (see p. 110). You can utilize a similar approach for recognizing external events and circumstances that might be influencing how you and other people feel. Start by articulating the feeling state you want to better understand in yourself or another person: "I am feeling embarrassed and ashamed" or "She appears to be worried about something." Then "stop and rewind" to the period of time right before the emotion arose, asking yourself: "What were the objective factors in play at that moment in time?"

It is important to note: This is different from asking "WHY did the emotion end up arising when it did?" As we have discussed, in BPD, you might not have a clear understanding of what led the emotion to come up, or you could endorse a more "cognitive" explanation of the emotion that does not take into account the full complexity of factors impacting the feeling in question. So in MBT, we suggest temporarily "pressing pause" on any "why?" questions at this stage of the process, instead simply itemizing all objective elements unfolding at the moment in time before the emotion emerged.

Examples of such external factors include:

- An interpersonal interaction with one or more people in some life domain: family, romantic relationships, parenting, friendships, work or school, hobbies, and so on.
- The *absence* of some interpersonal interaction in one of these domains, for instance involving social isolation, spending the holidays alone, your friend not texting you back, or a potential romantic partner failing to respond on a dating app.
- Work-related events: getting promoted, fired, or laid off from a job; taking medical or family leave; being assigned to a new project or responsibility; receiving some positive, negative, or neutral evaluation of your work performance

- Scenarios related to pets or animal companions: medical illness, death or loss of a pet, acquiring a new pet, alteration in your pet's behavior
- Situations in academics, school, or training: being accepted, rejected, or waitlisted at an academic institution; receiving some positive, negative, or neutral evaluation of your school performance; change in academic status (e.g., being suspended or expelled, taking medical leave)
- Financial events: monetary losses or gains; loss of possessions
- Getting into an accident
- Shift in body, health, or appearance: medical illness, physical ailments, gaining or losing weight, becoming healthier in some way
- Housing-related events: moving, getting evicted, or changing one's living situation; selling or purchasing a home
- Impersonal circumstances in the immediate environment, for example involving objects, sound, weather, or physical location
- Time and chronology: time of day, time of year, or anniversaries
- Events happening in broader society and culture (e.g., related to politics, public health, popular culture, or world events)
- Encountering objective factors (e.g., sounds, smells, visual stimuli) that remind you of past traumatic or stressful experiences

Utilizing the "Stop and Rewind" Mentalizing Toolkit, list all of the external circumstances that were unfolding in the period of time before the feeling state arose. Then for each one of these events, ask yourself the mentalizing question, "Could that scenario have influenced the feeling state under discussion?" If you think it potentially could, do not stop there. Work to *deepen* your reflection on the emotion by wondering, "What internal process potentially 'links' the external situation to the feeling state?"

Let me explain this point further, as it is so important. If you have BPD, it probably feels like external situations directly *cause* you to feel a certain way. Your mother criticizes you, and that makes you feel angry. You get a really bad cold, so you feel stressed out and overwhelmed. However, while outside things can certainly influence how you feel, they can only do that because there are *other* processes inside you—that is, thoughts, assumptions, emotions, desires, values, or feelings about yourself—that make you susceptible to *both* the external factor and the emotion in question. MBT refers to this as the internal "link" between the situation and the feeling state (Drozek et al., 2023).

For example, if you feel angry when your mother criticizes you, the internal link could be your desire for your mother to validate you, your sadness that you do not have a closer relationship with her, or your broader feelings of insecurity about your ability to function effectively in your life. When you reflect on these various processes, you are elaborating on the personal *meaning* that you ascribe to your mother's criticism, thus "broadening the picture" of your angry emotional response.

Or suppose that your family has been thinking about moving to another town *[upcoming event]*, and you notice that your son has been feeling anxious and on edge *[feeling state]* ever since he learned about this. Here, the internal link between these two factors could be your son's sense of connection with his current friends, his emotions of sadness and loss about leaving your current home, or his concern about his ability to succeed academically in the new school system. Again, in reflecting on these internal processes, you are broadening and deepening your reflection about the meaning your son ascribes to this experience of moving, hence "explaining" his complex emotional response to this experience.

Like most of the mentalizing practice points, you can employ "Stop and Rewind" in order to mentalize either yourself or another person. See here for an example of the "Stop and Rewind" Mentalizing Toolkit, utilized by a patient who is trying to understand why she has been feeling so irritable recently.

"Stop and Rewind" Mentalizing Toolkit		
Working to Mentalize *(circle one)* ⬭Yourself⬮ OR Another Person:		
Feeling State *(emotion, desire, or feeling about the self)* Irritability and impatience with everyone		
External Events before Feeling Arose	Could event affect feeling?	How? *(Specify internal "link" between feeling and event)*
Got COVID	Maybe	Feeling physically drained and uncomfortable
Big argument with Dad—he never apologized	Yes	I feel resentful at him all the time, fantasizing about telling him off
My friend started dating Alex, hanging out with me less	Definitely	I feel hurt, left out by them, and alone—this could be showing up as anger
I got a raise at work	No	(not applicable)
No dates from the dating apps for a while	Probably	I feel hopeless about this part of my life, and angry at the world. It feels unfair.

In this example, the patient started by listing a range of events that happened in the period of time before she started becoming more irritable and impatient, including getting COVID, getting into an argument with her father, receiving a raise at work, her close friend starting a new relationship, and lack of activity on the dating apps. Note that she is including a wide range of life domains in this list, ranging from physical health, family relationships, work, and romantic relationships. In addition, she is appropriately recording *all* events from that time period, even "getting a raise at work," which is unlikely to account for her mood shift. This ensures that she is not leaving anything out which could provide valuable information about her recent difficulties with irritability. For the events that are potentially related to her shift in mood, she then proceeds to explore the internal processes that might "link" the events to her irritability: physical exhaustion, resentment at her father, feeling hurt and left out by her friend, and emotions of hopelessness and anger about her dating life.

In this way, the patient has successfully reflected upon the variety of objective factors that might be influencing her mood, as well as *how* they could be exerting that influence (i.e., through the internal links outlined). The aim here is not to arrive at some singular, definitive "truth" about what caused the emotion in question. Rather, by reflecting on the external and internal processes influencing emotions in yourself and other people, you gain a better understanding of yourself, the world around you, and your emotional relationship to that world. This helps you to feel less confused by your emotions, and to flexibly engage with others, in a manner that respects your feelings and the feelings of the people around you.

If you are up for it, try taking "Stop and Rewind" for a test-drive, using the blank toolkit below.

"Stop and Rewind" Mentalizing Toolkit		
Working to Mentalize *(circle one)* Yourself OR Another Person:		
Feeling State *(emotion, desire, or feeling about the self)*		
External Events before Feeling Arose	Could event affect feeling?	How? *(Specify internal "link" between feeling and event)*

Mentalize behavioral impact. MBT recommends a similar strategy for considering how YOU end up influencing mental states in yourself and other people. We refer to this as mentalizing *behavioral impact*—that is, the ways in which your own actions (or failure to take certain actions) can impact how you feel, how other people feel, and even how other people feel about *you*. As you reflect on your actions in these ways, you experience a greater sense of agency surrounding these behaviors: an increased ability to implement changes that positively impact your mood, your relationships, and other people's sense of well-being in their lives.

Broadly speaking, you can mentalize behavioral impact in two different ways: starting with the behavior, and starting with the feeling state you want to understand better. When starting with the behavior, first identify the behavioral tendency that is causing trouble for you, which usually falls under the heading of either interpersonal challenges or behavioral challenges. Interpersonal challenges are things you do in your relationships that negatively impact you and other people, such as reassurance-seeking, social isolation, or argumentativeness. Behavioral challenges are actions that you take that interfere with your ability to function effectively in your life, such as addiction, perfectionism, or avoidance and procrastination. You developed a comprehensive list of these behaviors back in Chapter 5, when you were developing your personal priorities for treatment (see Worksheets 5.2 and 5.3).

Utilizing the "From Behaviors to Feelings" Mentalizing Toolkit below, write down the behavior that you want to address, and then examine how the behavior affects you and other relevant parties in your life. Try to avoid exploring the behavior in general terms, for example by considering "difficulties with dishonesty." Instead, focus on a specific, recent instance when you engaged in the problem behavior, for instance "that time last week that I lied to my mother about my self-injury." This approach enables you to remain in closer emotional contact with the real-world "ripple effects" of the behavior in yourself and other people, thus laying the foundation for more durable behavioral change. See here for an illustration of the toolkit, completed by a patient struggling with talking extensively about her psychiatric issues in dating relationships.

"From Behaviors to Feelings" Mentalizing Toolkit	
Problem Behavior: *Talking about my depression and suicidality with Tom on our date last week*	
You	Other Person: Tom
What emotions did the behavior generate in you? I felt sad and desperate—more hopeless about my situation. I also felt worried about what Tom was thinking about me: Is he judging me for being so fucked-up?	*What emotions might your behavior have generated in the person?* I think that I made him feel uncomfortable and awkward. He probably felt anxious, like he did not know what to say, especially about all of the suicide stuff.
How did the behavior impact your desires, i.e., what you wanted? I wanted him to feel sorry for me, to say comforting things to me, and to validate me in my suffering. I was hoping that we would hook up and maybe have a relationship together.	*How did the behavior possibly affect the person's wishes and desires?* He seemed to want to end the date, since he yawned and said he needed to get up early for work. Is this because of what I was talking about, or was he really tired?

How did the behavior make you feel about yourself?	How could your behavior have made the person feel about themself?
Initially I felt good about myself, since it seemed like Tom was impressed with how much I have been through. But when he did not ask me out again, I started feeling really embarrassed, like I was pathetic and weak for sharing all of this personal information so soon.	I don't think he felt any particular way about himself. If anything, he probably felt confident and strong, compared to me being so fucked-up.
	How did your behavior potentially impact how the person saw you and felt about you?
	I know that he was attracted to me because he asked me out in the first place. But I think that I was "too much" for him, coming across as a psychiatric patient rather than relationship material. I don't think he wanted to see me again.

In this toolkit, the patient clearly identified a specific instance of her problem behavior ("talking about my depression and suicidality with Tom on our date last week"), then examining the feeling states that the behavior generated in her: sadness, desperation, worry, desire for comfort and validation, wish for a relationship, and some positive feelings about herself ("initially I felt good about myself"), followed by feelings of embarrassment and self-judgment. She also reflected on Tom's experience of her oversharing, which potentially included feelings of discomfort, awkwardness, anxiety, a desire to end the date, seeing her as psychiatrically ill, and a lack of interest in continuing to date the patient.

Of course the patient cannot definitively know how Tom is feeling about her, but that "knowing" is not really the point in MBT. By interrogating the various mental states arising from her oversharing, the patient increases the chance that she will engage in this sort of mentalizing *before* taking the action next time—reflecting rather than reflexing. Over time, this leads to decreased engagement in the problem behavior. Now try this yourself with one of your own problem behaviors, utilizing the "From Behaviors to Feelings" Mentalizing Toolkit below.

"From Behaviors to Feelings" Mentalizing Toolkit	
Problem Behavior:	
You	Other Person:
What emotions did the behavior generate in you?	*What emotions might your behavior have generated in the person?*

How did the behavior impact your desires, i.e., what you wanted?	How did the behavior possibly affect the person's wishes and desires?
How did the behavior make you feel about yourself?	How could your behavior have made the person feel about themself?
	How did your behavior potentially impact how the person saw you and felt about you?

The second way to mentalize behavioral impact is to start with the feeling state that you want to understand better. Employing the "From Feelings to Behaviors" Mentalizing Toolkit, write down the emotion in question, for example sadness in yourself or seeming irritation in another person. Then itemize all of the actions you were taking before the feeling state arose. Key categories of behaviors include:

- *Maladaptive or "problem" behaviors.* As we have been discussing, problem behaviors are actions that negatively impact your mood, self-esteem, relationships, or overall functioning. Examples include procrastination, addiction, criticism of others, attention-seeking, and so on. As outlined in the "From Behaviors to Feelings" Mentalizing Toolkit, these behaviors can significantly influence your own emotions (e.g., leading to depression, anxiety, shame, and so on), as well as other people's emotions, including how they feel about you in your interactions with them.
- *Non-verbal communications with other people.* Non-verbal communications involve facial expression, eye contact, bodily posture and movements, vocal tone, and voice volume. These communications encompass not just what you say, but how you say it. Such cues significantly impact how people experience you. For example, if you have a dour facial expression much of the time, others will likely mentalize you as feeling sad and depressed, which will then impact how they feel spending time with you. Interestingly, these non-verbal processes can also impact how YOU feel in yourself. If you speak in a loud voice, you are more likely to feel excited, amped up, or even angry. If you never make eye contact with people, you could start to feel more isolated, lonely, and different from others.

These observations are supported by extensive research linking decreased facial expressiveness to various forms of psychiatric illness (Bylsma et al., 2008; Davies et al., 2016; Kring & Moran, 2008), as well as decreased well-being and satisfaction in relationships (Chervonsky & Hunt, 2017). Relatedly, studies show that smiling more (and frowning less) can increase people's levels of happiness (Coles et al., 2022), decrease distress (Kraft & Pressman, 2012), and decrease depression (Magid et al., 2015; Schulze et al., 2021). I mention this research NOT to encourage you to misrepresent what you are feeling, but rather to underscore the mentalizing point that your non-verbal cues can notably affect how you feel, and how other people feel about you.

- *Positive, adaptive behaviors.* The list of positive behaviors is infinitely broad, essentially encompassing anything you do that is able to effectively facilitate your well-being, self-esteem, personal values, or life goals, as well as other people's sense of well-being and fulfillment. You could take these actions in any of the life domains discussed throughout this book: friendships, family relationships, work or school, romantic relationships, treatment, hobbies and interests, living situation, or religious communities. Examples of positive behaviors might include studying for a test, asking about your partner's day, engaging in self-care, or helping to clean the house when it is messy.

- *"Neutral" behaviors.* Neutral behaviors are actions that you take that you see as neither positive or negative; they are thus highly subjective, varying depending on the person's preferences and values. For me, neutral behaviors could include eating a meal, watching TV, scrolling Facebook on my phone, or running an errand. You might have an entirely different set of neutral behaviors, which generate feeling states unique to you and your particular circumstances.

- *Positive or neutral behaviors NOT taken.* There are times, of course, when you do not do the thing that you had planned or hoped you would do. You forget to call your favorite aunt to check in on her. You cancel your date, instead just staying at home and feeling despondent about the state of your life. You know that you need to do your dishes, but they just end up piling up for days. These "inactions" can lead to painful emotions in yourself and other people, while also stopping you from experiencing the sense of satisfaction that comes when you engage in behaviors consistent with your wishes and values.

- *Broader interpersonal patterns.* Interpersonal patterns are your more general tendencies in relationships, that is, what you *tend* to do with other people. Specifying your broader interpersonal patterns entails "zooming out" and asking yourself the question: "What is my typical manner of relating to this person, from a 'big picture' perspective?" Examples run the gamut: "helping out the other person and neglecting my own needs," "sharing a lot about my accomplishments and achievements," "withholding information about my feelings, if I think it will upset the person," "forgetting to ask the other individual questions," "repeatedly inviting the person to hang out with me, even though they keep saying no," and so on. You have already started to identify your own relational patterns in Chapter 8, "What is Your Attachment Style?" Feel free to review your responses to worksheets 8.1 and 8.2, to refresh your memory about salient patterns for you.

Reflecting on your relational patterns plays an essential role in mentalizing behavioral impact. Feeling states are not simply influenced by your actions at a specific moment in time. They are influenced by how you tend to relate to other people *across* time: what you regularly say and do with others, and what you refrain from doing in your relationships. These recurring actions can significantly impact your own mood and emotions, in a manner that is so subtle and pervasive it is often difficult to fully recognize. Your recurring actions can also significantly impact other people's moods and emotions, and especially how others feel about you as a person as the relationship unfolds and progresses. People are not simply reacting to what you *just* did; they are responding to the fact that you have done this before on many occasions, and (from their perspective) you are likely to do it again. This applies equally to seemingly "positive" interpersonal patterns (e.g., helping others, effectively communicating about your feelings), as well as more maladaptive tendencies (e.g., dishonesty and misrepresentation, dismissing others' perspectives).

Once you describe the actions you were taking before the feeling state arose in yourself or the other person, for each of these actions, ask yourself the question: "Could this action potentially have influenced the development of the feeling under consideration?" If you think that there could potentially be a connection between these two things, reflect on *how* the feeling and action are related—that is, what internal process "links" the action and the feeling. This is the same idea covered earlier in the chapter, when we discussed how events and situations can touch on certain internal processes in people (e.g., beliefs, desires, emotions, or self-states), thereby triggering an emotional response to the situation. Actions work in an analogous manner, making us feel certain ways because we have *other* feelings and beliefs about the behavior in question.

For example, if you notice that procrastinating on your schoolwork *[behavior]* makes you feel anxious *[feeling state]*, the internal "link" between these factors could be your desire for vocational and professional success, your negative view of yourself as lazy and unmotivated, or your rigid standards for yourself and your academic performance. Similarly, if your partner has been irritated with you *[feeling state]* due to you nagging them about household chores *[behavior]*, the internal link between these factors could be your partner's sense of feeling easily overwhelmed by additional responsibilities, their desire to spend their time playing video games and watching TV, or their sensitivity to feeling ashamed when other people talk down to them. By "putting words on" these internal processes, you deepen your reflection about the emotional meaning that the person ascribes to the behavior in question, thus explaining "why" they might have this particular emotional response to that behavior. See here for an example of the "From Feelings to Behavior" Mentalizing Toolkit, completed by a patient trying to understand why her boss (referred to as "Martin") has been coming across as colder and more irritable with her lately.

"From Feelings to Behavior" Mentalizing Toolkit		
Working to Mentalize *(circle one)* Yourself OR Another Person: Martin (my boss)		
Feeling State *(emotion, desire, or feeling about the self)* Colder and more irritable in his interactions with me		
Actions You Took before Feeling Arose	Could action affect feeling?	How? *(Specify internal "link" between feeling and action)*
Problem behaviors: Missing work, late on assignments	Definitely	He gets really anxious about deadlines and work quality—worries it will make us look bad.
Non-verbal communications: Raising my voice at him in that performance review	Yes	He might have been scared of me, or worried that I would flip out at him. He knows I have psychiatric issues.

Positive behaviors: Started mentoring that new employee	Probably not	Not applicable. If anything, this probably made him a little LESS angry at me.
Neutral behaviors: Had to request additional funds for that project	No	Not applicable.
Positive or neutral behaviors NOT taken: I don't make small talk with him anymore, or stop by his office to say "hi"	Possibly	This might have hurt his feelings, and made him feel like I don't like him anymore. He can be pretty sensitive sometimes.
Broader interpersonal patterns: Getting defensive whenever he gives me feedback; being critical of him (e.g., in e-mails, at staff meetings)	Yes	He could feel like I don't respect him. This probably makes him upset, and then he withdraws/acts cold because he does not want to deal with me anymore.

This toolkit offers a helpful illustration of one patient's effort to mentalize "her part" in contributing to another person's mental states. She itemized a wide range of actions she took prior to Martin's increased coldness and irritability: missing work, turning in assignments late, raising her voice, criticizing him, and responding defensively to feedback, as well as requesting funds for a project and starting to mentor a new employee. Then she considered which of these actions could have impacted Martin's short-temperedness, reflecting on relevant psychological processes in him (e.g., feeling anxious, hurt, afraid, upset, and sensitive; an assumption that the patient does not respect him; desire to avoid the patient) that might be fueling that emotion.

In this way, the patient examined not simply her behavioral contributions to Martin's irritability; she was reckoning with the *impact* of these specific behaviors on Martin's emotional experience of their relationship, thus arriving at a broader picture of her boss's internal world. It is important to note: By encouraging these forms of reflection, MBT is not suggesting that other people's feelings are 100% your fault, or that you are to blame when others treat you in a problematic manner. However, especially in close relationships, we usually play some role in how people feel about us, and how people treat us. This is a human thing, not a BPD thing.

By systematically looking at your own behaviors and interpersonal approaches in your relationships, you have the opportunity to evaluate IF your actions could be affecting how the other person is feeling. In any particular situation, you may end up concluding that the other individual's mental state is strictly related to them and has nothing to do with you. Nevertheless, by interrogating your own contribution to the interpersonal interaction, you increase the chance that you will start noticing the things you are doing (or not doing) that are impacting your dynamic with the person. This opens up the door for change.

To apply these ideas to your own life, try completing the "From Feelings to Behavior" Mentalizing Toolkit below, either for yourself or for someone else.

"From Feelings to Behavior" Mentalizing Toolkit		
Working to Mentalize *(circle one)* Yourself OR Another Person:		
Feeling State *(emotion, desire, or feeling about the self)*		
Actions You Took before Feeling Arose	Could action affect feeling?	How? *(Specify internal "link" between feeling and action)*
Problem behaviors:		
Non-verbal communications:		
Positive behaviors:		
Neutral behaviors:		

Positive or neutral behaviors NOT taken:		
Broader interpersonal patterns:		

Mentalize your current experience of agency. As we discussed earlier in the chapter, if you have BPD, you may sometimes struggle to experience a full sense of agency and autonomy in your life: feeling like there is nothing you can do about your difficulties, assuming that other people need to fix the problem for you, or just saying "fuck it" and going along with whatever is happening around you. In MBT, we rarely prescribe specific behavioral strategies to address your challenges. Rather, we encourage you to "press pause" on the situation that is upsetting you, and to mentalize your own sense of agency in the situation. This helps you to be less reactive in your relationships, opening up a bit of space between your initial impulse and your ultimate behavior. Over time, you end up making decisions that feel like *yours*—that is, reflecting your emotions, desires, and values, in a deep way consistent with who you are as a person.

What does this look like? On the most basic level, mentalizing agency involves simply considering what you should or could do, in response to whatever it is you are going through in the moment. For example, you might reflect on the range of options available to you in a situation, whether in the past or the present.

- *Regarding past situations:* "Can I imagine other things that I could have done or said in that moment? What would that have looked like, and what impact could that have had on how things unfolded?"
- *In the current moment:*
  - "What should I do about all of this?"
  - "Where do I go from here? What are the pathways open to me?"
  - "How do I make my way through this situation?"

Or you could reflect on your sense of agency in relation to specific mental states, in yourself and other people.

- *Desires:* "What do I want to do most in this situation? What are my desires telling me to do?"
- *Emotions:* "Of all the options, what feels like the best course of action here? What is my gut telling me to do?"
- *Personal values:* "What is the right thing to do in this situation? What action feels most consistent with my values—with who I want to be as a person?"
- *Consequent mental states in yourself:* "What approach do I think would make me feel the most stable, the most grounded in myself?"
- *Consequent mental states in other people:* "What actions would help other people feel best here—in themselves, and about themselves?"

As you consider these questions, you will likely identify specific actions that you want to take in your life. You might feel strongly that you should apply to a new job, spend more time with your friends, get back on the dating apps, or communicate more openly about your feelings in your family relationships. Once you have identified one of these new behaviors, try reflecting more broadly on your experience of moving forward in this way.

- "What would that look like for me to take this action, or to relate to people in this way?"
- "How would I go about trying to do this?"
- "What makes this action important to me? What is the draw here?"
- "What would it feel like to engage in this behavior? What would that be like for me?"
- "If I started doing this, how would this make other people feel? What would it be like for them?"
- "Over the longer term, if I were able to make this change, what would the impact be—on me and the people in my life?"
- "How motivated do I feel to pursue this?"
- "What would be the biggest internal barriers to trying this? What might get in the way for me?"

Similarly, in exploring the above questions, you might identify actions that you want to *stop* taking: abusing substances, engaging in self-injury, yelling at your kids, or pursuing emotionally unavailable people. You can reflect on analogous questions surrounding these "stop" behaviors:

- "What would it look like for me to stop taking this action, or to refrain from engaging with people in this way?"
- "If I were not doing this thing, what could I do instead? What would *that* look like?"
- "How would I go about trying to curb this behavior?"
- "What makes me want to stop doing this? What is important to me about changing this pattern?"
- "What would it feel like, to shift this tendency in myself? What would that be like for me?"
- "If I stopped taking this action, how might that make other people feel? What would it be like for them?"
- "Over the longer term, what would the impact be of discontinuing this behavior—on me and the people in my life?"
- "How motivated do I feel to alter this approach?"
- "What are the biggest internal barriers to reducing this behavior? What might get in the way for me?"

Earlier in the chapter, we considered MBT's strategies for mentalizing behavioral impact—that is, how your actions and inactions can affect feeling states in yourself and other people. Along similar lines, there is tremendous value in reflecting on your own sense of agency in your interpersonal interactions and relationships. You can do this in the context of interpersonal challenges or conflicts, or also just more generally, when you are curious about how you approach and engage in your relationships. Some prompts for interpersonal mentalizing include:

- "How have I been approaching my interactions with this person? How have I been treating them?"
  - "What has this been like for the other person? How might this affect their emotions, desires, and feelings about themself?"
- *In situations of interpersonal tensions or conflict:*
  - "What is my part in all of this?"
  - "How might I be contributing to how things are going in this relationship?"
  - "Am I taking any actions that could be wrong, unwise, or inconsistent with my values? If so, could this be playing any role in the difficulties we are experiencing?"
  - "What might the other person say about anything problematic I am doing? Is there anything valid in that perspective?"

In wrestling with these questions, if you end up identifying any behaviors or interpersonal approaches you would like to shift in yourself, revisit the queries reviewed earlier this section, in order to further mentalize how to implement those changes in your life.

A word of caution about the mentalizing prompts in this section. As we have discussed throughout this book, there is a fine line between mentalizing and *ruminating*. In considering "what to do" in specific situations, it might be tempting to worry, obsess, or intellectualize about the different options available to you. *That is not the intention of these mentalizing practice points.* When you are reflecting on these questions, do your best to remain connected to your emotions and desires about the issue in question, rather than just what you *think* you should do (or could do—or might do—what are you going to do?!!) in the situation.

To the degree that it is in your power, do not put any pressure on these deliberations, and *whatever* you do, do not try to "figure anything out." As always with mentalizing, the goal here is curious, flexible, and emotionally grounded reflection about mental states in yourself and other people. As long as you bring this attitude into your deliberations, over time, you will learn how to make decisions that do justice to your best self, and to what other people deserve in their relationships with you.

Expand the emotional picture. We have been considering MBT's strategies for helping you to reflect on the broader context of people's feeling states, including situations and behaviors. Another key part of that context is *other psychological processes*—that is, additional emotions, desires, and feelings about the self that could be impacting what you or another person is feeling. For example, you notice yourself feeling surprisingly happy one day, but the happiness is not just some isolated emotion. You also realize that you have been feeling excited about this new person you met *[another emotion]*, hopeful that this could turn into a real relationship *[a desire]*, and more confident in yourself *[a self-state]*, given that this person really seems to like you. Or you are aware that your co-worker has been more irritable and impatient lately. Upon further reflection, you recognize that she also might feel hurt that she did not get that promotion *[another emotion]*, embarrassed about some recent mistakes that she made *[a self-state]*, and a desire for people to appreciate and admire her for her contributions to the team *[a desire]*.

By reflecting more broadly on the range of feeling states unfolding inside of you, you will feel more grounded and centered in yourself, and you will gain a greater sense of agency surrounding your emotions. When you are able to "see" the various internal processes influencing how you feel, you are less likely to be blindsided by your feelings, and more able to make choices that reflect your unique emotional investment in the situation. Similarly, as you consider the various things that other people might be feeling, they become more multifaceted to you, opening up the door for greater empathy and connectedness in your relationships.

Utilizing the "Expand the Emotional Picture" Mentalizing Toolkit, start by identifying the "evident" emotion that you or another person might be experiencing. As my colleagues and I have discussed elsewhere (Drozek et al., 2023), an evident emotion is the feeling state that is most apparent and obvious when you are looking at the situation—the emotional "star of the show," so to speak. Once you have described the evident emotion, work to "expand the emotional picture" by reflecting upon the other internal processes that could be in play for the individual: emotions, desires, and feelings about the self. These additional feelings might have been operating before the evident emotion arose, for example if you are feeling hopeful and excited about applying to graduate school, and then you start to feel inferior and inadequate, comparing yourself to the other applicants. Or these additional feelings might be unfolding at the exact same time as the evident emotion, for example if your best friend is feeling frustrated with you for your emotional instability, but they could also be experiencing hurt, sadness, and anxiety in the relationship.

When you are itemizing these other mental states, note that the person does not have to be *aware* that they are feeling the thing at the time. In many cases, if you are struggling in a situation, there are often emotions happening inside of you of which you are not aware, which are playing a pivotal role in what is making the situation so difficult for you. We will return to this key point in the next section, "Recognize your biases in mentalizing your own emotions."

For each additional emotion you pinpoint, ask yourself the question, "Could this feeling be influencing the evident emotion in any way?" If you suspect that the two feelings could be connected, reflect on *how* they are related—that is, the internal process that "links" the evident emotion to the other feeling state you have identified. For example, if you are feeling worried that your friend is upset with you *[evident emotion]*, and you are also struggling with a sense of shame and worthlessness *[self-state]*, the internal link between these feelings could be your desire for support and validation from her, in order to help you feel good about yourself. Or if you notice that your partner is feeling sad and depressed lately *[evident emotion]*, and you also recognize that she has felt quite rejected and hurt by her parents *[additional emotion]*, the internal link between these emotions might be her tendency toward self-blame—her assumption that it must be *her* fault that her parents are so hurtful and invalidating. As you reflect on these internal links between an individual's various feelings, you deepen your reflection about the individual's emotional life, explaining "why and how" a particular feeling state might impact the emotion that is most apparent in the person.

See here for an example of the "Expand the Emotional Picture" Mentalizing Toolkit, completed by a patient who was upset with his therapist for not replying to his text messages.

"Expand the Emotional Picture" Mentalizing Toolkit		
Working to Mentalize *(circle one)* (Yourself)　　OR　　Another Person:		
Evident Feeling State *(emotion, desire, or feeling about the self)* Anger at my therapist for not responding to my texts		
What other feelings could be present?	Could this feeling affect the evident feeling state?	How? *(Specify internal "link" between evident feeling and other feelings)*
Emotions: Hurt—I feel like she does not really care about me	Yes	The hurt feels weak to me. When I am angry, I feel strong, and powerful.
Desires: Desire for her to like me. I want to be her favorite patient.	Yes	When I am angry at her, it hurts less—I don't care what she thinks.
Feelings about Self: Insecure, worthless	Definitely	When I focus on her defects, it feels like SHE is the bad one, not me. It makes me feel better about myself.

In this toolkit, the patient worked to "expand the emotional picture" of his feelings of anger toward his therapist. He did this by describing his other additional mental states surrounding the situation (e.g., hurt, insecurity, desire to be her favorite patient), falling into the categories of emotions, desires, and feelings about himself. He ended up concluding that all of these feelings could be influencing his anger, examining the internal mechanics of this. When he feels angry with her, he feels stronger, he cares less about what she thinks, and he feels superior to her. This all helps him to feel less pain around the situation, mitigating his feelings of hurt and insecurity in their relationship. With these forms of mentalizing, the patient is clearly expanding his reflection beyond simply his feelings of anger—the emotion that is initially most prominent in the scenario. In this way, the patient deepens his sense of connectedness to his own internal world, and the highly personal meaning that this relationship holds for him.

To practice these principles in your own life, try working on the "Expand the Emotional Picture" Mentalizing Toolkit, either for yourself or another person.

"Expand the Emotional Picture" Mentalizing Toolkit		
Working to Mentalize *(circle one)* Yourself OR Another Person:		
Evident Feeling State *(emotion, desire, or feeling about the self)*		
What other feelings could be present?	Could this feeling affect the evident feeling state?	How? *(Specify internal "link" between evident feeling and other feelings)*
Emotions:		
Desires:		
Feelings about Self:		

Recognize your biases in mentalizing your own emotions. When mentalizing yourself, once you have identified a broader range of emotions in yourself, you can notice something quite curious: Most likely, you have different "levels of awareness" of these various feeling states in the situation under consideration. For example, you might be quite in touch with your anxiety about your work performance, but less attentive to your feelings of frustration toward your boss, or your dissatisfaction about your career trajectory more broadly. Or you clearly recognize that you are angry at your neighbor for parking in your driveway, but you could be less focused on your worries about what your other neighbors think about you, or your feelings of guilt for being too rigid and controlling around your living situation.

This is the "biases in mentalizing" problem that we discussed in Chapter 9, where you can easily notice some feelings in yourself, while neglecting and overlooking others. MBT refers to feelings you have not yet recognized or represented in yourself as *nascent emotions* (Drozek et al., 2023), or alternatively as "sub-dominant themes" (Bateman et al., 2023). Sometimes emotions are nascent because you are simply unaware of them; perhaps no one has ever seen or validated these feelings, and so you have never had the opportunity to be attuned to them in yourself. At other times, emotions might be nascent because you do not really *want* to experience them. Maybe they make you feel anxious, uncomfortable, or ashamed, or you might judge the emotion as "wrong" or "weak" in some way. In other words, you have painful feelings *about* your feelings, which then makes you want to stay away from them. As you reflect on your own biases in emotional experience, you are better able to work through these tendencies in the moment, recognizing and accessing the full range of feelings that are making the situation so difficult for you.

To start recognizing these biases in yourself, utilize the Biases in Mentalizing Toolkit. Begin by describing the concrete situation or moment in time that you would like to explore, ranging from "That argument with my partner about our holiday plans" to "Yesterday afternoon when I felt really depressed" to "Getting really upset with myself for forgetting my dad's birthday." Usually this process works best when you have already identified the various emotions you were experiencing in the situation—for example, after you have utilized the Content-mentalizing Toolkit (pp. 164–167), the Mentalizing from the Outside In Toolkit (pp. 167–169), or the "Expand the Emotional Picture" Toolkit (pp. 204–206)—and you want to take things further by considering your different levels of awareness of the feelings in question. Accordingly, the current toolkit is a bit more "advanced" from the perspective of mentalizing, presuming that you have already done the preliminary work of recognizing the full range of your feelings.

Once you have described the scenario, list all of the emotions, desires, and self-states that you have mentalized in yourself involving that situation: anger, sadness, anxiety, shame, and so on. Then rate your level of attentiveness to each feeling state, with "0" meaning "not attentive at all" and "10" meaning "fully attentive" to the emotion. Make sure to rank your attentiveness levels *at the time of the circumstance under consideration*, not at the moment that you are completing the toolkit itself. For instance, you might be *aware* that you feel hurt and sad about how your mother speaks to you, but in the moment of your argument with her, you were not especially *attentive* to these emotions, instead just noticing your anger and criticisms toward her. In that case, you would probably rate your attentiveness level to your anger as a 10 but your attentiveness to your hurt and sadness as a 2 or 3.

Finally, consider the question: "What is it like for you to feel this feeling, when you happen to access it?" Or stated somewhat differently: "What are your feelings *about* this feeling?" For example, you might notice that you feel empowered and confident *[self-state]* when you are enraged, you experience panic *[emotion]* when you feel hurt or rejected by someone, or you want to avoid or minimize *[desire]* your feelings of shame. When completed, this toolkit often reveals what MBT calls *biases in mentalizing*:

- You have different levels of attentiveness to your various emotions;
- You may find it easier to mentalize those feeling states that are more comfortable for you; and finally,
- You might struggle to mentalize feelings that you find upsetting or aversive in some way.

To illustrate these ideas, review the Biases in Mentalizing Toolkit below, which was completed by a patient who was feeling upset with her boyfriend for continuing to text with his ex-girlfriend.

Biases in Mentalizing Toolkit		
Situation or Moment in Time: Emmett texting with his ex-girlfriend, even though I have told him I don't like it		
List all feeling states that could be present in you *(emotions, desires, feelings about the self)*	Rate your "level of attentiveness" to feeling at the time *(0 = not attentive at all, 10 = fully attentive)*	What is it like for you to feel this feeling? Specify emotions, desires, and feelings about yourself.
Angry—he should not be texting with her when we are in a relationship	10	I feel like I am in the right, so I feel confident, and superior to him.
Jealousy. She is hot, and arguably more attractive than me.	6	Uncomfortable. I don't like feeling jealous; it feels gross, and pathetic.
Worried that he still has feelings for her	2	Panicked, terrified. I want to stay away from this feeling at all costs.
Desire for a more "official" relationship: getting engaged, moving in together	0	Embarrassed, needy. I'm afraid that I care more about him than he does about me.
Humiliated and ashamed. **SHE** knows that he is texting her even though we are in a relationship.	3	A horrible pit in my stomach, like I want to hide and be invisible. I feel disgusted with myself.

In this toolkit, the patient described the upsetting situation (i.e., her boyfriend Emmett texting with his ex-girlfriend), itemizing the various feelings she has noticed surrounding this: anger, jealousy, humiliation and shame, worry that Emmett is still invested in that past relationship, and desire for a more formal relationship status. The patient then reflected on her levels of attentiveness to these feelings, which represents a more "advanced" form of mentalizing than simply identifying what she is feeling. She noticed that, at the time in the situation, she was quite focused on her feelings of anger and jealousy (ranking them a 10 and a 6, respectively), far less attentive to her feelings of worry and shame (rating them a 2 and a 3, respectively), and completely inattentive to her desire for a more "official" relationship with Emmett (ranking this a 0). Finally, the patient considered her "feelings about these feelings," recognizing that, whereas she feels a sense of superiority and confidence in her anger, she experiences a range of more painful feeling states (e.g., discomfort, self-judgment, panic, embarrassment, worry, self-disgust, desire to hide) surrounding her other emotions, to which she was less attentive in the scenario.

It is important to note that these points will not always apply. Sometimes you might be largely unaware of highly positive emotions in yourself, or acutely attuned to intensely painful emotions arising in you. However, by working to mentalize your emotional relationship to your different feeling states, you will experience a greater sense of agency and self-control over these feelings, and an increased ability to effectively navigate them in your relationships. With these ideas in mind, try completing the Biases in Mentalizing Toolkit below, around some recent situation where you have had different levels of awareness of your various emotions and desires.

Biases in Mentalizing Toolkit		
Situation or Moment in Time:		
List all feeling states that could be present in you *(emotions, desires, feelings about the self)*	Rate your "level of attentiveness" to feeling at the time *(0 = not attentive at all, 10 = fully attentive)*	What is it like for you to feel this feeling? Specify emotions, desires, and feelings about yourself.

<table>
<tr><td></td><td></td><td>.</td></tr>
<tr><td></td><td></td><td></td></tr>
<tr><td></td><td></td><td></td></tr>
</table>

Mentalizing Cool-down

Now that you have learned about MBT's strategies for considering the broader context of people's feelings, revisit William's story at the start of the chapter, on page 181. How could William apply these techniques to address his challenges with depression, interpersonal conflict, and poor functionality?

RETURNING TO WILLIAM

Recognizing William's profound lack of agency in his life, his therapist worked with William to identify his challenges reflecting on the broader context of mental states in himself and other people. For William, these difficulties included:

- Struggling to consider external/situational factors (e.g., estrangement from Catherine, lack of daily structure, social isolation) that could be contributing to his depression
- Failing to reflect on the impact of his own behaviors (e.g., excessive alcohol use, argumentativeness, defensiveness, self-injury by hitting himself) on his mood, emotions, and feelings about himself
- A pattern of blaming Catherine for their interpersonal conflicts, without taking responsibility for his own contributions to their contentious dynamics
- Ruminating on his feelings of annoyance and frustration with Catherine, while feeling less curious about how his other emotions (e.g., emptiness, self-hatred) might be impacting those feelings
- Similarly, the tendency to fixate on Catherine's overtly displayed feeling states (e.g., anger, desire to control William, wish for him to stop drinking), while

thinking less about the role that her other emotions might be playing in how she was feeling, and how she was engaging with him

- Focusing extensively on Catherine's anger and judgment toward him, without contemplating how these feelings could be a reaction to his own maladaptive behaviors—in the relationship and in his life more generally

As William's depressive symptoms continued, his therapist encouraged William to try practicing MBT's "stop and rewind" technique, in order to consider the things happening around him that might be influencing his mood. William shared that, while he was *always* depressed, he had been much more despondent over the past week, experiencing lethargy, feelings of emptiness, and intense shame and self-loathing. What had been happening in his life right before this all started? William acknowledged that he had commenced a week-long binge on alcohol, resulting in some especially debilitating detox symptoms, including nausea, tremors, and vomiting. This culminated in an intense argument with Catherine, where she expressed how overwhelmed she was by William's continued drinking and incapacitation, even mentioning the possibility of divorce for the first time: "I can't keep living this way."

This all struck the therapist as highly important. Did William see any connection between these events and his increased depression and self-hatred? William had not considered this possibility, but something felt right about it: "She has never said anything like this before. I love her more than anything, and I do not want to lose her. I feel really afraid, and even hopeless about my situation. What has my life come to, that the person closest to me is thinking about leaving me? That has to be playing some role in why I am feeling so bad." In this way, William was considering not simply the objective circumstances surrounding his depression (e.g., relapse on alcohol, detox symptoms, an intense argument with Catherine), but the emotional meaning that he ascribed to Catherine threatening divorce—namely, feelings of fear and hopelessness about the status of his relationship, which understandably could be contributing to his increased depression.

Now recognizing the impact of this argument on William's low mood, the therapist and William worked together to "expand the emotional picture" of the argument. While William initially just identified "frustration and anger" toward Catherine in the argument, he was gradually able to articulate a more complex array of feelings in play for him there: hurt and sadness that Catherine was contemplating divorce; guilt for his continued alcohol use and its impact on her; desire for care and nurturance from Catherine related to his medical symptoms; and a sense of shame and humiliation about Catherine "talking down" to him about his drinking: "It's like she doesn't respect me at all, and that makes me feel horrible about myself."

The therapist inquired: Was there any connection between these feelings of shame and William's anger and defensiveness in these arguments? William acknowledged that, whenever he felt angry with Catherine and focused on her problematic characteristics (e.g., her controlling and critical tendencies), he felt strangely *less bad* about himself. "It's like I'm not the only one in the relationship who is failing. That makes me feel a little better about myself in the moment, but it never lasts." William thus observed a particular "bias in mentalizing" when he felt criticized by Catherine: namely, his tendency to be especially attuned to anger and frustration in their interactions, while often overlooking feelings like hurt, sadness, desires for care, and especially humiliation and shame.

With this new understanding of his emotional landscape, William's approach to his arguments with Catherine gradually evolved. When Catherine would give William constructive feedback (e.g., about his alcohol use, stubbornness, approach to chores), William worked to access the full range of his emotions, including the "softer" and more vulnerable feelings that were less easily apparent to him. For reasons he could not fully explain, when he was accessing emotions like hurt and shame, he somehow felt less angry with Catherine. He thus gained an increased ability to "press pause" in these moments, rather than immediately jumping into the fray.

However, William continued to find it extremely challenging to *not* defend himself when he felt like Catherine was talking down to him: "It's like I'm trying to stop myself from breathing. After a while, I just have to say something, and I snap." The therapist highlighted William's problem behavior of "telling Catherine why she is wrong," inviting him to consider the emotional impact of this behavior on both Catherine and himself. William recognized that, when he itemized Catherine's problematic tendencies in their arguments, he felt increasingly angry, emotionally isolated, and discouraged about the state of their relationship, also experiencing a strong desire to withdraw from Catherine. In turn, when he was criticizing Catherine and dismissing her perspective, she likely felt hurt, frustrated, and defensive, thus resulting in continued bickering and arguments.

These reflections were all somewhat surprising to William. He had long conceptualized his arguments with Catherine as stemming from what he called Catherine's "critical nature," but these reflections suggested that *he* was likely playing a significant role in Catherine's manner of relating to him. Utilizing the "From Feelings to Behavior" Toolkit, William worked to examine his specific behaviors that might be impacting Catherine's feelings of distress and anger toward him. William identified the biggest culprit as his tendency to "criticize Catherine's criticizing," but he also arrived at several other important contributors:

- His continued drinking, despite her pleading with him to curb this pattern. William noted that this could make Catherine feel hurt, as if he did not care enough about her to pursue sobriety.
- His social and emotional isolation, such that he would avoid Catherine for extended periods of time, and not share in any meaningful way about his internal experience. This might lead Catherine to feel lonely and isolated herself, as if she was "living alone" without a full, emotionally present partner.
- Some tendencies toward self-centeredness, where William would forget to ask Catherine about her day. In light of this, William acknowledged that Catherine might feel a bit insecure—worried that William did not desire intimacy and closeness with her, and that *she* might be deficient in some way.
- His intellectualized, "problem-solving" approach to communication with Catherine. Rather than empathize with Catherine at an emotional level about her experiences, he would give advice about how she should respond to the situation in question, becoming upset if she rejected that advice. Here William considered that Catherine might have a desire to connect with him in a deeper way, and she could potentially feel sad that they did not consistently have that in their relationship.
- More broadly speaking, William's lack of engagement in any meaningful, productive activity: work, volunteering, spending time with friends, attending mutual help groups, and so on. Along these lines, William knew that Catherine genuinely loved him, cared about him, and wanted him to prosper in his life. Catherine might thus feel afraid for William—concerned that he was stagnating in his life, and that he might further regress in his mental health and overall functionality.

Considering these behaviors and their potential impact on Catherine, William felt like he attained a much broader perspective on Catherine's emotional experience. Not only was he probably making Catherine more angry with him, but his manner of relating to her was generating a wide range of feelings in her, including sadness, loneliness, fear, and insecurity. Catherine thus seemed less like a villain to him, and more like a three-dimensional person who could be simultaneously angry, loving, and vulnerable herself.

Interestingly, when William was mentalizing Catherine in this way, he found it much easier to "hold his tongue," and to not respond defensively and aggressively to her. He shared in his therapy sessions: "I know that I am not the easiest person to live with, and I put her through a lot. Should she be kinder when she is talking to me sometimes? Absolutely. But I think she is just really overwhelmed by everything I am putting her through, and it is much easier for her to express her frustration with me than to be talking about her feelings of sadness, hurt, and insecurity. I guess that is one thing that we have in common!"

Over time, as William became less defensive and argumentative with Catherine, the quality of their relationship dramatically improved. They argued less, became more affectionate with each other, and had longer stretches of time when they were able to enjoy each other's company without conflict. William actively worked to ask Catherine about her experiences during her workday, and to empathize with her emotions rather than trying to problem solve around concrete situations. This all led Catherine to feel more "seen" by William, like he was more emotionally present with her and her experiences.

With William now experiencing far less turmoil at home, his therapist encouraged him to consider the life that he most wanted for himself. In order to maintain all of the progress he had made in his relationship, William knew that he needed to finally do something about his drinking. Utilizing MBT's techniques for mentalizing issues of agency, the therapist inquired: "What would it look like for you to try to decrease your drinking? How would you go about trying to make this change?" William had never been able to stop drinking on his own, so he suspected he would need more support around this, probably by attending mutual help meetings like Alcoholics Anonymous or SMART Recovery. He also just had so much time on his hands, so he needed to find something to do with himself. Maybe he could find some volunteer work, or even get a part-time job?

William started attending mutual help groups, ultimately finding a meeting specifically for first responders. Despite his history of feeling like an outsider in most social environments, he was able to make several friends there, including two members who were retired like himself. They attended meetings together, went out for coffee during the day, and got dinner together sometimes, all while actually sharing with each other about their lives and relationships. William's alcohol use significantly decreased, from approximately 20 days per month to 2–4 occasions each month. William also found several jobs that interested him, and he ended up applying for a role as a part-time dispatcher at a local ambulance company. In the job interview, the administration was so impressed by him that they offered him a job as a supervisor in the dispatch department, which he accepted. William excelled in that role, attending work consistently and not under the influence of alcohol.

After several years in MBT, William expressed feeling a much greater sense of stability and agency in his life. Rather than life just "happening" to him, he was able to play an active role in generating meaning and purpose for himself, and in implementing changes that had a positive impact on his relationships and the world around him.

Chapter Review 10.1
Challenges Understanding "Why" People are Feeling Something

What is Context-mentalizing?

- Context-mentalizing involves reflecting on the relationship between some feeling state and the broader "context" of the feeling itself, namely situations, behaviors, and other psychological processes.

- Context-mentalizing encompasses the "why?" as well as the "what's next?" of mental states

- **The "why?":** Includes considering why a person might be feeling a certain way—that is, how some situation, behavior, or other internal state (e.g., belief, desire, emotion, value) is affecting the person's emotions.

- **The "what's next?":** Also entails reflecting on how the emotion influences other aspects of experience: what actions the person takes, other things the person might feel, and how these behaviors and feelings then impact other people.

Difficulties Identifying "Why" You are Feeling Something

- With yourself, problems with context-mentalizing include:

  - Feeling unsure about "why" you are feeling a certain way

  - Difficulty identifying situational/environmental factors that might be influencing your mood and emotions

  - Trouble recognizing your other psychological factors (e.g., specific thoughts or emotions) that might be influencing your mental states

  - Challenges discerning how your emotions impact your behaviors

  - Difficulties understanding how your behaviors impact your mood, emotions, and desires

  - Tendency to focus on your discrete behaviors, and to "miss"/fail to recognize your broader patterns in relationships

  - A "passive," non-proactive stance toward your own problems and behaviors

- These difficulties mentalizing yourself can lead to significant challenges in borderline personality disorder (BPD):

  - You feel like your emotions just happen to you, with no rhyme or reason. This can feel scary and overwhelming.

  - You feel confused about what you need to do to address your emotional and interpersonal problems, or to get your needs met in your relationships.

  - You are more likely to blame other people for your instability, to keep repeating the same interpersonal patterns, and to feel like a victim in your life.

[continued on next page]

- You overlook behaviors that might help you to experience a greater sense of agency, fulfillment, and well-being.

- You feel like there is nothing you can do about your problems—assuming that other people need to fix your problem for you, or just saying "fuck it" and going along with whatever is happening.

Difficulties Identifying "Why" Another Person is Feeling Something

- Problems with context-mentalizing other people include:

  - Difficulty identifying situational/environmental factors that might be influencing other individuals' mood and emotions

  - Trouble recognizing other psychological factors (e.g., emotions, desires, feelings about themselves) that could be affecting what other people are feeling

  - Challenges understanding the connection between others' mental states and their behaviors, for example, how other people's feelings motivate their actions, or how their actions impact their mood

  - Problems recognizing how **YOU** are often the context of other people's mental states. For instance, you might "miss" that others' feelings/attitudes are a *reaction* to how you are treating them.

- These difficulties mentalizing others can lead to notable impairments in BPD:

  - You take things personally, presuming that others' feelings are "about" you in some way.

  - You sometimes struggle to understand and empathize with others—to really "see" what is happening in their life, and what they are going through.

  - You could make snap judgments of other people, leading to difficulties with reactivity, naivete, and paranoia.

  - You feel more confused and overwhelmed in your relationships, finding it challenging to figure out how to effectively relate to others.

  - You can feel perpetually victimized and mistreated in your interactions with other people.

Chapter Review 10.2
Mentalizing Practice Points: Considering External Events
Impacting People's Emotions

"Stop and Rewind" the Emotional Experience

Itemize all objective factors unfolding at the moment in time before the emotion emerged:

- Interpersonal interactions (or lack thereof)
- Events in school, work, housing, or finances
- Health issues
- Traumatic reminders
- Circumstances in the immediate environment
- Time of day or year
- Situations in broader society and culture

If you think these events could affect the emotion in question, ask yourself, "What internal process potentially 'links' the external situation to the feeling state?"

Examples of internal processes include thoughts, assumptions, emotions, desires, values, or feelings about the self.

"Stop and Rewind" Mentalizing Toolkit		
Working to Mentalize *(circle one)* Yourself OR Another Person:		
Feeling State *(emotion, desire, or feeling about the self)*		
External Events before Feeling Arose	Could event affect feeling?	How? *(Specify internal "link" between feeling and event)*

[continued on next page]

Chapter Review 10.3
Mentalizing Practice Points:
Exploring Other Feelings Impacting People's Emotions

Expand the Emotional Picture

First identify the "evident" feeling the person is experiencing—that is, the feeling state that is most apparent and obvious to you.

Then reflect upon the other internal processes that could be in play for the individual: emotions, desires, and feelings about the self.

If you think these additional feelings could be impacting the evident emotion, consider *how* they are related—that is, the internal process (e.g., thought, assumption, emotion, desire, value, or self-state) that "links" the evident emotion to the feeling state in question.

"Expand the Emotional Picture" Mentalizing Toolkit		
Working to Mentalize *(circle one)* Yourself OR Another Person:		
Evident Feeling State *(emotion, desire, or feeling about the self)*		
What other feelings could be present?	Could this feeling affect the evident feeling state?	How? *(Specify internal "link" between evident feeling and other feelings)*
Emotions:		
Desires:		

[continued on next page]

Feelings about Self:		

Recognize Your Biases in Mentalizing Your Own Emotions

Once you have identified the various emotions you were experiencing in a scenario, rate your level of attentiveness to each feeling state at the time of the situation.

Then consider the question: "What is it like for you to feel this feeling, when you happen to access it?" This exercise helps you to examine your emotional relationship to your different feelings—the ways in which you might be drawn to experience certain emotions and uncomfortable experiencing others.

Biases in Mentalizing Toolkit		
Situation or Moment in Time:		
List all feeling states that could be present in you *(emotions, desires, feelings about the self)*	Rate your "level of attentiveness" to feeling at the time *(0 = not attentive at all, 10 = fully attentive)*	What is it like for you to feel this feeling? Specify emotions, desires, and feelings about yourself.

[continued on next page]

Chapter Review 10.4
Mentalizing Practice Points: Examining Behaviors Impacting People's Emotions

From Behaviors to Feelings

Describe a specific, recent instance when you engaged in some problem behavior.

Then reflect on the specific mental states—emotions, desires, feelings about the self—the behavior generated in you and the other individual. Make sure to consider how your behavior could impact the other person's feelings about YOU.

"From Behaviors to Feelings" Mentalizing Toolkit	
Problem Behavior:	
You	Other Person:
What emotions did the behavior generate in you?	*What emotions might your behavior have generated in the person?*
How did the behavior impact your desires, i.e., what you wanted?	*How did the behavior possibly affect the person's wishes and desires?*

[continued on next page]

| How did the behavior make you feel about yourself? | How could your behavior have made the person feel about themself? |
| | How did your behavior potentially impact how the person saw you and felt about you? |

From Feelings to Behaviors

Identify some feeling state that you want to understand better, in yourself or another person.

Then itemize all of the actions you took before the feeling state arose. If you suspect the action could have impacted that feeling state, consider *how* they are related—that is, the internal process (e.g., thought, assumption, emotion, desire, value, or self-state) that "links" the behavior to the feeling in question.

"From Feelings to Behavior" Mentalizing Toolkit		
Working to Mentalize *(circle one)* Yourself OR Another Person:		
Feeling State *(emotion, desire, or feeling about the self)*		
Actions You Took before Feeling Arose	Could action affect feeling?	How? *(Specify internal "link" between feeling and event)*
Problem behaviors:		

[continued on next page]

Non-verbal communications:		
Positive behaviors:		
Neutral behaviors:		
Positive or neutral behaviors NOT taken:		
Broader interpersonal patterns:		

Chapter Review 10.5
Mentalizing Practice Points: Mentalize Your Current Experience of Agency

Mentalizing Agency

Mentalization-based treatment (MBT) rarely prescribes specific behavioral strategies to address your challenges.

Rather, we suggest that you "press pause" on the situation that is upsetting you, and mentalize your own sense of agency in the situation.

Mentalizing agency is not the same thing as ruminating, worrying, or intellectualizing. When considering "what to do" in some situation, do your best to remain connected to your emotions and desires about the issue, rather than just what you *think* you should do.

Reflect on the Range of Options Available to You

Consider what you should or could do, in response to whatever you are going through in the moment.

- *Regarding past situations:* "Can I imagine other things that I could have done or said in that moment? What would that have looked like, and what impact could that have had on how things unfolded?"

- *In the current moment:*

    - "What should I do about all of this?"

    - "Where do I go from here? What are the pathways open to me?"

    - "How do I make my way through this situation?"

Mentalize Your Experience of Trying Out New Behaviors

If you identify a particular action you want to start taking, reflect on your experience of moving forward in this way.

- "What would that look like for me to take this action, or to relate to people in this way?"

- "How would I go about trying to do this?"

- "What makes this action important to me?"

- "What would it feel like to engage in this behavior?"

- "If I started doing this, how would this make other people feel?"

- "Over the longer term, if I were able to make this change, what would the impact be—on me and the people in my life?"

- "How motivated do I feel to pursue this?"

- "What would be the biggest internal barriers to trying this?"

[continued on next page]

Mentalize Your Experience of Curbing Problem Behaviors

If you decide that you want to stop engaging in some maladaptive behavior, reflect on the process of working on this issue.

- "What would it look like for me to stop taking this action, or to refrain from engaging with people in this way?"

- "If I were not doing this thing, what could I do instead? What would *that* look like?"

- "How would I go about trying to curb this behavior?"

- "What is important to me about changing this pattern?"

- "What would it feel like, to shift this tendency in myself?"

- "If I stopped taking this action, how might that make other people feel?"

- "Over the longer term, what would the impact be of discontinuing this behavior—on me and the people in my life?"

- "How motivated do I feel to alter this approach?"

- "What things inside of me could get in the way of reducing this behavior?"

Mentalize Your Own Agency in Interpersonal Relationships

In specific relationships:

- "How have I been approaching my interactions with this person? How have I been treating them?"

- "What has this been like for the other person? How might this affect their emotions, desires, and feelings about themself?"

In situations of interpersonal tensions or conflict:

- "What is my part in all of this?"

- "How might I be contributing to how things are going in this relationship?"

- "Am I taking any actions that could be wrong, unwise, or inconsistent with my values?"

  - "If so, could this be playing any role in the difficulties we are experiencing?"

- "What might the other person say about anything problematic I am doing? Is there anything valid in this perspective?"

11

Rebalancing the
Dimensions of Mentalizing

Grace was in her early 20s when she sought out mentalization-based treatment (MBT) to address her challenges with self-injury and destructive patterns in romantic relationships. A PhD student in chemistry, Grace spent most of her time engaged in "productive activities": reading research, facilitating experiments in her lab, writing academic papers, training for marathons, and managing her financial investments. Grace prioritized competence and efficiency above all else. She felt like she always had to be performing well in these tangible pursuits, feeling highly uncomfortable and "stressed" if she was not consistently and effectively working toward some concrete goal.

Grace had never had a stable, long-term romantic relationship. While she wanted a partner, she had a longstanding pattern of becoming addictively fixated on emotionally unavailable women. These could be women in her profession (e.g., professors, other graduate students), whom she saw as "above" her in some way, and from whom she craved attention, care, and emotional nurturance. Or these could be women she met on the dating apps, specifically women she saw as "cool" and attractive, but who were less interested in pursuing a relationship with her. Despite the lack of mutuality in these dynamics, Grace would become hyperfocused on securing the attention and interest of these women: imagining what she could do to make them like her; ruminating about past interactions with them, searching for signs of their potential interest; going to social events where they would "accidentally" run into each other; fantasizing about them being together as a couple; and continuing to ask them out "as friends" even after this lack of reciprocity was clear.

As this unrequited longing intensified, Grace felt increasingly empty and emotionally disconnected—a vague, dull ache that made it difficult for her to think and do her work. This is when she would break bottles in her bedroom, using the broken glass to cut herself on her feet. When she saw the blood and experienced the *physical* pain from the cutting, the longing dissipated almost instantaneously, such that Grace was finally able to focus on her work again, and to think again about other things—that is, until the next time when she came across these addicting women, and the same cycle of longing and emptiness would repeat again. Alternatively, when Grace would meet women who were actually interested in her, she felt utterly bored with them—unstimulated and emotionally disengaged in these dynamics.

In her first therapy session, Grace explained that she had attained a lot of insight and self-understanding about how her challenges had developed. Her father was controlling, emotionally removed, and highly self-centered, whereas her mother was warm, accessible, and intermittently nurturing to her. Grace hated her father, and she had long tried to convince her mother to leave him, to no avail. Now she felt like she was desperately seeking out some woman who could finally provide her with the nurturance she had never consistently received from her mother, but she could not figure out a way to get her needs met.

The therapist tried to explore Grace's emotions surrounding all of these matters. What was it like for her to consistently fall into these same dynamics, despite all of the insights

Mentalization. Robert P. Drozek, Oxford University Press. © Oxford University Press 2025.
DOI: 10.1093/oso/9780198916857.003.0011

she had attained about herself? What emotions did this bring up in her? Interestingly, Grace responded to these questions by sharing her theories about "why" she was drawn to each particular woman. The only emotion word that Grace utilized was this idea of *stress*, but when invited to elaborate on this feeling, she could not share anything about what it was *like* for her: "It's just stress. Like you know, a stressful feeling. Definitely not good." At other times, Grace pressured the therapist to prescribe some behavioral solution to these challenges: "So what I am supposed to *do* about all of this? You're the therapist: Aren't you supposed to be telling me how to fix myself?"

Grace thus remained trapped in a highly narrow range of experiences: repeating the same behaviors, the same interpersonal patterns, and even the same *words*, over and over, over and over again. How could she introduce something genuinely new into this unchanging, recycled system?

THE DIMENSIONS OF MENTALIZING

In Chapter 3, we reviewed the three different domains of mentalizing: reflecting on the *content* of mental states (the "what"), examining the broader *context* of these states (the "why"), and considering the *process* of how you relate to internal states (the "how"). These can be seen as the most fundamental forms or "types" of mentalizing you use in your everyday life, which we work to strengthen in MBT. However, research suggests that mentalization can be specified even further, along at least four different dimensions, also referred to in the MBT literature as "polarities" (Bateman & Fonagy, 2016; Bateman et al., 2023). These dimensions include:

- automatic vs. intentional mentalizing;
- Self vs. Other mentalizing;
- internal vs. external mentalizing; and
- intellectual vs. emotional mentalizing.

Neuroscientific studies on mentalizing reveal that these dimensions have neurobiological foundations, involving distinct neural circuits (for reviews, see Arioli et al., 2021; Luyten et al., 2020; Luyten & Fonagy, 2015, 2018). More recently, researchers have confirmed the validity of these dimensions in the general population, as well as among people with psychiatric challenges, eating disorders, and personality disorders (Gagliardini, Gatti, et al., 2020; Gagliardini et al., 2018; Gagliardini et al., 2023; Gagliardini, Gullo, et al., 2020; Gori et al., 2021; Gori & Topino, 2023), including people with borderline personality disorder (BPD). To mentalize effectively, individuals must be able to maintain a balance across these dimensions—not simply "switching" between each pole but moving flexibly along each dimension, in an adaptive way that is appropriate to the context or situation. See Table 11.1 for a summary of the dimensions of mentalizing and what they entail.

Research suggests that people with BPD are more likely to exhibit *imbalances* in the dimensions of mentalizing—that is, the tendency to become "stuck" at one mentalizing pole, to the relative exclusion of the other pole (Gagliardini et al., 2018; Gagliardini et al., 2023; see also Bora, 2021; D'Aurizio et al., 2023; Johnson et al., 2022; Németh et al., 2018; Sebastian et al., 2013). This can lead to negative consequences, as all of these poles are essential for maintaining stability in your emotions, self-esteem, relationships, and everyday functionality.

It is important to note that mentalizing imbalances are unique to the individual, and they tend to manifest themselves quite differently depending on what you are feeling, and the people with whom you are interacting at the time. For example, you might flexibly mentalize

Table 11.1 Dimensions of mentalizing: Automatic vs. intentional, Self vs. Other, internal vs. external, and intellectual vs. emotional.

Dimensions of Mentalizing	
Automatic The process of making implicit, reflexive, and quick assumptions about mental states; involves minimal attention, awareness, effort, and intention	*Intentional* A deliberate, careful, relatively slow process of reflection about mental states; typically verbal; requires attention, awareness, and effort
Self Reflecting and focusing on one's own experiences, including one's thoughts, emotions, desires, behavior, physical sensations, etc.	*Other* Considering and focusing on the experiences of other people, including their thoughts, emotions, desires, behavior, physical sensations, etc.
Internal Directing attention to subjective factors in people: thoughts, beliefs, emotions, desires, non-conscious processes, etc.	*External* Directing attention to visible, concrete factors (e.g., actions, appearance, facial expressions, posture/physicality, possessions, status and affiliations, events) when considering mental states
Intellectual Recognizing, naming, and reasoning about mental states; usually involves communicating thoughts and beliefs	*Emotional* Accessing, experiencing, and FEELING emotions and desires; can encompass authentic connection to your own feelings, or empathic resonance with others' feelings

both yourself and other people as long as you are feeling emotionally stable, but when you feel tired, overwhelmed, or dysregulated, you could revert to a more self-focused stance. Or you could be more intellectually oriented at work but more emotionally focused in romantic relationships. Accordingly, when you are applying the mentalizing dimensions to your own experience, MBT recommends that you consider the psychological and interpersonal conditions under which you experience balanced versus imbalanced mentalizing. This allows you to arrive at a more nuanced understanding of your own mentalizing abilities.

As you are proceeding throughout this chapter, try to keep the following principles in mind.

- Consider the psychological or interpersonal conditions under which you engage in more balanced mentalizing along a certain dimension. For example:
  - *Psychological conditions:* "I tend to consider both internal and external factors when I am feeling more confident and secure in myself."
  - *Interpersonal conditions:* "When I am meeting with my therapist, I am able to do a good job 'thinking things through,' while also being in touch with my emotions."
- Reflect upon the psychological or interpersonal conditions under which you experience imbalanced mentalizing along a certain dimension. For example:
  - *Psychological conditions:* "When I get angry, I focus mostly on other people (and what I think they are doing wrong), paying less attention to my own feelings and behaviors."

- *Interpersonal conditions:* "I revert to 'automatic mentalizing' in my relationships with my parents: I always feel like they are criticizing me, and I blow up at them whenever they give me any feedback."
- If relevant, feel free to specify *both* the psychological and interpersonal conditions under which you experience imbalanced mentalizing.
  - "When I feel insecure *[psychological condition]* in my friendships *[interpersonal conditions]*, I can get really self-focused—talking about myself in order to make myself feel better, but not thinking about what other people are going through in their lives."

With these ideas in your back pocket, let's consider the dimensions of mentalizing in greater depth: what they look like in everyday life, and how they show themselves in BPD.

Automatic versus intentional mentalizing. Most of the time, you are probably not "intentionally mentalizing." You look at the person with whom you are interacting, and without even thinking about it, you naturally make assumptions about what is going on inside of them. Similarly, at any given moment, you probably are making lots of reflexive assumptions about what *you* are thinking, feeling, and wanting. This is called *automatic* mentalizing. At the other end of the spectrum, you might decide to slow things down and really try to figure out what you or another person is experiencing. Your best friend seems withdrawn, and you feel curious: *What are they going through right now? Have I done something to upset them, or did something happen at work that could be weighing on them? How could I sort this all out?* MBT refers to these forms of reflection as *intentional* mentalizing—a deliberate, careful, relatively slow process of reflection about mental states (Bateman & Fonagy, 2016, Ch. 1).

Effective mentalizing entails the ability to flexibly move across the automatic/intentional dimension—to automatically "read" and interpret yourself and other people, and then as the situation demands, to be able to switch gears and carefully consider people's internal states. Getting "stuck" at either of these poles can lead to significant difficulties. For example, it would be odd, laborious, and exhausting to always carefully consider what people are feeling. You would probably come across as quite awkward, and you would not have time for anything else in your life!

On the other hand, automatic mentalizing can be seen as one of the central problems in BPD: You make reflexive assumptions about what other people are feeling, you fail to consider your own emotions and desires, and you can become quite "fixed" and certain in your beliefs about yourself and other people. You *are* worthless and deficient. You *need* this other person in order to feel OK. When dominated by these views, you are caught at the automatic pole of mentalizing—assuming that you are correct or accurate in your perception, and then just "going along with" however you are instinctively seeing things. In this state, you are more likely to experience instability in your emotions, self-esteem, relationships, and behaviors.

When we are introducing new patients to MBT, we ask them to self-assess where they fall along this automatic/intentional continuum. From one perspective, it is something of a trick question. As we discussed in Chapter 2, MBT suggests that most of the suffering and instability that you experience in BPD stems from disruptions in mentalizing, or in other words: getting "stuck" at the automatic pole of mentalizing in some domain of your experience, without slowing things down and trying to nudge yourself toward more intentional reflection about the issue in question. The entire point of MBT is to help you move toward the intentional pole of mentalizing—to "reflect rather than reflex" in the areas of your life where you tend to get stuck.

Mentalizing Self versus mentalizing Other. When you are mentalizing yourself, you focus and reflect on your own experiences, including your thoughts, emotions, desires, behavior, physical sensations, and so on. When you mentalize other people, you consider and focus on *their* experiences: their thoughts, beliefs, emotions, desires, behavior, physical sensations, personality traits, and so on. Adaptive mentalizing involves the capacity to flexibly shift between these two poles, depending on what you are going through, what other individuals are feeling, and what is happening in your interactions with others. For example, following a difficult day at work, you might be more self-focused, thinking about what made the day so challenging for you, how you are feeling about it, and what you want to happen to resolve the situation. But then when you get home and learn that your partner got into a big argument with their mom, you are able to temporarily "suspend" your self-mentalizing, shifting instead to focus on your partner's experience: what happened in the argument, how it impacted them, and how they plan to move forward.

In BPD, you may find yourself getting temporarily stuck at one end of the Self/Other dimension of mentalizing. At times, you might be highly focused on yourself, your emotions, and your way of seeing things, such that it can become challenging to fully "hold others in mind." You could be less curious about what other individuals are feeling, struggle to empathize with them, or fail to recognize the validity of their perspectives, especially if those perspectives contradict your own beliefs. This prioritization of "Self over Other" can lead other people to feel hurt and neglected by you, resulting in conflicts and estrangement in your relationships. It can also make *you* feel more lonely and isolated, since you lack a full sense of connectedness with others' internal worlds.

On the other hand, you might significantly prioritize other people's experiences: focusing on what other individuals are doing and feeling, ruminating about how they are feeling about you, assuming that others are seeing things the "right" way, feeling like your emotions are significantly determined by other people's emotions, and believing that you need other people in order to function in everyday life. Here you can lose contact with your *own* emotions and desires, your personal opinions about things, the validity of those opinions, and your own sense of agency in directing your life. This imbalance of "Others over Self" can lead to difficulties with dependency, low self-esteem, poor functionality, and abuse and exploitation in your relationships.

Internal versus external mentalizing. Balanced mentalizing involves the ability to flexibly attend to both internal and external elements of life, in both yourself and other people. At times, you focus on the more "visible" components of experience:

- other people's actions, appearance, non-verbal cues (e.g., facial expressions, eye contact, bodily posture and movements), possessions, circumstances, academic or vocational status, and affiliation with certain people or groups;
- your own behaviors, appearance, bodily experience, possessions and material wealth, life circumstances, academic or vocational status, and affiliation with certain people or groups; or
- concrete events, objects, and states of affairs in your life, or in the broader world.

You are able to consider all of these things, and to adaptably utilize them as one of many factors in how you interpret what you are feeling, and what other people are feeling.

You also focus on and imagine the more "internal" facets of experience: thoughts, beliefs, emotions, desires, needs, attitudes, values, feelings about the self, and personality traits. When mentalizing successfully, neither the external nor the internal world exerts inordinate sway; you regard *both* poles of experience, allowing each to enrich and influence how you understand what you and other people are going through.

In BPD, however, you might sometimes get "psychologically stuck" at either the internal or external pole of mentalizing. When caught at the external pole, you are primarily focused on concrete things: how another person is treating you, what someone said (or didn't say!) to you, their non-verbal expressions, your own appearance and life circumstances, your bodily experience (including medical symptoms), or some action that you feel like you have to take, no matter what. In that state, you often feel controlled and dominated by these external things. You feel certain that the other person's actions prove that they do not care about you enough, and that the only way for you to feel OK is for the person to *do* something else. Or you feel convinced that your own insufficiency in some domain (e.g., work, school, attractiveness, life status, ability to "perform well" in some activity) means that you are not good enough, so you need to do whatever you can to get *better* in the area in question. This can lead to tremendous suffering in BPD, in the form of anxiety, depression, instability in relationships, and rigidity and demandingness with yourself and other people.

On the other hand, when you are caught at the internal pole of mentalizing, you significantly attend to what is going on *inside* of people: others' thoughts and emotions (including how they see you and feel about you), as well as your own beliefs, emotions, and feelings about yourself. You might then be less attentive to external reality, including events, actions, and characteristics of yourself and others that bear significant relevance to your life and relationships.

For example, you assume that someone is a good friend, but you ignore the fact that they have often treated you unkindly, and they tend to talk mostly about themself whenever you spend time together. Or you feel certain that you are not good enough at your job, but you focus less on external factors like your recent promotion, positive feedback from your boss, and your history of successfully meeting your responsibilities. Alternatively, you might focus extensively on your feelings of sadness and depression (internal experiences), but you devote less energy to the things you could *do* to make yourself feel better: spending time with your family, going for walks, and applying for a new job (all external factors).

When prioritizing internal processes in these ways, you operate like you are in a bubble, separated from factors in external reality that might "pop the bubble" and lead you to see or approach things in more productive ways. You thus become trapped in patterns and relationships that prevent you from reaching your full potential, and from achieving greater fulfillment and flourishing in your life.

It is important to note that most people with BPD do not neatly fit into discrete categories of being entirely "internally focused" or completely "externally focused." Rather, the internal/external dimension often intersects with the Self/Other dimension, such that many people tend to focus more on concrete versus psychological factors with themselves, as compared to other people. For example, you might be more externally focused with yourself (e.g., focusing on your actions, appearance, and vocational success) and more internally focused with other people (e.g., ruminating about how they are feeling, or what they think about you). Or you might be internally focused with yourself (e.g., spending a lot of time thinking about your mood, emotions, and your ideas about how to feel better), and externally focused with other people (e.g., attending to their non-verbal cues, and what they are doing/ not doing in their interactions with you).

We refer to these as *orientations* of mentalizing: the aspects of experience that you tend to prioritize when you are engaging with yourself and others. When you get "stuck" in these ways, you can overlook important parts of yourself and others (e.g., your behaviors, feeling states in other people) that can significantly impact how you feel, and how you approach your relationships. Take a look at Table 11.2: Where do you place yourself in these orientations for mentalizing yourself and other people?

Intellectual versus emotional mentalizing. When mentalizing effectively, you balance elements of intellectual mentalizing with emotional mentalizing. Intellectual mentalizing involves *thinking* about mental states: identifying, labeling, and reasoning about what you or another person is experiencing. This sort of mentalizing focuses more on thoughts and beliefs—your own thoughts and ideas, as well as your opinions about other people's behaviors, circumstances, and internal processes. Emotional mentalizing involves not

Table 11.2 ORIENTATIONS FOR MENTALIZING.

Orientations for Mentalizing		
Mentalizing Poles	Self	Other
Internal	*Self-Internal* When mentalizing yourself, you focus more on your own subjective states: your thoughts, beliefs, emotions, moods, desires, and feelings about yourself.	*Other-Internal* When mentalizing other people, you focus more on their subjective states: their thoughts, beliefs, emotions, moods, desires, self-states, and how they think and feel about you.
External	*Self-External* When mentalizing yourself, you focus more on visible factors: your actions, appearance, academic/vocational status, bodily experience, life circumstances, possessions, and affiliation with certain people or groups.	*Other-External* When mentalizing other people, you focus more on visible factors: their actions, academic or vocational status, appearance, life circumstances, possessions, and affiliation with certain people or groups.

simply "putting words on" mental states ("I think that I probably feel sad and disappointed," "He appears to be angry with me"), but actually *feeling* those states—accessing and authentically experiencing your own emotions and desires, and also empathizing, caring about, and feeling motivated by other people's emotions and desires. When flexibly utilizing both forms of mentalizing, you are able to feel your feelings while also reflecting on them, a psychological state that Elliot Jurist refers to as mentalized affectivity (Greenberg et al., 2017; Jurist, 2018). Similarly, you are able to see things from other people's perspectives—a psychological construct known as *cognitive* empathy—while also empathically resonating with what other people are going through, referred to as *emotional* empathy (Salgado et al., 2020).

In BPD, you might find yourself getting stuck at either the emotional or intellectual poles of mentalizing. When caught at the emotional pole, you could feel overwhelmed by your emotions, such that it becomes difficult to "think things through" and respond to people in a balanced and thoughtful manner. You could be constantly *focused* on what you are feeling, and your behaviors can be significantly dictated by your emotions and impulses in the present moment—to seek out pleasure and relief, and to do whatever you can to "get rid of" the feelings that you find painful and uncomfortable. With other people, you might feel overwhelmed and "emotionally hijacked" by their feelings, finding it challenging to think, reason, and reflect in the presence of their intense emotions.

For readers familiar with dialectical behavior therapy (DBT), this prioritization of emotions corresponds with DBT's concept of emotion mind, in which "you are ruled by your moods, feelings, and urges to do or say things. Facts, reason, and logic are not important" (Linehan, 2015a, p. 50; see also Hollander, 2017). As you probably know first-hand from your own life, this imbalanced mentalizing can lead to difficulties with emotional dysregulation, impulsivity, and the "unstable and intense" interpersonal relationships that are a hallmark of BPD (American Psychiatric Association, 2022, pp. 752–757).

In contrast, when you are fixed at the intellectual pole of mentalizing, you are more "in your head," rather than "in your heart." You focus on your thoughts and beliefs, and without even knowing it, you could be more disconnected from your emotions and desires. Or you might be intellectually aware that you are feeling a certain way, but you do not fully *inhabit* the feeling. Along similar lines, you have cognitive empathy without emotional empathy: You accurately "read" other people's emotions, but you may not empathically resonate with those emotions or care about what other people are going through. In addition, you could emphasize your ideas about what you or others "should" be feeling and wanting, leading you to disregard those emotions that are not fully rational or logical.

This overly intellectual approach can take different shapes in BPD. You might gravitate to this state as your baseline manner, or you might "switch" to this intellectual orientation after falling into states of emotional unrest, in order to regain your emotional stability. As we will discuss further in Chapter 14, when you prioritize cognition over emotion, you feel more separate from yourself, as if you are hollow inside and missing a huge chunk of your experience. This leads to an unstable sense of self, feelings of emptiness, and a lack of purpose and meaning. You also feel more separate from other people, resulting in difficulties with loneliness, social isolation, and a lack of depth in your relationships. You may be around people, but they feel so far away from you, as if they are behind a thick glass wall.

Mentalizing Warm-up

With these ideas in mind, revisit Grace's story at the start of the chapter, on page 227. Where do you see the mentalizing imbalances in Grace's experience? These could fall into the categories of automatic vs. intentional, Self vs. Other, internal vs. external, and intellectual vs. emotional. What negative consequences do these imbalances create in Grace's mood, self-esteem, relationships, and overall functionality?

Now that you have learned about the dimensions of mentalizing, dive into Worksheet 11.1, which walks you through how to apply these concepts to your own life and relationships.

Worksheet 11.1
Mapping Out Your Imbalances in Mentalizing

Automatic versus Intentional Mentalizing

Automatic	*Intentional*
The process of making implicit, reflexive, and quick assumptions about mental states; involves minimal attention, awareness, effort, and intention	A deliberate, careful, relatively slow process of reflection about mental states; typically verbal; requires attention, awareness, and effort

(1) Review the description of automatic vs. intentional mentalizing above. When you are mentalizing in a balanced manner, you are able to flexibly shift from one pole to the other, as the situation requires. What are the psychological and interpersonal conditions under which you are able to engage in more "balanced" mentalizing along this dimension?

(2) When you are mentalizing in an imbalanced manner, you can get "stuck" at one pole and find it challenging to flexibly switch to the other pole. Along the automatic/ intentional dimension, draw a circle around the pole that tends to be your default— your most common manner of experiencing your life and relationships. Outline at least three examples of this.

(3) Describe the psychological and interpersonal conditions under which you are most likely to get stuck at that pole. What negative consequences have you experienced from this imbalance?

[continued on next page]

Mentalizing Self versus Other

Self	*Other*
Reflecting and focusing on one's own experiences, including one's thoughts, emotions, desires, behavior, physical sensations, etc.	Considering and focusing on the experiences of other people, including their thoughts, emotions, desires, behavior, physical sensations, etc.

(4) Review the above description of mentalizing yourself vs. mentalizing other people. What are the psychological and interpersonal conditions under which you are able to engage in "balanced" mentalizing along this dimension?

(5) Along the Self/Other dimension, draw a circle around the pole that tends to be your default—your most common manner of experiencing your life and relationships. Outline at least three examples of this.

(6) Describe the psychological and interpersonal conditions under which you are most likely to get stuck at that pole. What negative consequences have you experienced from this imbalance?

[continued on next page]

Internal versus External Mentalizing

Internal Directing attention to subjective factors in people: thoughts, beliefs, emotions, desires, non-conscious processes, etc.	*External* Directing attention to visible, concrete factors (e.g., actions, appearance, facial expressions, posture/physicality, possessions, status and affiliations, events) when considering mental states

(7) Review the description of internal versus external mentalizing above. What are the psychological and interpersonal conditions under which you are able to engage in "balanced" mentalizing along this dimension?

(8) Along the internal/external dimension, draw a circle around the pole that tends to be your default—your most common manner of experiencing your life and relationships. Outline at least three examples of this.

(9) Describe the psychological and interpersonal conditions under which you are most likely to get stuck at that pole. What negative consequences have you experienced from this imbalance?

[continued on next page]

Intellectual versus Emotional Mentalizing

Intellectual Recognizing, naming, and reasoning about mental states; usually involves communicating thoughts and beliefs	*Emotional* Accessing, experiencing, and FEELING emotions and desires; can encompass authentic connection to your own feelings, or empathic resonance with others' feelings

(10) Review the description of intellectual versus emotional mentalizing above. What are the psychological and interpersonal conditions under which you are able to engage in "balanced" mentalizing along this dimension?

(11) Along the intellectual/emotional dimension, draw a circle around the pole that tends to be your default—your most common manner of experiencing your life and relationships. Outline at least three examples of this.

(12) Describe the psychological and interpersonal conditions under which you are most likely to get stuck at that pole. What negative consequences have you experienced from this imbalance?

MENTALIZING PRACTICE POINTS: REBALANCING THE DIMENSIONS OF MENTALIZING

As you have learned throughout this book, the aim of MBT is to stimulate reflection about mental states, especially in the areas where you tend to get "stuck" in your thinking, feeling, and behavior. So when you get caught at a particular pole of mentalizing, MBT helps you to achieve more *balance* in your reflectiveness, so that you are able to flexibly consider a broader range of factors in your experience, and in the experiences of other people.

When you reflect in these ways, your psychological world gets bigger. You start to notice things you had overlooked before—in the outside world, but also inside of you, and in the people that matter to you. Rather than feeling like you have to "choose" between prioritizing yourself and prioritizing others, you learn how to be true to yourself, while simultaneously respecting and valuing the other person who is sitting right in front of you. You are able to think things through while also *feeling* things through, so that you remain emotionally connected to yourself and other people. You feel a greater sense of self-control, able to "press pause" in intense moments while also naturally putting yourself in other people's shoes as you move throughout your life. As you mentalize across these different dimensions, you approach your relationships in new ways, and you make decisions that *themselves* are more balanced, flexible, and fulfilling to yourself and others.

MBT's practice points for the dimensions of mentalizing involve just two steps:

(1) Determine where you stand along these dimensions in the present moment. And then

(2) Work to shift yourself along those dimensions, in order to reflect more broadly on the experience in question.

Let's consider these strategies in turn.

"Find your location" on the dimensions of mentalizing. If you ever get lost in a new city, or if you are hiking in the wilderness and do not know where you are, most mapping or navigation apps have a "find my current location" function. With the tap of your finger, the app can tell you where you are in geographical space, so that you can make your way to safer territory. With the dimensions of mentalizing, MBT wants *you* to serve as your own navigation app—to learn how to assess where you are getting stuck along these dimensions, as the first step in moving toward greater balance in your thinking. In order to get where you want to go, you first need to know where you are starting from!

To help with this, try utilizing the "Find Your Location" on the Dimensions of Mentalizing Toolkit on the next page. There are a handful of statements listed for each mentalizing pole, which broadly summarize the experience associated with the pole. After reading the description of both poles of a mentalizing dimension, ask yourself the question: "Which pole best describes where I am at right now?" Keep in mind that everyone's experience is unique, so no summary statement will reflect the full complexity of what it is like to be you. However, for most of us, we are more aligned with one type of mentalizing at any given moment in time, so do your best to "place yourself" somewhere on each dimension.

"Find Your Location" on the Dimensions of Mentalizing Toolkit	
Automatic "I feel certain that I am seeing things (e.g., myself, other people, the situation) accurately. I want something to change, or I need to DO something, in order for things to get better."	*Intentional* "I am curious about what I and other people are feeling. I feel tentative about my perspective, and open-minded about other ways to see the situation. I feel flexible and accepting of myself, other people, and the world around me."
At this moment, I identify more with . . . *(circle one)*	
Automatic Mentalizing	Intentional Mentalizing
Self "I am primarily focused on my own experiences: my own thoughts, opinions, emotions, desires, behavior, and physical states. I feel less curious about other people, less able to 'put myself in others' shoes,' and perhaps less empathically connected to them."	*Other* "I am more focused on other people: their thoughts, emotions, desires, behavior, personality traits, and feelings about me. I feel dependent on others, like their feelings determine my experience. I feel less connected to myself, my opinions, and my own sense of agency."
At this moment, I identify more with . . . *(circle one)*	
Mentalizing Myself	Mentalizing Other People
Internal "I am primarily focused on the things going on inside myself and other people: thoughts, emotions, desires, needs, attitudes, values, feelings about the self, and personality traits. I feel less attentive to external reality, what is going on around me, and my own actions."	*External* "I am more focused on visible, concrete things in myself and others: behaviors, appearance, non-verbal communications, circumstances, possessions, status, and affiliation with certain people or groups. I am less focused on 'the inside stuff': thoughts, emotions, and desires."
At this moment, I identify more with . . . *(circle one)*	
Internal Mentalizing	External Mentalizing
Intellectual "I am more 'in my head' right now, focusing on my thoughts, beliefs, explanations, analysis, and abstract concepts. Even if I am 'aware' of emotions in myself and others, I feel less authentically connected to my own emotions, and less emotionally resonant with others' feelings."	*Emotional* "I feel overwhelmed by my own emotions and desires, as if THEY are running the show, not me. I might also feel besieged by other people's feelings— I cannot get away from them! It is more challenging to 'think things through,' to reflect on all of the feelings that are barraging me."
At this moment, I identify more with . . . *(circle one)*	
Intellectual Mentalizing	Emotional Mentalizing

For example, if you have been spending all day obsessively cleaning and organizing your house, all the while paying less attention to what you are feeling, you might identify more with "external mentalizing." Or perhaps you are feeling ashamed and humiliated after a difficult social interaction: You know that you made a fool of yourself in front of those people, and you feel convinced that they want nothing to do with you. This feels more consistent with "automatic mentalizing," since you are highly certain about how things unfolded, and less curious about other ways to interpret the situation.

Once you have identified where you stand along a particular dimension of mentalizing, work to privately "put words on" the specific type of mentalizing you are noticing in yourself. You can do this by articulating simply the mentalizing pattern itself ("I am feeling overwhelmed by my emotions, and finding it challenging to reflect on what this is about for me"), or by framing that pattern in terms of the specific situation happening in the moment: "I am feeling enraged at my mother, but I have no interest in trying to understand what is making me so upset. I just want to say something to hurt her, and to punish her." See here for examples of how to express particular imbalances in mentalizing:

- *Automatic over intentional mentalizing:* "I think that I am operating more 'automatically' right now, and not really engaging in any intentional reflection about this situation."
- *Internal over external mentalizing:* "I have only been considering my husband's internal experience, especially how he is feeling about me. I have not really been thinking about how he is treating me, and how he is living his life more generally."
- *Mentalizing others over Self:* "I am focused more on other people's thoughts and feelings, and less attentive to what *I* am feeling and wanting."
- *Intellectual over emotional mentalizing:* "I have really been intellectualizing a lot today: trying to analyze all of my problems and how to fix them, but not actually *feeling* my difficult emotions, especially my hurt, insecurity, and worry that everyone is upset with me."

If you have followed the above suggestions, you have taken important steps toward "finding your location" on the dimensions of mentalizing. Now you are in a position to *rebalance* these dimensions, in order to achieve greater flexibility and openness in your experience.

Practice "contrary moves" along the mentalizing dimensions. When you find yourself stuck at a particular pole of mentalizing, MBT recommends that you employ "contrary moves" in order to move toward the alternative pole. *Contrary moves* involve simply "slowing things down," and directing your attention to the aspect of experience that is less prominent in your current thinking (Bateman et al., 2023; Drozek et al., 2023). As Bateman and colleagues (2023) explain, "In MBT, becoming comfortable with moving across all of the mentalizing dimensions is the key. Good mentalizing involves using the dimensions fluently to ensure optimal adaptation to each social context" (p. 194). See the Contrary Moves Mentalizing Toolkit for a summary of MBT's contrary move strategies.

Contrary Moves Mentalizing Toolkit	
I am stuck in . . .	**Contrary Move**
Automatic Mentalizing	**From Automatic to Intentional:** "Press pause" on the moment. Try to not do or say anything, at least for now. Work to "reflect rather than reflex," by asking yourself: • "What am I feeling right now?" • "What might this other person be feeling?" • "Are there any ways in which I feel quite certain in this situation?" • "Can I imagine any OTHER ways to see this issue?" • "What could my part be in all of this?" • As relevant, utilize any other mentalizing practice points in this book!
Mentalizing Myself	**From Self to Other:** "How is the other person experiencing this? What is their view of the situation?" "What is the person feeling and wanting in all of this? How are they feeling about themself?" "Is there anything valid or reasonable in how they are feeling, and how they are seeing the situation?"
Mentalizing Other People	**From Other to Self:** "What are my emotions, desires, and feelings about myself?" "What do **I** think is going on here? What is my opinion about this?" "How are my feelings valid, reasonable, and understandable, in light of my own history and the facts of the situation?"
Internal Mentalizing	**From Internal to External:** Try to "take in" what is going on around you: your immediate environment, other people's behaviors and non-verbal cues, your own actions, your bodily experience, and other external events and circumstances. "Are there any external factors (e.g., my actions, characteristics, circumstances, recent or remote history) that challenge how I am seeing myself?" "Are there any external factors related to the other person (e.g., their actions, characteristics, circumstances, manner of treating me) that contradict my current view of them?" "What actions could I take that might improve how I have been feeling?"

External Mentalizing	**From External to Internal:** Shift your focus to the "inside" of people: thoughts, beliefs, emotions, desires, needs, attitudes, values, feelings about the self, and personality traits. Do this with yourself, and with other people. "Can I imagine myself being OK, and feeling OK, even without this outside thing?" Consider the possibility that you might have value and worth, independently of your circumstances and behavioral "performance." "Even though the other person did this thing, what OTHER feelings and motives might be happening inside of them?"
Intellectual Mentalizing	**From Intellectual to Emotional:** Get out of your head, and into your heart: Work to access, inhabit, and authentically FEEL your emotions and desires. Try to empathize with the other person—to resonate with them, and to truly care about what they are going through.
Emotional Mentalizing	**From Emotional to Intellectual:** Attempt to "put words on" what is happening inside of you and other people. • "I have the thought that _____." • "I am feeling an emotion of _____." • "I am experiencing a desire to _____." • "He/she/they could be feeling _____." Consider your thoughts and beliefs about the situation. • "What is leading me to feel this way? Why might the other person be feeling this way?" • "What do I think is going on right now?" • "What do I make of all this?"

The first contrary move is the most fundamental technique in all of MBT: moving from automatic to intentional mentalizing. First "press pause" on the present moment, doing your best to refrain from taking any actions or making any comments. This helps you to not add any fuel to the fire, when you are trying to cool things down. Meanwhile, at an internal level, work to *reflect rather than reflex* in the situation. For example, you might examine internal processes in yourself and other people (Chapter 9), identify and address any areas of certainty in yourself (Chapter 12), or consider your own interpersonal or behavioral contributions to the situation (Chapter 10). In addition, if any of the other mentalizing practice points outlined in this book seem potentially relevant to the circumstances, feel free to try these out as well—all of these techniques are especially designed to promote intentional mentalizing!

When you are focused more on yourself, try to consider other people's feelings and experiences, as well as how it might be valid and reasonable for them to have this response. If you are prioritizing other people, shift back to your *own* emotions and perspective: How are YOU feeling in the situation, and how might that be completely understandable and valid? (See Chapters 5, 9, 14, and 15 for more on all of these strategies.)

When you are thinking more about internal processes in yourself and others, try to take in the *external* dimensions of experience: your immediate environment, other people's behaviors and non-verbal cues, your own actions, your bodily experience, and other external events and circumstances. Then consider the question: Do any of these factors potentially "challenge" your current view of yourself or other people? For example, if you are feeling certain that you are a failure who has not achieved enough in your life, consider some of the objective things in your history that undermine that narrative: your academic successes, professional accomplishments, people you have helped, as well as positive things that other people have said about you as a person. Or if you are feeling worried that your partner is pulling away from you, search for external evidence *against* that idea, including affectionate comments your partner has made, positive aspects of your sexual life, the fact that you recently moved in together, and recent moments of emotional connectedness in your relationship. Finally, drill down on the importance of your own behavior (a key external factor) in the situation, considering things that you could actually *do* to make yourself feel better, improve your own circumstances, and help other people.

On the other hand, if you are already privileging external factors in your life, turn your attention to the *internal* facets of yourself and others: thoughts, beliefs, emotions, desires, needs, attitudes, values, feelings about the self, and personality traits. If you are making any assumptions about what certain external factors "say" about you or another person, work toward an interpretation or viewpoint that decouples the external thing from the internal experience. For example, if you are feeling like you need your mother to apologize to you *[external factor]* in order to feel OK *[internal factor]*, imagine yourself feeling centered in yourself even if she never takes responsibility for how she treated you. Or if you are putting a lot of pressure on yourself to "perform" in some way *[external factor]*, consider the possibility that you could have worth and value in yourself *[internal factor]*, independent of any success or achievement. In addition, if you are assuming that your friend cancelling plans on you *[external factor]* means that they do not really care about you *[internal factor]*, reflect on other feelings and motives (e.g., work stress, need for self-care, guilt about taking time away from their family) that might explain this behavior. As we will discuss further in Chapter 13, all of these contrary moves expand the range of mental states potentially associated with the concrete things, thus shifting your focus to the internal pole of mentalizing.

Along the intellectual/emotional dimension, if you are more "in your head," try to get into your heart (see Chapter 14). Work to access, inhabit, and authentically FEEL your emotions and desires. Or strive to empathize with other people in your life—to resonate with them, and to truly care about what they are going through. Alternatively, if you are overwhelmed by your or others' emotions, attempt to "put words on" what is happening inside of you and other people. This is essentially the "taking inventory" technique that we discussed in Chapter 9: "I am experiencing an emotion of anger, and a strong impulse to 'tell him off'" (see Harris, 2022). "I suspect that she might be feeling sad and lonely, as if there is no one there to help her." Then take a step back and consider your thoughts and beliefs about whatever is happening at the time: "What is leading me to feel this way? Why might the other person be feeling this way?" "What do I think is going on right now?" "What do I make of all this?"

In different ways, all of the above techniques help you to get "unstuck" in your thinking and behavior. As you learn how to flexibly move across these dimensions, you gain access to a wider range of experiences in yourself and other people, while also responding more effectively in your life and relationships.

Mentalizing Cool-down

Now that you understand more about how to rebalance the dimensions of mentalizing, turn back to Grace's story at the start of the chapter, on page 227. How might Grace apply these ideas in her treatment, in order to address her difficulties with perfectionism, self-injury, and unfulfilling relationships?

RETURNING TO GRACE

In the earliest phases of MBT, the therapist introduced Grace to the dimensions of mentalizing, exploring how these concepts might apply to Grace's life. Grace identified several forms of automatic mentalizing in her experience:

- her certainty that she always needed to be engaged in productive activities, and that she had to be competent and effective in these endeavors;
- her compulsive need for attention and care from emotionally unavailable women, as well as her instinctive boredom with women who actually liked her;
- the powerful impulse to cut herself in order to regulate her emotions; and
- the automatic assumption that the therapeutic solution to her challenges was concrete and behavioral in nature.

Grace also acknowledged that she was almost exclusively focused on other people, finding it much more challenging to reflect on herself and her experiences. When considering herself, she was much more externally oriented, attending primarily to her actions, appearance, and ability to effectively pursue her concrete goals. With other people (and especially with the women she was pursuing), she fixated on their internal states, especially their feelings about *her*—the possibility that they could be attracted to her and want to be with her.

Grace assessed herself as being primarily intellectually organized. She lived in her *ideas* about herself and other people, struggling to say much about her feeling states. This applied especially to her approach to her psychiatric challenges, where she would attempt to intellectually "explain" why she was struggling, rather than fully accessing her painful emotions in the present moment. One exception to this was Grace's overwhelming longings for these unavailable women, which would become so intense that she found it impossible to think about anything else.

With this new understanding of her mentalizing imbalances, Grace started trying to catch herself when she got stuck in these ways. Grace had been cutting quite frequently, and she agreed with her therapist that it was important to curb this behavior. In order to help Grace shift from automatic to intentional mentalizing around this issue, Grace and her therapist developed an MBT Crisis Plan together (see Chapter 5), and Grace attempted to "press pause" when she wanted to break bottles in her room. Rather than just going along with these impulses, Grace started trying to mentalize: What was coming up for her internally, which might be leading these impulses to overwhelm her? Grace observed that she felt dead, empty, and disconnected from herself, and she desperately wanted to get rid of these feelings—to "reset" her brain so that she could focus on other things again. She also identified a key form of certainty that appeared to be fueling these desires: namely, that hurting herself was literally the *only* way that she could make herself feel better. Nothing else would do the trick.

Continuing with this movement toward more intentional reflection, Grace considered if there was any OTHER way for her to relate to these impulses. "I don't really know. As long I am feeling so numb and disconnected, I feel like I *have* to cut myself in order to feel OK again. I guess the only way to avoid this if I didn't feel so numb in the first place. But how am I supposed to make that happen?" While Grace did not have a clear answer to this question, the act of *asking* it—that is, of becoming curious about these feelings in the very moment when she wanted to cut—made her feel quite different, as if there was a little bit more "space" between herself and the impulse. She started feeling a greater sense of agency around her need to self-injure, and the frequency of her cutting dramatically decreased.

At the time, Grace was especially focused on securing the attention of another graduate student at her university, Anna. Grace felt like Anna was everything that she was not: highly attractive, creative and stylish in her fashion choices, socially magnetic, and operating at a level of coolness and desirability that was somehow "above" everyone around her. Grace had once had coffee with Anna in the graduate student lounge, and now Grace was continuously thinking about this interaction, scrutinizing every detail for signs that Anna might have been attracted to her, or impressed with her. Noticing a prioritization here of "others over self," Grace's therapist attempted a contrary move, inviting Grace to consider what it would mean to her if Anna wanted to be with her.

For the first time in the treatment, Grace gave voice to her negative feelings about herself. While she was highly confident about herself as an academic, she felt perpetually anxious and insecure in interpersonal relationships. She never knew what to say when she was relating to people, and she constantly worried that others were going to "see through" her and judge her for her deficiencies. Grace thus carried around an inescapable sense of shame and inadequacy, as if there was something fundamentally broken about her that she was unable to fix. Anna, on the other hand, was confident, self-assured, even effortless in her interactions with others. She felt good about herself, and people were instinctively drawn to her. This gave her a sense of power that Grace herself perpetually lacked. So when Grace fantasized about Anna wanting to be with her, it felt like she was almost "partaking" in Anna's value: "If someone like that could like me, then maybe I am not so bad. This makes me feel so much better about myself even talking about it, like I am gaining a sense of worth and value that I could never find on my own."

Grace thus arrived at a broader perspective on her romantic obsessions—namely, that she was somehow using these women not simply to fulfill some unmet need from childhood, but to attain a fundamental element in her sense of self right now. This made sense to her, and made her feel even more motivated to alter this pattern. Given her significant emphasis on Anna's feelings about her, Grace attempted a contrary move from internal to external: "In my obsessions about Anna, are there any objective facts that I have not been considering?" Grace arrived at an idea that she really did not like contemplating: that she had actually asked Anna to hang out again when they were having that coffee date, and Anna had declined the offer, on the grounds that she was "too busy" with her schoolwork. This happened again on several occasions afterwards, where Grace asked Anna out, and Anna never responded to her messages. Similarly, when they would see each other in social occasions, Anna rarely initiated interactions with Grace, instead directing her energy to other women at the event, often people she was pursuing sexually. Considering this broader range of external factors, it was difficult for Grace to keep focusing onto the possibility that Anna secretly wanted to be with her. It felt much more likely that Anna simply liked Grace as a person, but she did not seem to be interested in Grace romantically, or else she would have taken at least some steps to move their relationship forward.

In subsequent sessions, Grace expressed a range of emotions surrounding the loss of Anna as a romantic possibility: sadness, loneliness, and especially shame and embarrassment for being so focused on someone who, in hindsight, was so clearly not interested in her. Her therapist observed Grace's significant progress in articulating her own emotions, rather than just focusing on other people's feelings about her, indicating greater balance in the Self/Other dimension of mentalizing. That said, her therapist also gave Grace feedback that she continued to communicate these emotions with a largely flat and deadpan expression, as if she were reading a grocery list with a bunch of boring ingredients. This resonated with Grace: She *knew* she was feeling these painful emotions, but they still felt distant and far away from her. She thus attempted a contrary move from intellectual to emotional mentalizing, working to access and *feel* her emotions, in a deeper and more authentic manner.

This started with Grace accessing her emotions surrounding the loss of Anna (e.g., sadness, loneliness, shame, longing), which she found intensely painful, and highly distracting. "This is just too much. I have to do my work, but whenever I start to feel these feelings, I just want to cry, and I can't focus on anything else." Grace stuck with it, ultimately learning how to experientially "walk the tightrope" between intellectual and emotional mentalizing. Whenever she felt overwhelmed by her emotions, she would attempt a contrary move toward intellectual mentalizing, namely by trying to put words on her feelings, and to reflect on "why" they were arising in her. Then when she started to feel more disconnected and dissociated, she worked to nudge herself back to actually *inhabit* what she was feeling, by thinking of topics (e.g., Anna, her desire for romantic connection, her relationships with her parents) that sparked an immediate affective response in her.

As treatment progressed, Grace developed the ability to fully experience her emotions and desires, while also being able to identify, verbalize, and reflect upon what she was feeling in the present moment. She started to feel more connected to herself, as if she had a solid core of something that was fundamentally *her*, to which she could return regardless of what was happening around her. Interestingly, Grace also experienced a shift in her emotional relationship to these emotionally unavailable women. They felt slightly less compelling to her, and she became more interested in cultivating more mutual dynamics with other people—friends as well as potential romantic partners.

Now acutely aware of her tendency to become addictively focused on other people's internal states, Grace created a little "mentalizing test" that could alert her to these unhealthy dynamics, before they ended up developing. When she met someone new, or when an existing relationship was starting to progress, she would ask herself the following questions.

- "Does the person seem to be genuinely, spontaneously interested in me?"
- "Do our interaction feel mutual and reciprocal—with each of us asking each other questions, and trying to spend time with each other?"
- "Do I feel centered and emotionally safe with this person? Or do I feel a constant sense of lack, like I have to 'work' to get them to like me and care about me?"

By reflecting in these ways, Grace worked to cultivate relationships based on mutuality and collaboration, where she could maintain a healthy balance between valuing herself and valuing other people. Her friendships deepened, and she started dating romantic partners who were as invested in her as she was in them. "Before, I was so focused on whether or not the person liked me, but I wasn't paying attention to how they were *treating* me. I can still feel pretty insecure sometimes, and worried about how people are seeing me. But I feel like, as long as I stay connected to myself and try to remember what I actually deserve in my relationships, I am going to be OK."

Chapter Review 11.1
Rebalancing the Dimensions of Mentalizing

The Dimensions of Mentalizing

- Mentalization can be specified along at least four different dimensions, also referred to as "polarities."

- Mentalizing dimensions are the focus or "form" of mentalizing in which an individual can engage. These include:

  - automatic vs. intentional mentalizing;

  - Self vs. Other mentalizing;

  - internal vs. external mentalizing; and

  - intellectual vs. emotional mentalizing.

- When mentalizing effectively, individuals maintain a balance across these dimensions—not simply "switching" between each pole but moving flexibly along each dimension, in an adaptive way that is appropriate to the context or situation.

- Research suggests that

  - These dimensions have neurobiological foundations, involving distinct neural circuits.

  - These dimensions are present in the general population, as well as among people with psychiatric challenges, eating disorders, and personality disorders, including people with borderline personality disorder (BPD).

[continued on next page]

Dimensions of Mentalizing	
Automatic The process of making implicit, reflexive, and quick assumptions about mental states; involves minimal attention, awareness, effort, and intention	*Intentional* A deliberate, careful, relatively slow process of reflection about mental states; typically verbal; requires attention, awareness, and effort
Self Reflecting and focusing on one's own experiences, including one's thoughts, emotions, desires, behavior, physical sensations, etc.	*Other* Considering and focusing on the experiences of other people, including their thoughts, emotions, desires, behavior, physical sensations, etc.
Internal Directing attention to subjective factors in people: thoughts, beliefs, emotions, desires, non-conscious processes, etc.	*External* Directing attention to visible, concrete factors (e.g., actions, appearance, facial expressions, posture/physicality, possessions, status and affiliations, events) when considering mental states
Intellectual Recognizing, naming, and reasoning about mental states; usually involves communicating thoughts and beliefs	*Emotional* Accessing, experiencing, and FEELING emotions and desires; can encompass authentic connection to your own feelings, or empathic resonance with others' feelings

Imbalances in Mentalizing in Borderline Personality Disorder

- People with BPD are more likely to exhibit *imbalances* in the dimensions of mentalizing—that is, they can become "stuck" at one mentalizing pole, to the relative exclusion of the other pole.

- These imbalances lead to significant instability in emotions, self-esteem, relationships, and everyday functionality.

- Mentalizing imbalances are highly unique to the individual, manifesting themselves differently depending on what you are feeling, and the people with whom you are interacting at the time.

- When working to identify your own mentalizing patterns, specify the psychological and interpersonal conditions under which you experience balanced versus imbalanced mentalizing.

  - *Psychological conditions:* "When I get angry, I focus mostly on other people (and what I think they are doing wrong), paying less attention to my own feelings and behaviors."

  - *Interpersonal conditions:* "When I am meeting with my therapist, I am able to do a good job 'thinking things through,' while also being in touch with my emotions."

[continued on next page]

Orientations for Mentalizing

- *Orientations* for mentalizing are the aspects of experience that you tend to prioritize when you are engaging with yourself and others.

- You might focus more on internal states in Self or Other, or you could attend more to external factors in Self or Other, as summarized in the following table.

Orientations for Mentalizing		
Mentalizing Poles	Self	Other
Internal	*Self-Internal* When mentalizing yourself, you focus more on your own subjective states: your thoughts, beliefs, emotions, moods, desires, and feelings about yourself.	*Other-Internal* When mentalizing other people, you focus more on their subjective states: their thoughts, beliefs, emotions, moods, desires, self-states, and how they think and feel about you.
External	*Self-External* When mentalizing yourself, you focus more on visible factors: your actions, appearance, academic/vocational status, bodily experience, life circumstances, possessions, and affiliation with certain people or groups.	*Other-External* When mentalizing other people, you focus more on visible factors: their actions, academic or vocational status, appearance, life circumstances, possessions, and affiliation with certain people or groups.

Chapter Review 11.2
Mentalizing Practice Points: "Find Your Location" on the Dimensions of Mentalizing

In order to achieve greater balance in your thinking, first work to determine where you are getting "stuck" at particular mentalizing polarities.

After reading the description of both poles of a mentalizing dimension, ask yourself the question: "Which pole best describes where I am at right now?"

"Find Your Location" on the Dimensions of Mentalizing Toolkit	
Automatic "I feel certain that I am seeing things (e.g., myself, other people, the situation) accurately. I want something to change, or I need to DO something, in order for things to get better."	*Intentional* "I am curious about what I and other people are feeling. I feel tentative about my perspective, and open-minded about other ways to see the situation. I feel flexible and accepting of myself, other people, and the world around me."
At this moment, I identify more with . . . *(circle one)* Automatic Mentalizing Intentional Mentalizing	
Self "I am primarily focused on my own experiences: my own thoughts, opinions, emotions, desires, behavior, and physical states. I feel less curious about other people, less able to 'put myself in others' shoes,' and perhaps less empathically connected to them."	*Other* "I am more focused on other people: their thoughts, emotions, desires, behavior, personality traits, and feelings about me. I feel dependent on others, like their feelings determine my experience. I feel less connected to myself, my opinions, and my own sense of agency."
At this moment, I identify more with . . . *(circle one)* Mentalizing Myself Mentalizing Other People	

[continued on next page]

Internal	External
"I am primarily focused on the things going on inside myself and other people: thoughts, emotions, desires, needs, attitudes, values, feelings about the self, and personality traits. I feel less attentive to external reality, what is going on around me, and my own actions."	"I am more focused on visible, concrete things in myself or others: behaviors, appearance, non-verbal communications, circumstances, possessions, status, and affiliation with certain people or groups. I am less focused on 'the inside stuff': thoughts, emotions, and desires."
At this moment, I identify more with . . . *(circle one)*	
Internal Mentalizing	External Mentalizing
Intellectual	*Emotional*
"I am more 'in my head' right now, focusing on my thoughts, beliefs, explanations, analysis, and abstract concepts. Even if I am 'aware' of emotions in myself and others, I feel less authentically connected to my own emotions, and less emotionally resonant with others' feelings."	"I feel overwhelmed by my own emotions and desires, as if THEY are running the show, not me. I might also feel besieged by other people's feelings—I cannot get away from them! It is more challenging to 'think things through,' to reflect on all of the feelings that are barraging me."
At this moment, I identify more with . . . *(circle one)*	
Intellectual Mentalizing	Emotional Mentalizing

Once you have identified where you stand along a particular dimension of mentalizing, work to privately "put words on" the specific type of mentalizing you are noticing in yourself. You can do this either by

- Articulating the mentalizing pattern itself: "I am focused more on other people's thoughts and feelings, and less attentive to what I am feeling and wanting" *[mentalizing others over Self]*

- Framing the pattern in terms of the specific situation happening in the moment: "I feel enraged at my mother, but I have no interest in trying to understand what is making me so upset. I just want to say something to hurt her, and to punish her." *[automatic over intentional mentalizing]*

Chapter Review 11.3
Mentalizing Practice Points: Practice "Contrary Moves" along the Dimensions of Mentalizing

When you find yourself stuck at a particular pole of mentalizing, MBT recommends that you employ "contrary moves" in order to shift toward the alternative pole.

Contrary moves involve "slowing things down," and directing your attention to the facet of experience that is less prominent in your current thinking.

Contrary Moves Mentalizing Toolkit	
I am stuck in . . .	Contrary Move
Automatic Mentalizing	**From Automatic to Intentional:** "Press pause" on the moment. Try to not do or say anything, at least for now. Work to "reflect rather than reflex," by asking yourself: • "What am I feeling right now?" • "What might this other person be feeling?" • "Are there any ways in which I feel quite certain in this situation?" • "Can I imagine any OTHER ways to see this issue?" • "What could my part be in all of this?" • As relevant, utilize any other mentalizing practice points in this book!
Mentalizing Myself	**From Self to Other:** "How is the other person experiencing this? What is their view of the situation?" "What is the person feeling and wanting in all of this? How are they feeling about themself? "Is there anything valid or reasonable in how they are feeling, and how they are seeing the situation?"
Mentalizing Other People	**From Other to Self:** "What are my emotions, desires, and feelings about myself?" "What do I think is going on here? What is my opinion about this?" "How are my feelings valid, reasonable, and understandable, in light of my own history and the facts of the situation?"

[continued on next page]

Internal Mentalizing	**From Internal to External:** Try to "take in" what is going on around you: your immediate environment, other people's behaviors and non-verbal cues, your own actions, your bodily experience, and other external events and circumstances. "Are there any external factors (e.g., my actions, characteristics, circumstances, recent or remote history) that challenge how I am seeing myself?" "Are there any external factors related to the other person (e.g., their actions, characteristics, circumstances, manner of treating me) that contradict my current view of them?" "What actions could I take that might improve how I have been feeling?"
External Mentalizing	**From External to Internal:** Shift your focus to the "inside" of people: thoughts, beliefs, emotions, desires, needs, attitudes, values, feelings about the self, and personality traits. Do this with yourself, and with other people. "Can I imagine myself being OK, and feeling OK, even without this outside thing?" Consider the possibility that you might have value and worth, independently of your circumstances and behavioral "performance." "Even though the other person did this thing, what OTHER feelings and motives might be happening inside of them?"
Intellectual Mentalizing	**From Intellectual to Emotional:** Get out of your head, and into your heart: Work to access, inhabit, and authentically FEEL your emotions and desires. Try to empathize with the other person—to resonate with them, and to truly care about what they are going through.
Emotional Mentalizing	**From Emotional to Intellectual:** Attempt to "put words on" what is happening inside of you and other people. • "I have the thought that _____." • "I am feeling an emotion of _____." • "I am experiencing a desire to _____." • "He/she/they could be feeling _____." Consider your thoughts and beliefs about the situation. • "What is leading me to feel this way? Why might the other person be feeling this way?" • "What do I think is going on right now?" • "What do I make of all this?"

12

Addressing Problems with Certainty and Rigidity

INTRODUCTION TO THE NON-MENTALIZING MODES

Over the last several chapters, we have been reviewing the challenges in mentalizing commonly associated with borderline personality disorder (BPD): difficulties reflecting on the content of mental states in yourself and others (Chapter 9), problems understanding the broader context of these states (Chapter 10), and trouble with imbalanced thinking when you are considering what people are feeling (Chapter 11). This brings us to the final set of mentalizing challenges in BPD—*process-related* deficits in mentalizing, or disruptions in "how" you relate to mental states in yourself and others. Mentalization-based treatment (MBT) refers to these disruptions as *non-mentalizing modes*, also dubbed "pre-mentalizing" or "low" mentalizing modes (Bateman & Fonagy, 2016; Bateman et al., 2023; Drozek et al., 2023). There are three different non-mentalizing modes:

- **Psychic equivalence mode**, or excessive certainty and rigidity in your thinking (Chapter 12);
- **Teleological mode**, or tendencies toward concreteness and externalization (Chapter 13); and
- **Pretend mode**, or significant disconnection and dissociation (Chapter 14).

According to MBT's theory of child development, these difficulties with reflectiveness "have parallels with the ways in which young children behave before they have developed full mentalizing capacities (hence, they may also be termed *prementalizing* modes)" (Bateman & Fonagy, 2016, p. 16; see also Fonagy et al., 2002). For example, young children tend to focus extensively on external and physical reality, relying mostly on visible factors to interpret what they and others are feeling *[teleological mode]*. They feel quite certain in their perspectives, assuming that other people see things in the same way they do *[psychic equivalence mode]*. They also engage in elaborate fantasy and pretend play, which is often significantly disconnected from their emotions and experiences in the real world *[pretend mode]*. As development unfolds and children hopefully develop the capacity to mentalize, they are able to flexibly move between adaptive mentalizing and these developmentally "earlier" ways of being, and the non-mentalizing modes become less prominent in their thinking.

Not so for people with BPD, who suffer from *attachment-related disruptions in mentalizing*. As we discussed in Chapter 2, when your need to connect with other people gets stimulated or threatened, your "good" mentalizing can go offline. The good mentalizing is essentially all of the adaptive forms of reflection that we have been encouraging over the past several chapters: considering what people are feeling, contemplating why they are feeling that way, and doing so in a balanced manner.

When you stop mentalizing in these ways, there is no buffer for the challenging and painful tendencies unfolding inside of you, and the "bad" mentalizing starts to creep in. Non-mentalizing

Mentalization. Robert P. Drozek, Oxford University Press. © Oxford University Press 2025.
DOI: 10.1093/oso/9780198916857.003.0012

modes are the maladaptive forms of experience that can grip, paralyze, and control people with BPD, such that it feels almost impossible to do or see things in more effective ways. You become highly certain in your perspective *[psychic equivalence mode]*; you focus excessively on external things *[teleological mode]*; and you lose contact with yourself and other people *[pretend mode]*. When these forms of thinking take hold, you experience all of the instability in mood, self-esteem, relationships, and behavior that are endemic to BPD. On this view, non-mentalizing modes are a primary driver of the symptoms of BPD—the "breeding ground" for your instability and suffering. See Figure 12.1 for a visual rendering of these ideas—a slightly more "advanced" theory than the bare bones model we reviewed in Chapter 2.

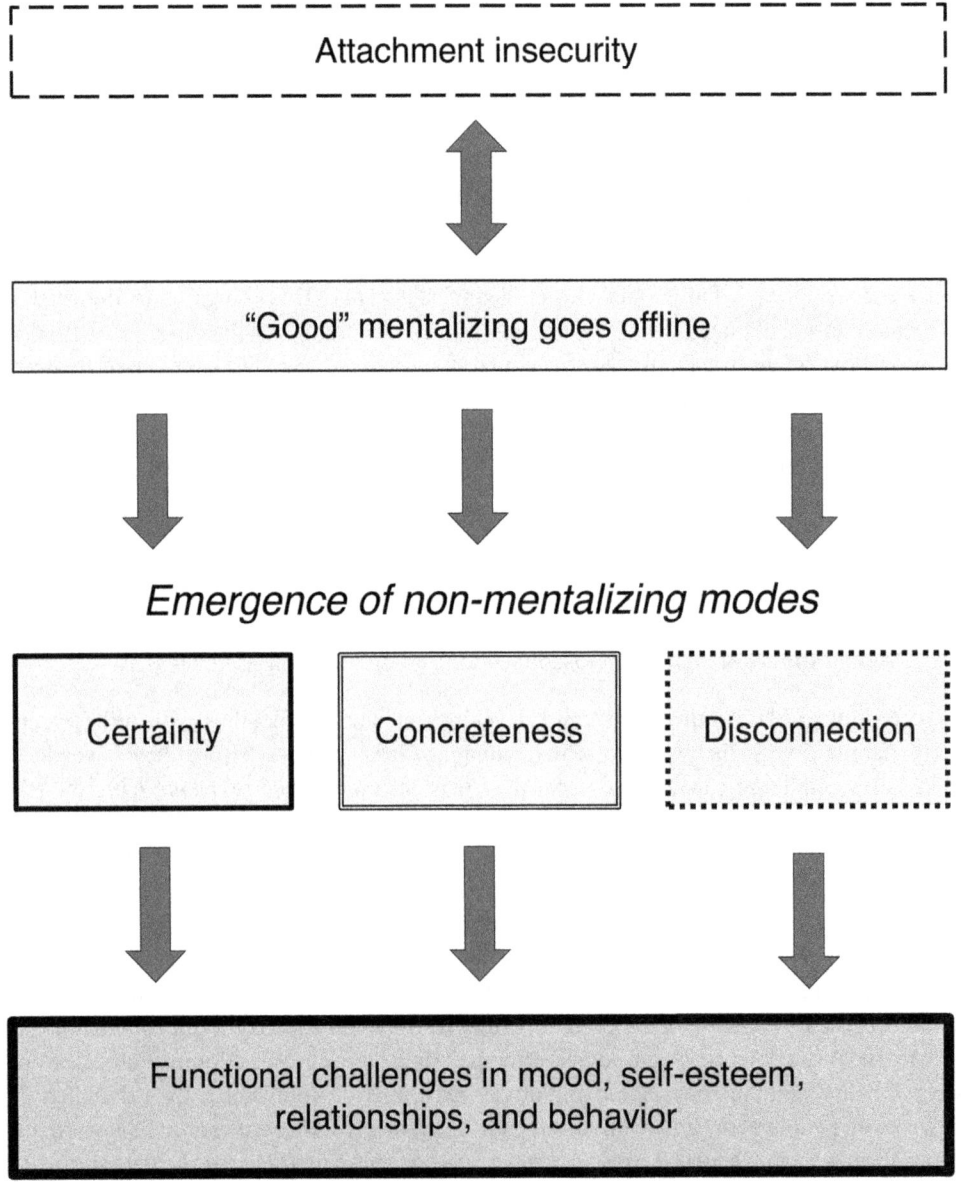

Figure 12.1 MBT's theory of non-mentalizing modes in borderline personality disorder (BPD). When encountering experiences of rejection, criticism, or abandonment, people with BPD struggle to mentalize in effective ways, instead reverting to three maladaptive forms of thinking and experience: certainty and rigidity, concreteness and externalization, and disconnection and dissociation. These "non-mentalizing modes" then lead to the functional difficulties associated with BPD: instability in mood, self-esteem, relationships, and behavior.

By helping you to continue mentalizing when you are under emotional stress, MBT tries to prevent you from falling into these non-mentalizing modes, in this way enabling you to achieve greater stability in your life. However, while this all sounds lovely on paper, as you probably know all too well, it is easier said than done. Even if you read, memorize, and implement every suggestion in this book, you will still slip into the non-mentalizing modes—that is, you will become highly certain, concrete, or disconnected in some important area of your experience. But rest assured: This is not just a "you" problem, or something unique to BPD. It is part of being human! According to MBT, wherever there is significant psychological or interpersonal stress, the non-mentalizing modes are usually somehow in play, impacting how we feel and engage in the situation. By starting to recognize these forms of mental stuckness, and by learning how to "reflect rather than reflex" when you are caught up in them, you will gain the ability to usher yourself out of the non-mentalizing modes, to move toward solid footing in your mood and relationships. Over the next three chapters, we will consider what these modes look like in BPD, as well as MBT's evidence-based techniques for treating them.

Before we proceed, a word about terminology. The idea of "non-mentalizing" can sound misleadingly black-and-white, as if MBT is proclaiming, "There is definitely no mentalizing going on here!" However, in everyday experience, we see mentalizing processes much more along a continuum. At any given moment, there are ways in which you are probably employing ineffective forms of thinking (e.g., rigidity, concreteness, disconnection), while simultaneously also engaging in more helpful, adaptive reflectiveness about mental states in yourself and others. Accordingly, when we talk about the non-mentalizing modes, we aim to describe the areas where you tend to get "stuck" in your life, without ignoring all of your other healthy tendencies, and without implying that you are somehow bad or problematic for having these problems.

Along similar lines, when we make distinctions between the different non-mentalizing modes, we are not proposing that you only experience "one mode at a time." Not to stress you out, but in many cases, you might be struggling with all three modes simultaneously! For example, you may conclude that your best friend not texting you back means that they are upset with you *[teleological mode]*, you might then feel certain that they are not a good enough friend to you *[psychic equivalence mode]*, and this could lead you to feel less empathy and compassion for them *[pretend mode]*. So as you are making your way through the next few chapters, rather than forcing your experience into a single (non-mentalizing) box, it is usually most helpful to consider *when and how* these processes show themselves in your life, so that you can flexibly apply the specific MBT techniques that are best suited to address them.

Now let's consider the first non-mentalizing mode in BPD: psychic equivalence mode, or difficulties with certainty and rigidity in your thinking.

INTRODUCING ELEANOR

Eleanor struggled with a long history of self-loathing, self-injury, and risky sexual behavior. During her childhood, her father was an active alcoholic, verbally and physically abusing Eleanor, Eleanor's mother, and her siblings. While Eleanor felt deeply connected to her mother, she lived in constant fear of her father's outbursts, and she coped with this by keeping quiet and staying in her room, in the hopes that she could avoid his rage and criticism. This anxiety carried over into her social relationships, where she felt deeply inadequate, trying to avoid doing or saying anything that would make others see her in a negative light. Eleanor compared herself to other people constantly, and she always found herself coming up short: She was not smart enough, not attractive enough, not interesting enough, and too timid and shy to ever relate to people in a "normal" way.

Eleanor was able to make it through college, graduating with a degree in education and securing a job as a teacher's aide at a middle school. She loved reading and literature, and her dream was to become a high school English teacher, so that she could read and discuss books with students, and help them learn to express themselves through their writing. But Eleanor knew that this "dream" was just a fantasy. She was not intelligent enough to ever succeed in graduate school, and she was far too anxious to stand in front of a classroom full of adolescents, trying to communicate information that she did not really understand herself.

Now in her early 30s, Eleanor lived alone and spent most of her time by herself—reading, cleaning her apartment, and eating small but healthy meals. In the evenings, she would drink wine and inevitably find herself on the dating apps, where she connected with anonymous partners for risky, unprotected sex. Here Eleanor finally had something to offer—namely, herself as a sexual object, who could inspire desire and pleasure in men. This gave her a temporary sense of self-esteem, while also validating her negative views of herself: She was *just* a sexual object, something to be used, discarded, and forgotten. As Eleanor's self-hatred grew, so did her desires to harm herself. What was the point of being alive, if she was so worthless that nothing would ever get better? She began to cut and burn herself, as a form of self-punishment. Before walking across the street, she would take a deep breath and close her eyes, in the hopes that she would "accidentally" get hit by a car, and this could all finally end.

There was only one person Eleanor hated more than herself: her father. While he had stopped drinking when Eleanor was a teenager, he continued to be a critical, disapproving presence in Eleanor's life, and in the life of her family. To Eleanor, he remained the same larger-than-life villain that he was in her childhood: angry, powerful, cruel, and always ready to take pleasure in making her squirm. When she was forced to be around him, she felt panicked, humiliated, and *small* in relation to him, as if he could obliterate her with a single glance.

This is where Eleanor found herself at the start of MBT: paralyzed by an overwhelming sense of her own badness, weakness, and futility.

CERTAINTY AND RIGIDITY IN YOUR BELIEFS ABOUT YOURSELF

As reviewed earlier, psychic equivalence mode involves excessive certainty and rigidity in your thinking, beliefs, and viewpoints. "If I think it, that makes it true." But even that way of describing psychic equivalence does not do it justice, since when you are caught in this mode, you usually do not even see yourself as "making an assumption" or "drawing a conclusion" about anything. You feel like you are accurately perceiving reality, in an objective sense. *I am seeing things accurately. This is actually what's going on.*

Sometimes you might simply presume that other people see things exactly the same way you do. At other times, you recognize that others see things differently, but you also recognize that they are wrong! So when you are in psychic equivalence mode, you find it very challenging to consider alternative perspectives. *This is the only way to see the situation.* Even if you cognitively recognize that your views could be incorrect, extreme, or unhelpful, you cannot use that intellectual knowledge to change what you deeply FEEL is true. For those of you who are familiar with acceptance and commitment therapy (ACT), MBT's concept of psychic equivalence shares significant similarities with ACT's concept of cognitive fusion, defined as "getting caught up or entangled in our thoughts, or holding on to them tightly" (Harris, 2009, pp. 17–18). When you relate to your thoughts in this way, they do not quite feel like "thoughts"—for all intents and purposes, they are FELT FACTS.

You can hold psychic equivalent beliefs about a wide range of topics: yourself; other individuals; groups of people or organizations; concrete events and occurrences in the world; and even abstract concepts or principles. Chronologically, these beliefs can concern the past ("I was not a good enough—that is why my partner left me"), the present ("I am still not good enough: I am boring, weak, and overly emotional . . . "), or the future ("I will never be good enough, so there is no hope for me"). Given the attachment-related challenges associated with BPD, the most important psychic equivalence in BPD tends to center on two main themes: yourself and other people. Let's consider these topics in turn.

In BPD, your rigid, overly certain beliefs about yourself could variously focus on:

- *Your own characteristics or abilities:* You might feel highly certain that you are accurately perceiving your personal characteristics, for example regarding physical appearance ("I am ugly, unattractive"), cognitive functioning ("I am so stupid"; "My brain is broken"; "I cannot concentrate on anything"), knowledge and competence ("I am the only person at this job who knows what they are doing"; "I am so behind in this class—I have no idea what the professor is talking about"), and task-specific abilities ("I am a horrible driver"; "I am so socially awkward. I don't know how to relate to people").
- *Your psychology and internal states:* You could also feel quite certain about your own psychological processes, including your psychiatric issues ("There is no way that I could work full-time, given my history of trauma"; "I can only really connect with people who are neurodivergent like me"), psychological vulnerabilities ("I am too needy and emotionally sensitive"; "I am so fucked up"), and your personality ("I'm a caretaker. I always put other people in front of myself"). You also might feel confident that you are NOT feeling a certain emotion ("I definitely only like him as a friend. We would never be right together"; "I don't really get angry at people—it is a waste of time"), or you could experience judgments or criticisms about your different feeling states ("This is so stupid—I should not be so upset about this").
- *Your actions and behavior:* You could also endorse inflexible beliefs about your own actions and behavior. These could include positive or negative evaluations of your actions ("I never should have sent those texts"; "I knocked it out of the park in that presentation"), views on your broader behavioral tendencies ("I am so passive, I just let everyone walk all over me"; "I always say the wrong thing"; "I am the first person to arrive at work, and the last to leave"), or thoughts about your own role or responsibility in a situation ("I did not do anything wrong in that relationship"; "What have I done? Now I have destroyed everything").
- *Your concrete life circumstances:* You might experience certainty and rigidity surrounding your life circumstances, for example your possessions or finances ("There is no way that I can support myself on this salary"), work or school ("This job is killing me"; "My grades are not good enough to get into a good college"), medical issues ("I have a bad cold, so I cannot go to work today"), or living situation ("This place is so toxic, stifling, and oppressive").
- *Negative evaluations of yourself:* In BPD, perhaps the most painful and debilitating forms of psychic equivalence involve how you see yourself, especially the ways in which you affirm your own badness and insufficiency. These views could involve your views of yourself in general ("I'm not good enough"; "I'm a loser";

"I am worthless and unlovable. I just drive people away from me"), in specific roles or contexts ("I'm a bad parent/child/sibling/friend"; "I am doing such a terrible job in therapy"), or related to particular tasks or qualities ("I made a fool out of myself in that conversation"; "I am so bad at sex"; "I am lazy and unmotivated").

- *Positive evaluations of yourself:* While this probably occurs far less frequently than your self-criticisms and self-judgments, you might occasionally find yourself rigidly holding a more *positive* view of yourself. These beliefs could involve thinking positively about yourself in general ("I am killing it"; "I have come so far, and made so much progress in my life"), in specific roles or contexts ("I am much more talented than the other people in this play"; "I am doing so well—I don't really need treatment anymore"), or related to particular tasks or qualities ("I can read people like a book"; "I am an amazing leader").
- *Standards or expectations for yourself:* You also might affirm inflexible standards or expectations for yourself—in other words, ideas about what you "should" or "should not" be doing or feeling. These "shoulds" can variously concern your actions ("I should have gotten more done today"; "I need to be true to myself, even if it alienates other people"; "I should never have told her about my diagnosis"), internal experiences ("I just have to stay positive"; "I should not want attention from other people. It is weak and pathetic"), or life circumstances ("At this point in my life, I should be married, have a career, have a house, etc.").
- *Experiences of self or identity:* You also might feel highly attached to particular conceptions of identity and self-esteem. These self-concepts can feel definitively *true* about you, exerting significant influence over how you feel about yourself. Examples include ideas about "who you are" as a person ("I'm a caretaker. I always put other people in front of myself"), notions about your capacities or potential ("I am too sick to work, or to function independently in my life"), or beliefs about the conditions for your own identity or self-esteem ("I need to be in a relationship to feel OK"; "If other people are upset with me, I cannot feel good about myself").
- *Predictions about the future:* Psychic equivalent beliefs do not simply concern what you think *is* the case, or what "should" be the case; they also encompass your assumptions about what *will* be the case—the things you presume will (or won't!) happen in your future. The circumstances in question could involve your internal states ("I am never going to get better"; "I will never feel happy again"), your behavior ("There is no way I can go on that date"), your external circumstances ("I will never be able to succeed at this new job"), or "hypothetical" future scenarios ("If they reject me, I am not going to be able to function"; "I cannot make it through Thanksgiving dinner with those people").

The problem with the above beliefs is not that they are factually incorrect. In many cases of psychic equivalence, there will be a grain of truth to your perspective. For example, you might believe that you are a failure, and you could have a wealth of "evidence" to support that view: instability in relationships, problems at work, or difficulties with mood. According to MBT, what makes these views harmful is how tightly, rigidly, and confidently you are holding on to them. Or as I like to I say it, the problem with these beliefs is the *only-ness* of them: When you are thinking them, you feel quite strongly that this is the only viable way to see the situation. Under those conditions, your thoughts will dominate and control your life, significantly impacting your mood, self-esteem, relationships, and behaviors.

So in the case of believing "I'm a failure," you will likely feel depressed every time you think about these perceived failings, and anxious whenever you are confronted with situations where you might fail again *[mood]*. You will probably struggle with low self-esteem and self-worth, feeling ashamed and inadequate as you are moving through the world *[self-esteem]*. You then might engage in avoidance, withdrawal, and "hiding" of your imperfections, in order to prevent further debilitating feelings of humiliation and shame *[behaviors]*. This can all make you feel more separate from people, and you end up missing out on new opportunities (e.g., in work, friendships, romantic relationships) that could help you feel more fulfilled and connected in your life *[relationships]*. Here, as in many cases of BPD symptoms, this rigid and certain belief is a key driver of instability and functional impairment.

Mentalizing Warm-up

Now that you have a clearer sense of psychic equivalence mode and what it means, return to Eleanor's story on page 257. In what ways does Eleanor exhibit certainty and inflexibility in her thinking about herself? And how does this certainty affect her mood, self-esteem, relationships, and functionality?

Now let's use these ideas to consider your own experience. Where you have you struggled with certainty and inflexibility in your assumptions about yourself? Try tackling Worksheet 12.1, which helps you examine these matters.

Worksheet 12.1
Psychic Equivalence Mode: How Can You be Overly Certain in Your Beliefs about Yourself?

Psychic equivalence mode involves excessive certainty and rigidity in your thinking, beliefs, and viewpoints. See below for examples of areas where you might experience significant certainty. Try to provide at least three examples of your beliefs in these areas. In each category, how does this certainty affect your emotions, self-esteem, relationships, and behavior?

(1) Certainty about your own characteristics or abilities:

(2) Certainty about your psychology and internal states:

(3) Certainty about your own actions and behavior:

(4) Certainty about your life circumstances:

[continued on next page]

(5) Certainty in your negative evaluations of yourself:

(6) Certainty in your positive evaluations of yourself:

(7) Certainty about your standards or expectations for yourself:

(8) Certainty in your experiences of self or identity:

(9) Certainty in your predictions about your future:

CERTAINTY AND RIGIDITY IN YOUR BELIEFS ABOUT OTHER PEOPLE

In BPD, psychic equivalence does not simply affect how you see yourself; it can infect your experience of other people as well. Your rigid, overly certain beliefs about others could focus on:

- *Other people's characteristics or abilities:* You could feel highly certain that you are accurately perceiving other people's personal characteristics, for example regarding physical appearance ("He is one of the most attractive people I have ever seen"; "She is so disgusting"), cognitive functioning ("He is such a stupid person"; "She is brilliant—so much smarter than I am"); knowledge and competence ("My co-workers have no idea how to do their jobs"; "My therapist is not helping me"), and task-specific abilities ("My parents never knew how to parent me"; "My boss is amazing—he always knows the right thing to say in every situation").
- *Others' psychology and internal states:* You could also hold inflexible beliefs about other people's psychological processes, including their psychiatric issues ("He is such a narcissist"; "Her OCD is so bad—she is impossible to work with"), psychological vulnerabilities ("He is a fundamentally lazy, unmotivated person. He does not care about anything"), self-concepts ("She sees herself as a leader, but nobody really respects her"; "He is deeply insecure, and he compensates for that by trying to sound smart"), and personalities or character ("She is the most caring, empathetic person I have ever met"; "He is so controlling; he always has to get his way"; "The customers here are so selfish and entitled"). You also might feel confident that other people are feeling certain emotions ("I know that they hate me and want nothing to do with me"; "She is clearly trying to sabotage me"; "I can tell that he still has feelings for me"), that other people are NOT feeling certain things ("He does not care about me—this is all about him"; "She does not have an angry bone in her body"), or that others *should* not be feeling certain things ("He has no right to be judging me"; "She should not be so pessimistic—everything is going to be fine").
- *Other individuals' actions and behavior:* You could also endorse inflexible beliefs about other people's actions and behavior. These could include positive or negative evaluations of others' actions ("My mom never should have said that to me"; "They failed miserably at managing this department"; "She did such a great job expressing herself in that conversation—I could never be that articulate"), views on people's broader behavioral tendencies ("He is extremely passive in the relationship, always deferring to me and my preferences"; "She just talks about herself constantly. She never asks me questions or follows up about things going on in my life"), or thoughts about other people's role or responsibility in a situation ("He ruined my life"; "Without my therapist, I would not be alive today"; "She has been completely avoiding her responsibilities—I had to make that complaint").
- *Other people's concrete life circumstances:* You might experience certainty and rigidity surrounding other people's life situations, for example others' possessions or finances ("She was born with a silver spoon in her mouth"), work or school ("Everybody in this class is doing better than me"; "He only got this job because of his family connections"), medical issues ("Her fibromyalgia is so bad—she cannot work or have a relationship"), and geographical location or living conditions ("This town is killing her. She is so much better than all of this").
- *Negative evaluations of other people:* As we discussed in Chapter 1, BPD is often characterized by "splitting" processes, or the tendency to experience other people as either "all good" or "all bad." Translated into the terms of psychic equivalence,

you might find yourself devaluing other people, focusing on their defects and feeling as if they are harming you in some way. This could involve devaluing others in general ("She is a worthless, toxic person"; "He is such an asshole"; "They are so horrible—I cannot stand to be in the same room as them"), in specific roles or contexts ("He has been a terrible friend to me, right when I needed him the most"; "She is the worst boss I have ever had"), or related to particular tasks or qualities ("He is so socially awkward. He is always putting his foot in his mouth"; "She is clueless—completely unable to manage her own life").

- *Positive evaluations of other people:* The other side of splitting is the "all good," or ascribing significant *positive* value to other people. These valuations could involve thinking positively about other people in general ("He is the most amazing person I have ever met"; "She is everything I want to be"), in specific roles or contexts ("They are the best partner I could ever hope for": "Everyone there is so much more competent and knowledgeable than me"), or related to particular tasks or qualities ("She is such a creative person. I envy that"; "He is so loyal, supportive, and dedicated to me—the only one who has stood by me in my difficulties").

- *Standards or expectations for others:* You might also affirm inflexible standards or expectations for other people, understood as ideas about what others "should" or "should not" be doing or feeling. These standards could concern other people's actions ("She should never have said that to me. It was so insensitive"; "He needs to get his shit together: get a job, move out of his parents' house, and start going to therapy"), internal experiences ("He has no right to be angry at me—I have not done anything wrong"; "My therapist thinks that I should get out of the relationship, but she does not know what she is talking about"), or life circumstances ("She is way underpaid, given how much she does for that company").

- *Predictions about other people in the future:* You also might find yourself making assumptions about what other people will (or won't) experience in the future. These assumptions could involve other individuals' internal states ("She will be so mad at me, once she finds out that I have been lying to her"), behavior ("I know that he is going to break up with me"), external circumstances ("It's only a matter of time before they move away"), and "hypothetical" future scenarios ("He would never agree to being in a monogamous relationship"; "If she keeps this up, she is going to get fired").

- *Tendency to base your own mental states on others' mental states:* In BPD, another facet of psychic equivalence is the pattern of basing your own feelings on how other people are feeling—or more accurately, on how you *think* that other people are feeling. This might include "absorbing" other people's emotional states ("If my parents are feeling anxious and worried, that makes me feel anxious and worried"), feeling like you can ONLY experience positive emotions if other people are feeling positively toward you ("I need my partner to be happy with me, in order to feel good about myself"), or reflexively experiencing painful emotions when others are seeing you in a negative light ("If my boss is upset with me, I feel panicked and ashamed, like I need to do whatever I can to win her approval again").

Like your psychic equivalent beliefs about yourself, the above beliefs about other people can significantly impact how you feel, and how you live. When you feel highly certain that a particular thing is true about another person, this does not feel like a "belief" or "viewpoint." Rather, the other person *becomes* the thing—this is just how they are. This then sets off a whole cascade of consequences, significantly impacting your emotions, self-esteem, behavior, and overall relationship with the person. For example, if you feel convinced that your best friend does not care about you enough, you will likely feel more sad, lonely, and hurt in that dynamic *[emotions]*. To the degree that you end up basing your self-worth on your friend's feelings about you *[another form of certainty]*, you could also feel ashamed and worthless when you are with the person *[self-esteem]*. You might then become more irritable and impatient in your interactions with the friend, ultimately withdrawing from them, secretly hoping that they might notice you are upset and reach out to you *[behavior]*. Over time, your friend feels hurt, alienated, and distant from you; you grow apart from each other, which leads you to feel more isolated and lonely in your life overall *[relationships]*.

In this scenario, the culprit is not your belief that your friend does not care about you enough. Everyone has those sorts of beliefs sometimes! The problem is how tightly you are holding that belief. When in psychic equivalence mode, your beliefs do not *feel* like beliefs, and so they have inordinate control over your emotions and behavior.

Mentalizing Warm-up

Having considered these ideas about psychic equivalence mode in BPD, turn back to Eleanor's story on page 257. In what ways does Eleanor exhibit certainty and inflexibility in her thinking about other people? How does this certainty affect her mood, self-esteem, relationships, and functionality?

What about you: How have you struggled with excessive certainty and rigidity in your thinking about other people? Worksheet 12.2 helps you apply these ideas to your everyday life.

Worksheet 12.2
Psychic Equivalence Mode: How Can You be Overly Certain in Your Beliefs about Other People?

Psychic equivalence mode involves excessive certainty and rigidity in your thinking, beliefs, and viewpoints. See below for examples of areas where you might experience significant certainty. Try to provide at least three examples of your beliefs in these areas. In each category, how does this certainty affect your emotions, self-esteem, relationships, and behavior?

(1) Certainty about other people's characteristics or abilities:

(2) Certainty about others' psychology and internal states:

(3) Certainty about other individuals' actions and behavior:

(4) Certainty about other people's concrete life circumstances:

[continued on next page]

(5) Certainty in your negative evaluations of other people:

(6) Certainty in your positive evaluations of other people:

(7) Certainty about your standards or expectations for others:

(8) Certainty in your predictions about other people in the future:

(9) Tendency to base your own mental states on others' mental states:

MENTALIZING PRACTICE POINTS: DEVELOPING GREATER CURIOSITY AND FLEXIBILITY

As we have seen, excessive certainty is a core driver of instability and suffering in BPD. We have a saying in our MBT groups here at McLean: "Wherever there is suffering, there is certainty." If you feel excessively certain that you are accurately perceiving something, then that "something" will exert significant influence over your emotions, desires, and behaviors. In our experience, for many people with BPD who have insufficiently benefited from psychotherapy, there are often areas of certainty that have never been addressed in their treatment. *"I am bad, insufficient." "No one really cares about me." "I need this person's approval in order to feel OK."* Perhaps you have tried to treat the *manifestations* of these rigid beliefs (e.g., depressed mood, suicidal thinking, dependency and anxiety in your relationships), but the rigid beliefs themselves remain largely intact in your experience—pristine and untouched, and thus fully empowered to exert their destructive influence over your life. And so your suffering just continues unabated. Treatment can go on for years and years with no improvement, with everyone (e.g., your therapist, your loved ones, yourself) feeling confused, demoralized, and discouraged that you are not getting any better.

This is not your fault, and the situation is not hopeless. In MBT, you learn how to identify and address your difficulties with excessive certainty. This includes your "in-the-moment" certainty, for example when you feel convinced that your boss is judging you, or if you are confident that you embarrassed yourself in that social interaction. This also includes your more longstanding, pervasive forms of certainty—the beliefs that you always carry around inside of you that tend to pop up in your life whether you like it or not. "I am never going to have a successful relationship." "It is weak and pathetic to want attention from people."

So when you are suffering, MBT implores you to actively wrestle with the question:

"Where is the certainty?"

Work to ferret out and isolate the ways in which you are feeling overly certain about the issue in question. And then, rather than trying to change your feelings (a byproduct of the certainty), or attempting to change other people and the world around you (who are often the "focus" of the certainty), devote yourself to treating the certainty itself. Once *that* problem is resolved, you usually start to feel better, and to approach your life in a more flexible way. For the rest of this chapter, we are going to explore MBT's techniques for targeting and addressing your difficulties with certainty.

Let's make one thing clear, right out of the gate. **In MBT, we are not trying to get you to stop believing what you believe.** Let's try that one more time, just to make sure there are no misunderstandings: **In MBT, we are not trying to get you to stop believing what you believe.** You have probably experienced this a lot in your life—where a friend, family member, or therapist tries to convince you to see things more positively, or to feel a different way about something. How does this usually go? Perhaps it works in the moment, but usually the thought just comes right back, often more intensely the next time. This can make you feel even more discouraged and hopeless: "I can't even do therapy right! If only I could just see things more positively, then maybe I could get better."

So if MBT does not try to change the content of your beliefs, what the heck does it do? MBT's strategies for psychic equivalence simply aim to help you see your beliefs *as beliefs*— one of many ways to think about something, or to interpret reality. The goal here is addition, not subtraction. So rather than trying to get you to "delete" any thoughts from your mind, MBT helps you to

(1) Recognize that these are thoughts in your mind, not necessarily facts. This is essentially what mentalization means: to mental-*ize*, or to make something mental. This part of MBT dovetails significantly with ACT's techniques for cognitive defusion (Harris, 2022; Hayes, 2020), which work to "create space" between yourself and your thoughts.

(2) Consider other ways to see the situation. In this way, we are working to "add" some additional perspectives to your repertoire, rather than trying to get rid of your initial perspective. You will thus be able to stand right alongside your original belief, while also acknowledging the potential validity of other viewpoints.

In these ways, MBT helps you to achieve greater curiosity and flexibility in your thinking. Whatever else is happening around you, your thoughts are fundamentally *mental*—they come from your mind. This means that they underscore a facet of reality, rather than reality as it is in itself. Once you appreciate this, at a deep emotional level, you are able to become more curious about your thoughts. What makes me see things in this particular way? How does it impact me to feel so certain about this particular interpretation? And in light of all of this, are there any other valid ways of seeing this situation? You thus become more flexible in your thinking—more receptive and open to other perspectives and viewpoints. **This flexibility is the antidote to the symptoms of BPD.** Your mood improves, you begin to feel better about yourself, and you gain a greater sense of agency over your behavior, and how you relate to others. Over time, you notice that your relationships are improving: You feel more engaged and secure with other people, and they start to experience you in a more positive light.

With all of this in mind, let's consider the techniques for addressing excessive rigidity and certainty in BPD. While most of the mentalizing practice points reviewed in previous chapters can be utilized in any order, there is value in following these practice points in a more step-by-step fashion, especially when you are just getting started out. This is because, when you are feeling highly certain about something, it is often counterproductive to just "jump ahead" and try to shift your perspective. This can feel invalidating and threatening, paradoxically leading you to dig in your heels and cling more tightly to your original view.

Step 1: Articulate the rigid assumption you want to address. The first step in addressing certainty is "putting words on" the specific viewpoint that is causing you trouble. Here it is important to explicitly frame the perspective *as a belief state*—that is, as a psychological, verbal construction about some person, place, thing, or concept. For example, you might affirm:

- "I am believing that _____."
- "I am having the thought that _____."
- "I am assuming that _____."
- "I feel certain/convinced/confident that _____."
- "My view/perspective/attitude is that _____."
- "I have concluded that _____."

The content of these beliefs (i.e., whatever you would insert into the spaces above) could essentially be any of the forms of certainty that you itemized in Worksheets 12.1 and 12.2. So try writing out your rigid assumption in the first section of the Mentalizing Your Certainty Toolkit on the following page. For now, don't skip ahead to the additional sections—we're going to take this one step at a time.

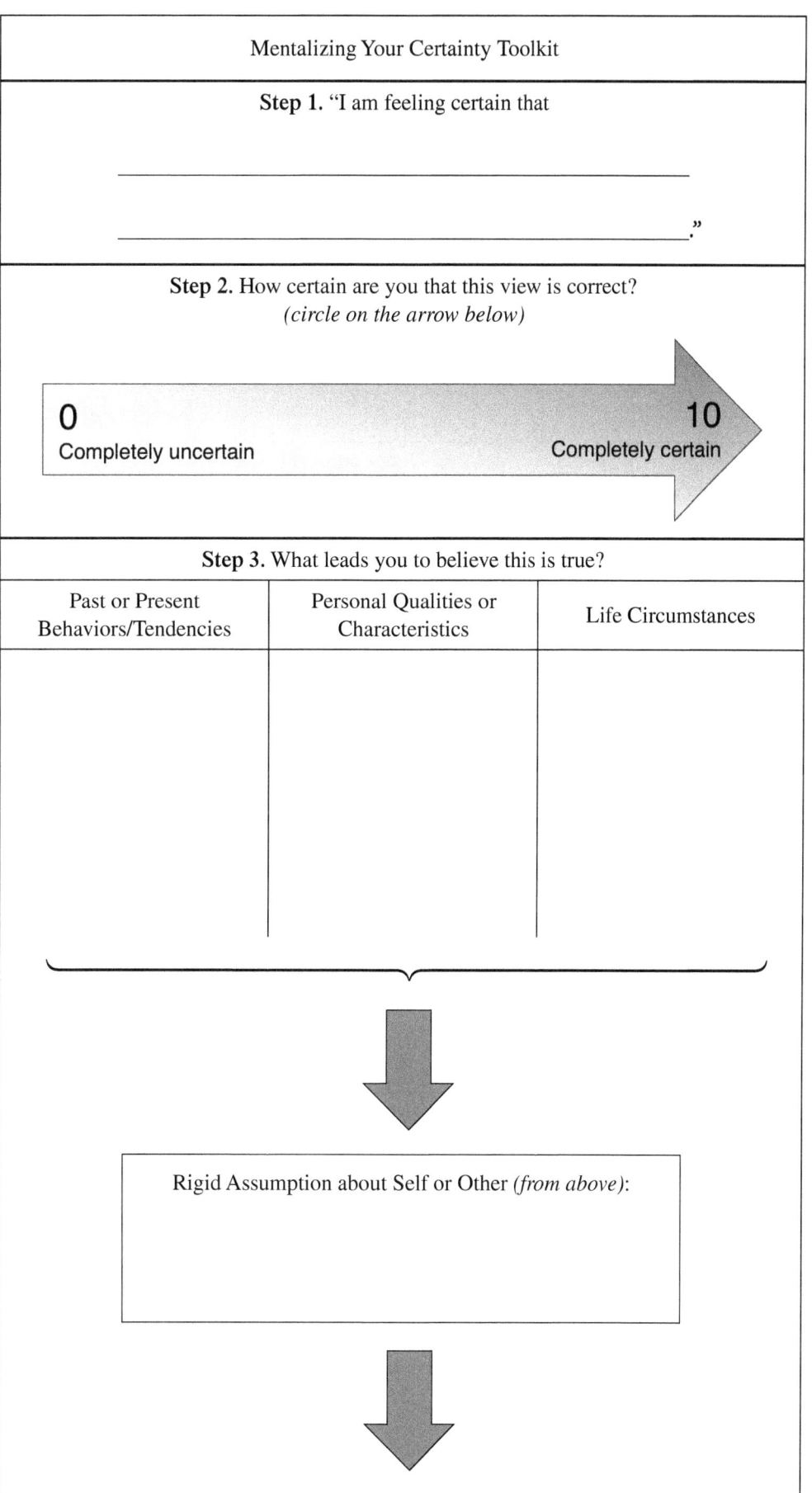

Mentalizing Your Certainty Toolkit

Step 1. "I am feeling certain that

_____

_____."

Step 2. How certain are you that this view is correct?
(circle on the arrow below)

0
Completely uncertain

10
Completely certain

Step 3. What leads you to believe this is true?

Past or Present Behaviors/Tendencies	Personal Qualities or Characteristics	Life Circumstances

Rigid Assumption about Self or Other *(from above)*:

Step 4. What are the consequences of this certainty?		
Your Emotions, Desires, and Self-states	Actions You Take	Impact of Your Actions on Relationships/ Other People

By defining your rigid assumption at the outset, you shift the focus from the perceived "fact" under discussion (e.g., about yourself, other people, or the world) to *your own mind*—your belief or interpretation about that potential fact. And by spelling out the content of your belief, you clarify the focal point of the remaining steps. This prevents confusion, while also increasing the effectiveness of MBT's techniques. In order to pursue greater curiosity and flexibility, you need to first (a) understand *what* you are thinking, and (b) be focused on your *thinking*.

Step 2: Rate your level of certainty in this assumption. Once you have articulated your assumption, ask yourself the question: "How confident am I that this presumption is correct?" To nail this down more fully, challenge yourself to "rate" your level of certainty in your belief state. If zero means "I am not certain at all," and ten means "I am completely certain, believing this with every ounce of my being," how would you rank yourself? Try using the Certainty Meter on Step 2 of the toolkit, in order to place yourself somewhere along the certainty continuum.

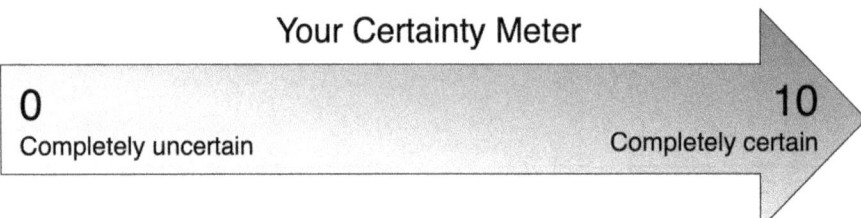

By reflecting on your level of certainty in your belief, you consider not simply "what" you believe, but HOW you are relating to that belief in yourself. Or stated somewhat differently, utilizing the domain-based theory of mentalizing introduced in Chapter 3: You start to mentalize your own psychological processes (e.g., flexibility versus rigidity), in addition to identifying the content of your thoughts. This approach offers a new opportunity for cultivating curiosity and flexibility. If the problem is your degree of certainty in your perspective, then perhaps you can work to decrease the intensity of that certainty, without having to surrender the thoughts and beliefs that feel so true to you.

Step 3: Examine support for the assumption. Now spend some time examining your support for your viewpoint. What leads you to believe that this thing is true? If you were a lawyer arguing a case in front of a judge, this is the "evidence" you would present to justify your argument. Assuming that your rigid belief centers on yourself or other people, such support tends to include past or present actions (i.e., things that you or the other person has done), personal qualities or characteristics, or life circumstances. Check out Step 3 on the toolkit, where these categories are laid out. So if you feel certain that your boss is incompetent, in considering support for that view, you might reflect on his disorganization and forgetfulness *[personal qualities]*, specific poor decisions he has made at your company *[past actions]*, and increased frustration among you and your co-workers *[life circumstances]*. Or if you feel certain that you are unlovable, you could acknowledge your challenges with emotional dysregulation *[personal qualities]*, patterns of instability in romantic relationships *[life circumstances]*, and certain actions you have taken in those relationships that make you feel ashamed *[actions]*.

This "compiling evidence" might seem like a strange technique to use, in a therapy that is supposed to be addressing excessive certainty. Isn't this just adding fuel to the "certainty fire," and thus just making you feel worse? On the contrary, MBT suggests that exploring support for your perspective is an essential step in helping you approach your difficulties in a more flexible way. Flexibility entails seeing things from *multiple* perspectives, including the perspective you are currently endorsing. When you hold some belief in psychic equivalence, there is always some valid, understandable reason why you are feeling so invested in your position. By taking the time to review these reasons, you are honoring the part of you continues to affirm that belief. You thus feel validated and "seen" in your certainty, which paradoxically helps you to become more willing to consider other views on the situation.

Interestingly (and perhaps sneakily on MBT's part), when you examine the support for your perspective, you are implicitly relating to it *as a perspective*, rather than just a brute fact. In other words, you have already begun mentalizing! In many cases, as you take stock of this support, you start to notice holes in your own case: "As I say this now, it starts to sound a little bit foolish. It doesn't really make sense." Or you find that you cannot fully explain *why* you feel so convinced of your view. "I'm not really sure why I believe this. It's like someone asking, 'What makes you think the sky is blue?' It just feels obvious to me." If this happens, hold on to these reflections for later. They will be useful in Step 5, when you consider other views or perspectives on your belief state.

Step 4: Explore the consequences of your certainty. Once you have examined the support for your rigid assumption, shift your attention to the *consequences* of relating to your belief in this way. When you are feeling so certain about the belief in question, how does that affect you and other people in your life? As outlined on the toolkit, such consequences include your own feeling states (e.g., your mood, emotions, desires, and feelings about yourself), your actions and interpersonal tendencies, and the impact of those actions on other people: their emotions, desires, feelings about themselves, overall well-being, feelings about you, and ultimately their manner of treating you (which is usually influenced by all of those internal states).

Returning to the aforementioned examples, if you feel confident that your boss is incompetent, you might end up feeling annoyed and impatient with him *[your feelings]*, sometimes speaking to him dismissively and disrespectfully when you are discussing work projects *[your actions]*. This might make him feel hurt and insecure, but it also places your job at risk, since he could write you up for unprofessional behavior *[impact of your actions on others]*. Or if you feel convinced that you are unlovable, you feel anxious and ashamed *[your emotions]*, desperately crave approval in your relationships *[your desires]*, and relate to other people in a more "needy" and dependent manner *[your actions]*. This can lead other people to feel overwhelmed by you, pulling away from you *[impact of your actions on others]* and leaving you feeling rejected and abandoned *[your subsequent feelings]*.

This step is important for several reasons. When you reflect on the consequences of your certainty, you are implicitly relating to that certainty as a belief state. This underscores that the problem is a *psychological process* in you, rather than simply an objective fact in the world. While this idea might feel invalidating at first, from a therapeutic perspective, it is ultimately good news: You can't usually change the fundamental nature of reality, but you *can* work toward greater curiosity and flexibility in your perspective.

Furthermore, since the consequences of excessive certainty are usually negative in nature, considering these consequences can help you to feel more motivated to address your rigid thinking. In the psychotherapy world, we call this "problematizing" a pattern or tendency: The pattern starts to *feel* like a problem in your life, and so you feel more personally invested in altering the pattern. Even if you feel like you are 100% justified in seeing things a specific way (e.g., that your psychiatric issues are not going to get better, or that some other person has mistreated you), if that belief causes significant distress and suffering for yourself and other people, that is a big strike against it. Over time, as you reflect on the destructive impact of your certainty, you will feel increasingly invested in developing more flexible, curious forms of thinking.

For an illustration of these steps so far, see here for a completed version of the Mentalizing Your Certainty Toolkit, focused on the rigid assumption that your boss is incompetent.

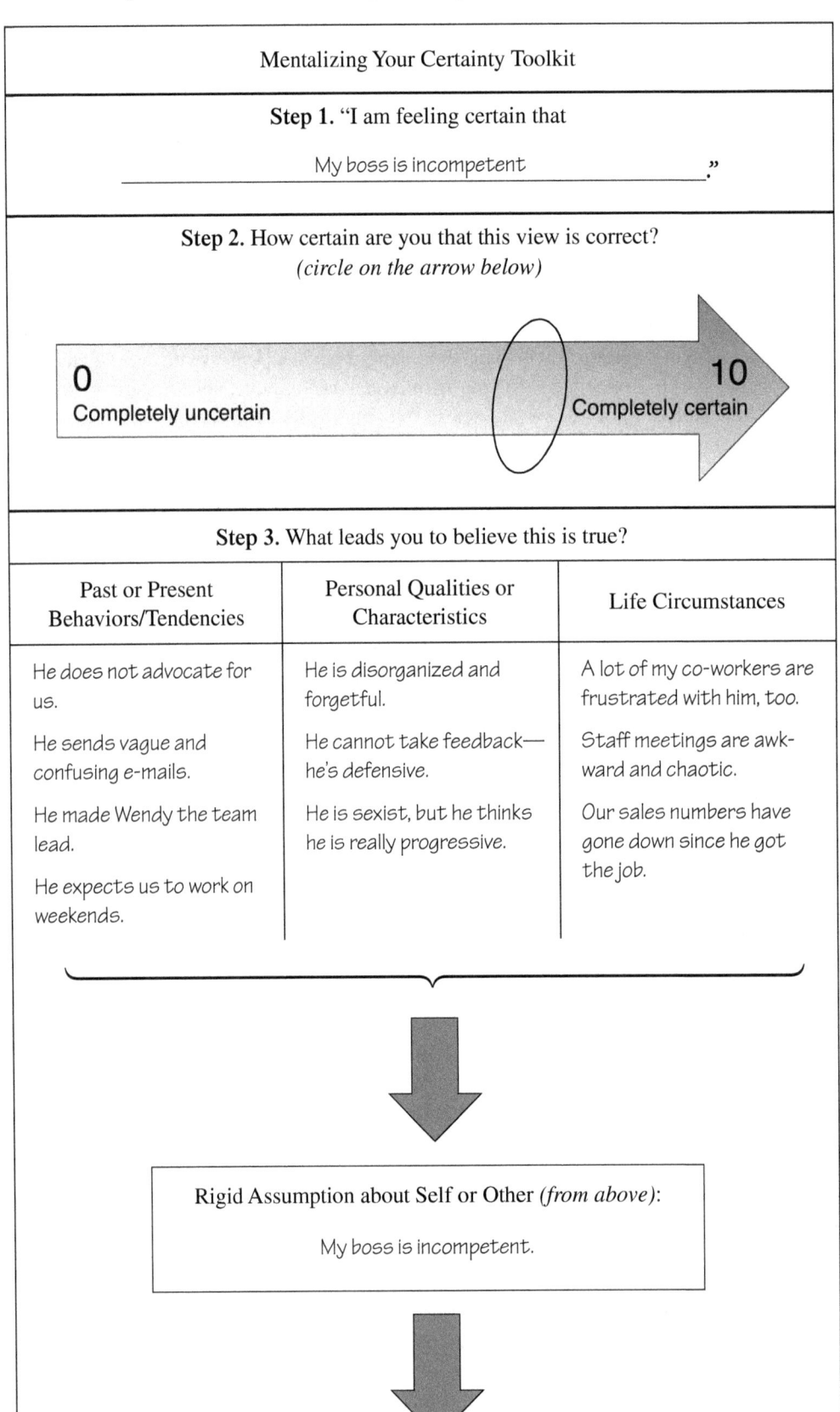

| Mentalizing Your Certainty Toolkit |

Step 1. "I am feeling certain that

My boss is incompetent   "

Step 2. How certain are you that this view is correct?
(circle on the arrow below)

0
Completely uncertain

10
Completely certain

Step 3. What leads you to believe this is true?

Past or Present Behaviors/Tendencies	Personal Qualities or Characteristics	Life Circumstances
He does not advocate for us. He sends vague and confusing e-mails. He made Wendy the team lead. He expects us to work on weekends.	He is disorganized and forgetful. He cannot take feedback—he's defensive. He is sexist, but he thinks he is really progressive.	A lot of my co-workers are frustrated with him, too. Staff meetings are awkward and chaotic. Our sales numbers have gone down since he got the job.

Rigid Assumption about Self or Other *(from above)*:

My boss is incompetent.

Step 4. What are the consequences of this certainty?		
Your Emotions, Desires, and Self-states	Actions You Take	Impact of Your Actions on Relationships/ Other People
I feel annoyed and impatient with him. I end up feeling superior to him, and looking down on him. I desperately want a new job, always fantasizing about quitting and telling him off.	I have spoken to him dismissively and disrespectfully. I delay handing in my work, since I don't really respect him. I spend hours each day looking for new jobs. This gets me behind on my work projects.	He could feel hurt and insecure—I am sure he can tell that I don't like him. My co-workers could feel annoyed with me, since they have to pick up my slack. He could write me up for being a jerk, which puts my job at risk.

Step 5: Consider other views or perspectives on the issue in question. Now that you have mentalized your certainty itself, you are ready for what is perhaps the most challenging step in addressing the psychic equivalence: considering other ways to think about the topic that is occupying you. This is probably the part of MBT that overlaps most significantly with cognitive-behavioral therapy (CBT), the form of therapy that devotes itself to examining alternative perspectives, in order to modify your current maladaptive thoughts (Beck, 2020; Greenberger & Padesky, 2016). But there is a key difference between CBT and MBT: MBT is not suggesting that you try to "get rid of" or alter your original assumption. In contrast, while keeping that assumption right alongside you, look around and try to "take in" other viewpoints on the issue at hand. Our focus is on stimulating a *process* of reflection, rather than on changing the content of your thoughts. As you learn how to reflect on other vantage points in the *exact moment* that you are feeling rigidly attached to some assumption, you increasingly feel less controlled by your thoughts, as well as all of the forms of instability (e.g., in mood, self-esteem, relationships, and behavior) that spring from them.

See below for some mentalizing prompts for contemplating additional perspectives. While these new views sometimes directly challenge your rigidly held belief, often these views simply focus on some additional facet of reality, which does not inherently contradict your original assumption: another person's take on the issue, your perspective at a different moment in time, your own psychological processes, and so on. By "adding in" these new perspectives to your original assumption, you arrive at a more flexible, nuanced, and multi-faceted outlook on the matter at hand.

- Consider other people's outlooks:
  - *Your loved ones' perspectives:* "How would someone I care about view the issue? Can I notice anything valid in this perspective?" Try doing this for a range of important people in your life: your parents, romantic partner, best friend, siblings, and so on. Since you know these people quite well, it is often easier to "put yourself in their shoes" and envision how they might regard the matter. And given that the people in question care about you, their views often introduce a kinder, more benevolent attitude into the reflective process.
  - *Close but not the same:* "Can I imagine someone who would see things in a similar (but not identical) manner as I do? What slight differences can I notice between their view and mine?" Since it is often easier to consider a viewpoint that is

closer to our own, this prompt "takes it slow" by inviting you to regard someone's experience that is almost completely aligned with your own. However, since there will inevitably be *some* differences between the other person's standpoint and yours, you are still working toward a broader array of outlooks on the topic.

- *Reckon with difference:* "Can I imagine someone who would see the situation quite differently from me? What would they think, and what differences can I observe between their view and mine? What feels valid and reasonable about their perspective to me?" This prompt takes it up a notch by encouraging you to grapple with a belief state that significantly departs from your own, AND to simultaneously reflect on the potential validity of this position. This can feel difficult and even threatening, especially when you feel highly invested in your own assumption. However, remember that you do not have to assume or adopt the other person's view, only to truly contemplate the question: "Is there at least some grain of truth to their outlook?"

- *Put yourself in the other person's shoes:* When you are upset or angry with someone, one of the most difficult things to do is to try to put yourself in their shoes. But once you have validated and reviewed the consequences of your certainty (steps 1–4 in the techniques of psychic equivalence), MBT recommends that you do just that, specifically by asking yourself: "How is the other person experiencing the situation? What is their opinion about all of this? Is there anything valid, reasonable, or understandable in their perspective?" When engaging in this inquiry, it is easy to inadvertently interpret the other person's experience through the lens of your own judgment, for example by concluding things like "He just wants to control me" or "She hates me, and she is trying to sabotage me." In contrast, do your best to imagine how the *other* person would describe their experience—from their own standpoint, and in their own words. "If the person were standing right in front of me, what would they say about what they believe, and why they believe it? Is there any part of their perspective that rings true, even in the smallest way?"

- *Import the other person's situation:* Sometimes it feels genuinely impossible to mentalize another individual, either because you are so angry or upset with them, or because you simply cannot imagine what they are feeling. In such cases, MBT recommends that you temporarily skip "putting yourself in the other person's shoes" and instead try bringing the other person's situation to *you.* "If I am struggling to understand what another person is going through, can I try to imagine what it would be like for me if similar things were happening to me in my own life? What would I be feeling and wanting, and what might I think about this whole thing?"

  These queries require less "heavy lifting," at the level of mentalizing. Rather than requiring you to see things from the other person's perspective, they bring the person's situation to *you,* and then you just have to consider your own perspective! This is another way of asking, "How would you feel if the roles were reversed?" For example, if you feel like your therapist is making too big a deal about you being late to your appointments, rather than trying to reflect on your therapist's feelings, consider how YOU feel when people are consistently late when spending time with you. You might notice that you feel hurt, frustrated, and insecure . . . is it possible that your therapist might experience similar emotions? In this way, you can utilize your own self-mentalizing to attain a new perspective on other people's feeling states.

- *Export your own situation:* At other times, you may find it extremely challenging to see your own life situation from a different perspective. Perhaps you are viewing yourself in a highly negative light, or you are struggling with anger and resentment toward others, feeling like they are mistreating you. In moments like this, try imaginatively "exporting" your own circumstance onto someone else, namely by asking yourself: "If another person were experiencing what I am going through, how would I be viewing the situation? What would I say to them, if they were struggling in this way?" In many cases, you will find that you are able to adopt a much more flexible and balanced perspective on the other person's challenges, as compared to your own.

For example, if you are feeling ashamed for relapsing on substances, you might consider how you would view a family member who fell back into their addiction, recognizing your feelings of warmth, care, and concern toward them: "They have been doing such a great job in their recovery. Everybody makes mistakes, and this does not say anything about who they are as a person." Or if you are angry at your partner for not paying enough attention to you, you could imagine what you might say to your close friend who struggles with similar issues: "You often forget to directly communicate your emotions. Have you told Isaac about how you are feeling, and asked him to spend more time with you? He might have no idea that you are so upset."

As a follow-up to these musings, consider: "What differences do I notice between my viewpoint on my scenario, and my viewpoint on the other person in a similar situation? What do I make of these differences?" By reflecting in these ways, you often notice your own natural biases about the situation in question—the ways in which your personal investment in the issue might lead you to approach things in an overly certain, inflexible manner. You can thus become more open to reconsidering your original rigid viewpoint, and to "trying on" a more nuanced attitude toward yourself and your difficulties.

- Work toward greater nuance in your own viewpoint:
  - *"What am I missing?"*: "Are there additional aspects of the topic that are less prominent in my thinking? Is there anything that feels important in the situation that I have not been considering?" This prompt is intentionally broad, so as not to shut down any important forms of reflection. Examples of these "additional aspects" could be mental states in yourself and others, actions and interpersonal approaches, or events and circumstances on which you have not been focused. For example, if you have rigidly focused on the idea that your romantic partner has been acting colder toward you lately, additional elements in the situation could include your feelings of anger toward your partner *[mental states in you]*, your partner's expressed love and commitment to you *[mental states in others]*, or your partner stating that they want to resume date night, so that you two can have more one-on-one time together *[another person's actions]*. Note that none of these considerations necessarily "contradict" your assumption that your partner has been more emotionally removed. They simply highlight aspects of the scenario that are *also* in play, thus contributing to a picture of reality that is likely "broader" and more expansive than your original experience of your partner's attitude.
  - *Nuance across time:* "Can I remember times that I have seen this differently? Could I imagine ever potentially seeing this differently in the future?" These questions essentially invite you to mentalize yourself at different moments in time, by considering ways in which you *have* held an alternative view, or how you *might* hold an alternative view. For example, if you feel highly certain that you need to stop therapy, you might reflect on times in the past where you have really benefited from therapy, or you could consider areas where you

still struggle, which therapy might be helpful in addressing. Even if you find it difficult to attain a more flexible perspective in the present moment, when you reflect on these different perspectives in the past and future, you are broadening the array of outlooks under consideration.

- *Anger and control:* "If I am judging myself for something, are there any ways in which I do not have full control over the issue in question? If I am judging another person for something, how might they not have complete agency in the situation?" Whenever you are feeling judgmental or frustrated with someone, you are usually assuming that the person could be doing something differently (or could have done something differently) in the scenario (Strawson, 2008). This includes yourself! Interestingly, once you reflect on the parts of the experience that are *not* under the person's control, you often feel less upset at the person. Areas of life that are not under an individual's full control include their history, background, and childhood; having certain psychological tendencies (e.g., cognitive capacities, psychiatric diagnoses, emotional challenges); mental states operating outside of awareness; bodily experiences (e.g., physical appearance, medical illness, biology, or temperament); actions and internal states of other parties in their life; and events in the world, including situations of trauma and loss.

  So for example, if you are feeling ashamed about your own history of childhood trauma, you could consider your own lack of agency as a child, as well as the objective actions that other people took to harm you, which you could not have prevented given your real vulnerability. Or if you are feeling resentful at your mother for her intrusiveness and insecurity, you might reflect on her history of childhood neglect, undiagnosed psychiatric issues, and lack of self-awareness about her own emotions and motivations. She did not "choose" to have any of these experiences, and yet they likely play a powerful role in driving her off-putting interpersonal style. Without ignoring the person's own agency and responsibility, this approach broadens your perspective on the issue in question, namely by "adding in" additional reflections about the factors over which none of us have full control. This can open up the door for greater understanding, compassion, and empathy—for other people and also for yourself.

- *"What's my part?":* "Can I identify any of my actions or beliefs that might be contributing to my suffering in this situation? Is there anything I have done that is wrong, ineffective, or unwise that could be playing a role in these challenges?" In Chapter 10, we reviewed how to mentalize behavioral impact—to consider the actions you are taking that could be contributing to how you and others are feeling (see pp. 194–202). The "What's my part?" prompt covers similar conceptual terrain, encouraging you to reflect on your own role in the situation that is bothering you. Such reflections usually focus on two categories of experience: your actions and your beliefs. "Actions" include things you have done (or not done) that could be seen as wrong, ineffective, or unwise, while "beliefs" are your assumptions, expectations, or thought patterns that might be exacerbating your certainty (and thus your suffering) in the scenario.

  So if you are feeling certain that your romantic partner has not been carrying their weight in completing the household chores, you might reflect on your own history of communicating in a critical and aggressive manner toward your partner when talking about this *[actions]*, your lack of setting clear expectations about each person's responsibilities *[actions you have not taken]*, as well as your broader pattern of being hyper-focused on issues of fairness and equality in your relationships *[beliefs]*. Or if you are judging yourself for not being knowledgeable enough in your coursework, you could consider your overly harsh standards for academic performance *[beliefs]*, your tendency to explicitly criticize yourself when you are studying *[actions]*, and your procrastination on assignments when you feel like you are going to fail at them *[actions you have not taken]*. While these reflections do not directly contradict the aforementioned psychic equivalent viewpoints (e.g., that you are not knowledgeable enough, or that your partner is a freeloader), they broaden your perspective by emphasizing your own agency and responsibility in the areas in question.

- Contextualize the certainty:
  - *"What else has happened?"*: "Temporarily bracketing my 'case' for the rigid view, are there any OTHER events or circumstances in my life and history which could be making me feel more certain or attached to this viewpoint? If these things had not happened, how might I be seeing this issue differently?" As discussed in Step 3 in the strategies for psychic equivalence, when you are certain of something, you usually have a "case" or argument for why you are perceiving things correctly. However, your certainty can also be influenced by other events and circumstances in your life, which do not directly support your belief but still could be leading you to feel more attached to it, namely by influencing your expectations, biases, and emotional states. Examples of these events and circumstances include your childhood and developmental history (e.g., involving abuse, neglect, trauma, or other early interactions with caregivers); background in social, family, sexual, or romantic relationships; experiences in school, vocation, or hobbies; events in broader society and culture; and more recent situations in your life and relationships, including in your relationship with the person who is the "focus" of your rigid belief.

    For instance, if you are feeling worried that a romantic partner is cheating on you, you might consider the role that infidelity played in your parents' relationship difficulties, your own history of exes being unfaithful to you, and your partner telling you that they are not sure if they are ready to move in together, which has made you feel insecure about the status of the relationship. These experiences could be leading you to feel more suspicious of your partner, rather than feeling more naturally trusting and comfortable with them.

    Note that these reflections are not simply restating your case for the certainty in question, for example by noticing that your partner sometimes takes a couple of hours to text you back, or that they have been going on more "business trips" lately. By reflecting on *other* events and situations that might be increasing your certainty, you start to see your viewpoint as a somewhat arbitrary "side effect" of your unique personal history, rather than a definitive reflection of reality. This helps you feel more receptive to other ways of seeing the issue in question.
  - *"Where is my mind?"*: Events and circumstances are not the only triggers for your inflexible beliefs; these beliefs can be significantly impacted by *psychological* factors as well. So when you are feeling "stuck" on a certain thought, try asking yourself: "How might this rigid assumption be partially influenced by processes unfolding in my own mind, personality, or emotional life? Is this belief consistent with the symptoms of any of my psychiatric diagnoses or other psychological vulnerabilities?" At first glance, this

mentalizing prompt can come across as highly invalidating, as if it is saying, "You just think this because you are crazy!" However, it can be especially useful in contextualizing beliefs that are often associated with mental health issues or other psychological challenges.

For example, many people with BPD struggle with self-hatred and self-loathing, feeling convinced that there is something inherently bad or defective about who they are as a person. But as we discussed in Chapter 1, self-hatred is actually a *symptom* of BPD, falling under diagnostic criterion #3, "Identity disturbance: markedly and persistently unstable self-image or sense of self." So if you continue to struggle with feelings of self-loathing and worthlessness, this prompt would encourage you to (a) notice the overlap between these feelings and your BPD diagnosis, and to (b) consider the possibility that you might be hating yourself so much not because you *are* so objectively horrible, but because you happen to have a psychiatric diagnosis where people feel convinced that they are objectively horrible.

Feel free to use this prompt if you happen to have other psychiatric diagnoses associated with rigid thinking (e.g., posttraumatic stress disorder, body dysmorphic disorder, eating disorders, obsessive-compulsive personality disorder). "I feel convinced that I am ugly, and that my face looks weird and misshapen. Of course I am aware that people with body dysmorphic disorder get obsessed with flaws in physical appearance. Is it possible that this is just a symptom of my BDD, and I am feeling so disgusted with myself because I happen to have that diagnosis?"

- *Patterns of rigidity:* "Has this ever happened before, where I have felt highly convinced of this sort of thing? What are the similarities between these past scenarios and my current certainty?" When you feel certain about something, you feel like you are accurately perceiving the issue. This is not a "perspective" you are having—it is about the thing itself. However, when you consider other instances of your rigid perspective, you start to contemplate your broader *tendency* to become fixated on particular ideas, rather than whatever specific content is occupying you at the time. Here, the "additional perspective" is this recognition about your own psychology, which can interestingly make you more curious and reflective about your current inflexible assumption.

- *The MBT formulation:* "Does this rigid view resemble any forms of certainty outlined in my MBT formulation, or on Worksheets 12.1 and 12.2 in this book? Could this current situation be an example of me getting overly invested in one particular perspective?" If you happen to be in a formal MBT treatment, you likely already have an MBT formulation, or if you have made it this far in the book, you have completed the worksheets that itemize the forms of certainty with which you struggle. Once again, by considering parallels between your current viewpoint and your other challenges with rigidity, you are placing your certainty in a broader context—namely, the context of *your mind*, and its tendency to stubbornly attach to certain ideas.

- *Mentalize the consequences:* "When I was deeply wedded to my viewpoint in these other scenarios, how did things go—for me and for other people? Were there any negative consequences to my rigidity? If so, what are the chances that similar things could unfold in this current situation?" As reviewed earlier, your challenges with certainty can have a significant negative impact on yourself and other people, resulting in instability in your mood, self-esteem, relationships, and functionality. Sometimes it is easier to recognize these destructive consequences in your past experiences, whereas in your current life, you might be primarily focused on being "right" or justified in your viewpoint. As you notice parallels between your past and current certainty, you can consider the possibility that your present rigidity might lead to similar negative outcomes in your life. This can give you pause, helping you to feel more curious about your *approach* to your thoughts, rather than just their accuracy or validity.

- Take issue with your certainty:
  - *Dismantle the certainty:* "Can I notice any 'holes' in my own argument? Are there any facts or considerations that undermine my position?" This prompt calls upon you to actively work against the grain of your certainty, namely by reflecting on mental states (e.g., thoughts, emotions, desires, self-states), actions or interpersonal approaches, or objective events and circumstances that potentially contradict your own rigid position. For example, if you feel convinced that you are too "needy" and dependent on other people, you might reflect on your improved sense of confidence and self-esteem *[mental states]*, your decreased outreach to others when you are emotionally distressed *[actions]*, and this recent extended period of time when you have not been in a romantic relationship *[events and circumstances]*.

    Or if you feel certain that your boss is overly controlling and aggressive, you could ponder her apparent warmth and appreciation when you see her in the hallway *[mental states]*, her asking for your input on a recent work project *[actions]*, and the fact that many of your colleagues seem to have positive relationships with her *[events and circumstances]*. Remember that you do not have to fully adopt any alternative perspective about the issue in question. However, by actively searching for information that undercuts your rigid assumption, you are cultivating a more complex, multifaceted outlook on the issue under consideration.
  - *Find the exceptions:* "Are there any exceptions to my belief—any facts or considerations that contradict my more general assumption?" This mentalizing inquiry is especially useful when you are thinking in more black-and-white, categorical ways: "always," "never," "everyone," "no one," "completely," "not at all," and so on. So if you are feeling certain that no one has ever truly loved you, you might think about your best friend and your longer-term romantic partner, with whom you are deeply close. Or if you feel like you have never been an effective communicator, you might remember some of your successful presentations at work, or your positive experience expressing your emotions in therapy. When considering these exceptions, you are adding in additional perspectives to your more absolute thinking, which allow for a more nuanced view on the issue in question.
  - *Crack the crystal ball:* "If I am making assumptions about what will (or won't) happen in the future, is there any chance that things might unfold in some other way? What other options are possible here, and what supports these potential outcomes?" As discussed earlier in the chapter, some forms of certainty concern what will (or will not) happen in the future. When you are struggling with these rigid assumptions, try reflecting on other potential outcomes for yourself and others, specifically by considering internal states, actions, or circumstances that might result in these outcomes. For example, if you worry that you will never be able to support yourself financially, consider the strong possibility that this might

end up happening, given your internal motivation to work in your field *[mental states]*, all of your recent job search efforts *[actions]*, and the solid earning potential of your chosen profession *[circumstances and events]*. By imagining this alternative state of affairs, you are "adding in" another outlook to your certainty about the future.

- *Challenge splitting:* "If I am devaluing myself or other people, what facts or considerations contradict those assumptions? If I am rigidly ascribing positive value to myself or others, what facts or considerations undermine those ideas?" As reviewed earlier, when you have BPD, you can often become rigidly attached to highly positive or negative beliefs about yourself and other people—this is the idea of "splitting." In order to broaden your perspective in these moments, this prompt encourages you to reflect on factors (e.g., mental states, actions, events, and circumstances) that might challenge these rigid beliefs.

  So if you are judging yourself as being selfish and self-centered, you could acknowledge your feelings of empathy and compassion for people in emotional distress *[mental states]*, your history of helping out colleagues when they are behind on their work projects *[actions]*, and your active social world, where you regularly connect with friends and loved ones *[events and circumstances]*. Or if you are idealizing a romantic partner, you might reflect on their intermittent feelings of anger or impatience with you *[mental states]*, their history of blowing you off in order to hang out with their friends *[actions]*, and their lack of employment prospects *[events and circumstances]*. With these reflections, you are "adding in" these contradictory experiences to your original viewpoint, thus working toward a broader, more three-dimensional outlook on yourself and other people.

- *Test-drive other perspectives:* Even if you find it challenging to shift your rigid assumptions, there can be value in simply trying to *imagine* alternative perspectives on the topic. "Identify some other way of seeing the issue in question. Now try to imagine: What would it be like if I genuinely saw things in this way? How would I feel, what would I do, and how would my life be different? Would there be any positive consequences to this new perspective, for myself and the people around me?" This prompt invites you to enter into another outlook on the matter at hand, and to reflect on its implications for yourself and other people.

  For example, if you feel certain that you will never have a stable relationship, consider what it would feel like if you believed that you *will* find meaningful connectedness someday. You could picture yourself feeling decreased anxiety, an improved sense of hope, and an increased sense of confidence when interacting with potential romantic partners. In turn, this could lead other people to feel more attracted to you, and to see you in a more positive light. Interestingly, by simply envisioning the positive impact of these new perspectives, you can find yourself feeling more emotionally drawn to them. Over time, this helps you become more receptive to other ways of seeing things, and less devoted to your inflexible viewpoints, with all of their negative consequences.

As you work your way through the above prompts, try to keep track of the additional perspectives that come to you, recording them on the Mentalizing Additional Perspectives Toolkit on the next page. No pressure to respond to all of the prompts. Feel free to just "pick and choose" the ones that feel most interesting to you, or salient to the particular rigid viewpoint under discussion.

Mentalizing Additional Perspectives Toolkit	
Original Rigid Assumption:	
Consider Other People's Outlooks	
Your Loved Ones' Perspective	
Close but not the Same	
Reckon with Difference	
Put Yourself in the Other Person's Shoes	
Import the Other Person's Situation	
Export Your Own Situation	
Work Toward Greater Nuance in Your Own Viewpoint	
"What am I missing?"	
Nuance across Time	
Anger and Control	
"What's my part?"	

Contextualize the Certainty	
"What else has happened?	
"Where is my mind?"	
Patterns of Rigidity	
The MBT Formulation	
Mentalize the Consequences	
Take Issue with Your Certainty	
Dismantle the Certainty	
Find the Exceptions	
Crack the Crystal Ball	
Challenge Splitting	
Test-drive Other Perspectives	

Check out a sample version of the completed toolkit, focusing on the rigid assumption we discussed earlier, "My boss is incompetent."

Mentalizing Additional Perspectives Toolkit

Original Rigid Assumption:
"My boss is incompetent."

Consider Other People's Outlooks	
Your Loved Ones' Perspective	My spouse thinks I am being too hard on him—that he is not that bad.
Close but not the Same	My office mate agrees that our boss has no idea what he is doing. But she likes how much freedom he gives us to do things our own way.
Reckon with Difference	The other people on my team really like him. They say that he is a good person, and that he cares about his workers. I guess they are right about that, but "being a good person" does not make you good at your job.
Put Yourself in the Other Person's Shoes	I bet he is feeling frustrated with me, since I have not been as consistent with my work, and I have had an edge with him. I can understand that—this is not how I want to be acting.
Import the Other Person's Situation	If one of my employees were treating me this way, I would feel really upset, sad, and anxious. I would worry about it all the time. I guess he could be upset too, but he seems a lot more secure than me, so it is hard for me to imagine him getting that worked up about this.
Export Your Own Situation	If this were happening to my best friend and she was approaching it the way that I am, I would probably think she was making too big a deal out of all this. It is just a job, and there are a lot of positive things about the role (e.g., the pay, the hours, it's pretty easy), even if the people in charge kind of suck. I would tell her to chill out and try to enjoy the good parts of the job.
Work toward Greater Nuance in Your Own Viewpoint	
"What am I missing?"	I have not really been thinking about my feelings of insecurity interacting with my boss, the fact that he advocated for me getting a raise, and our improved workflow as a team since he started.

Nuance across Time	I remember really liking him when he first got promoted, and feeling like he was a kind, compassionate person. I could imagine feeling that way about him again, if he got more organized and started communicating better.
Anger and Control	It is not my boss' fault that many of my co-workers are lazy, and that the market was already taking a downturn before he started. He also seems like a naturally anxious person—this is probably not under his control.
"What's my part?"	I have never really tried to get along with my boss. I talk to him in a critical and dismissive way, and I gossip about him to my co-workers. I also probably place too much emphasis on knowledge and competence, rather than the other things that make for a good leader (e.g., integrity, empathy, flexibility).
Contextualize the Certainty	
"What else has happened?"	My father was really critical of me; this makes me feel more sensitive and on edge with men in power. I also got fired from my last job, and my boss gave me that negative performance review recently, so this all probably makes me more defensive and judgmental of him.
"Where is my mind?"	I know that people with BPD often struggle with anger issues, especially when other people reject or criticize them. I have definitely felt like my boss doesn't like me, so I guess my anger toward him could be a reaction to me feeling rejected by him.
Patterns of Rigidity	I have a long history of judging my bosses—feeling like they do not know enough and are doing a bad job. This has basically come up at every job I have ever had.
The MBT Formulation	In the "rigidity and certainty" section of my MBT formulation, my therapist wrote about how I get really angry at people in authority (e.g., bosses, teachers, therapists), devaluing them and getting into conflicts with them. I don't like to admit it, but I guess I could be falling into that same thing again.
Mentalize the Consequences	In those other situations, I have a history of getting angry, acting out, and creating drama at work. My bosses end up getting fed up with me, and I have lost several jobs because of this. It's totally possible that this could happen again, if I don't do something about this.

Take Issue with Your Certainty	
Dismantle the Certainty	He does know a lot about our programs and policies, and he is a good public speaker. Even though he is disorganized, he is charming and charismatic, and a lot of people like him. That probably makes him a more effective leader.
Find the Exceptions	He is not ALWAYS disorganized and incompetent. He did a good job responding to that crisis situation, and he has this bizarre ability to remember specific things going on in his employees lives. People seem to appreciate that.
Crack the Crystal Ball	Not applicable.
Challenge Splitting	He is certainly not "all bad." He really cares about his employees, and given how much he talks about his kids, he seems to be a good father. He is also good at relating to the higher-ups, which is superficial but I guess important.
Test-drive Other Perspectives	I could imagine believing that my boss is intelligent, kind, and knowledgeable in our field. If I saw him in that way, I would probably feel less resentful of him, more fulfilled in my work, and more motivated to do a good job on my assignments. I would treat him with more respect, which could lead him to like ME more.

Step 6: Revisit and reconsider your original assumption. Having reflected upon all of these alternative perspectives on the matter, you can now return to your original rigid assumption, utilizing the Mentalizing a Broader Perspective Toolkit on the next page. In light of these new perspectives, how do you see the issue now? What similarities and differences do you notice between your previous view and your current one? Continuing with the example of the rigid view that your boss is incompetent, you might reflect: "Well, 'incompetent' might be too strong of a word. It's probably more accurate to say that he is disorganized, spontaneous, and distractable, but I guess he also brings some strengths to the job, especially his ability to relate to management and his employees." In comparing this view and your original assumption, both perspectives acknowledge your boss's serious deficiencies, but the newer perspective presents your boss in a more three-dimensional light, with a range of vulnerabilities as well as strengths.

Mentalizing a Broader Perspective Toolkit
Original Rigid Assumption:
Having considered these additional perspectives, what is your view on your original assumption now? What similarities and differences do you notice between your previous view and your current one?
Revisit your initial assumption. How certain are you now that it is correct? Has your level of certainty changed from before? *(circle on the arrow below)*   0   **10**   Completely uncertain   Completely certain
Even if your original belief has not changed, has your outlook on the issue broadened or expanded in any way?   "I still feel strongly that   _____."   *[original rigid assumption]*   "At the same time, I recognize that   _____   _____."   *[new, additional perspective]*

You can also revisit your Certainty Meter. How certain are you now that your original view is correct? Has your level of certainty changed from before? Interestingly, by reflecting on other ways to see the topic in question, and by applying these perspectives to reconsider your original viewpoint, you will often notice yourself feeling slightly less certain about your initial assumption. But don't have too high of a bar here. You might still agree with your original belief, but even if you feel a *tiny* bit less confident in it, or if you feel less emotionally "revved-up" about that belief, that is a huge win from the perspective of mentalizing. This is a sign that you are moving into a stance of greater flexibility, where you can be more receptive and open to other ways of seeing things.

What happens if your original position does not shift in any way, and you still feel just as certain in your view? Remember, in addressing certainty, MBT does not aim to alter the initial belief, but to simply help you attain a more curious, flexible view of the issue in question. We are going for expansion, not negation. So as a final step in targeting your certainty, simply affirm your original view, and then "add in" one or more of the new perspectives you have considered throughout this process. For example, you might still feel like you are unlovable *[initial rigid assumption]*, but you can also acknowledge that perhaps this feeling could be intensified by your recent break-up, which has made you feel more overwhelmed and paralyzed by this experience *[response to the "What else has happened?" prompt]*. Or you could remain convinced that your boss is incompetent *[original rigid assumption]*, while recognizing that you have likely made the situation worse by criticizing him, gossiping with colleagues, and procrastinating with your work *[response to the "What's my part?" prompt]*.

In these ways, you are working toward a broader perspective on your certainty, even though your original position remains intact. Over time, this approach progressively dilutes the psychological power of your certainty, such that you feel less dominated and controlled by your original viewpoint, and more curious about other perspectives on the issue in question. For an illustration of these strategies, see below for a completed version of the Mentalizing a Broader Perspective Toolkit, applied to the rigid assumption we have been examining throughout this section.

Mentalizing a Broader Perspective Toolkit

Original Rigid Assumption:

My boss is incompetent.

Having considered these additional perspectives, what is your view on your original assumption now? What similarities and differences do you notice between your previous view and your current one?

Thinking about it now, "incompetent" might be too strong of a word. It's probably more accurate to say that he is disorganized, spontaneous, and distractable, but I guess he also brings some strengths to the job, especially in his ability to relate to management and his employees.

Revisit your initial assumption. How certain are you now that it is correct? Has your level of certainty changed from before?

(circle on the arrow below)

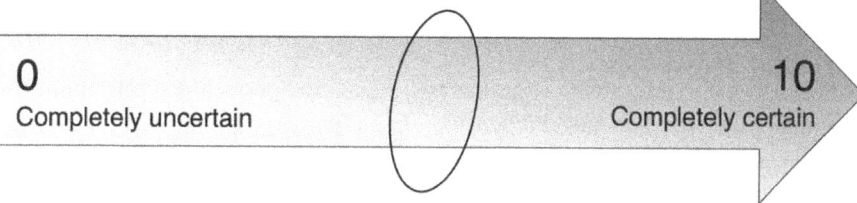

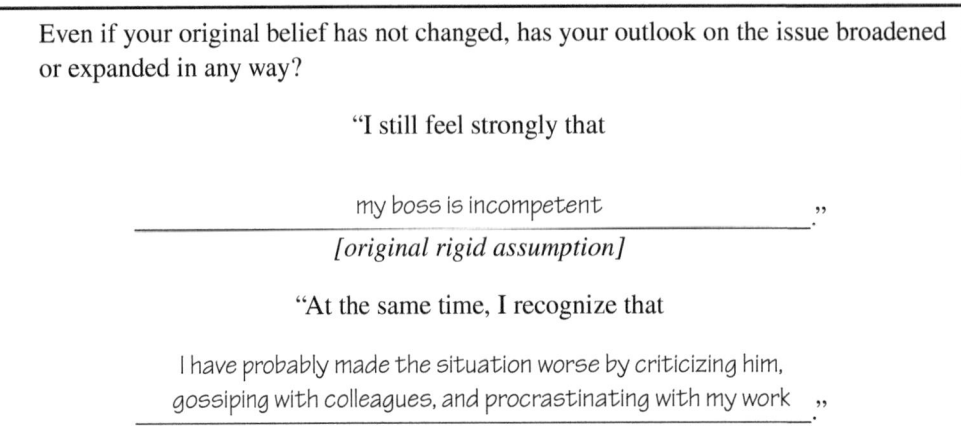

Even if your original belief has not changed, has your outlook on the issue broadened or expanded in any way?

"I still feel strongly that

my boss is incompetent   ,"
_____
[original rigid assumption]

"At the same time, I recognize that

I have probably made the situation worse by criticizing him,
gossiping with colleagues, and procrastinating with my work   ,"
_____
[new, additional perspective]

Mentalizing Cool-down

Now that you have learned the steps for addressing rigidity and certainty in BPD, return to Eleanor's story on page 257. How could Eleanor utilize these principles in her life, in order to address her challenges with black-and-white thinking, self-injury, and risky sexual behavior?

RETURNING TO ELEANOR

At the outset of treatment, Eleanor and her therapist worked together to develop her MBT formulation, outlining the various forms of certainty that would serve as the focus of treatment:

- a powerful sense of self-hatred, including a sense that she deserved to be mistreated and punished;
- the conviction that she was highly inadequate and inferior to other people across multiple domains: intelligence, attractiveness, and social abilities;
- a pattern of basing her sense of self-esteem on other people's views of her: feeling good about herself when men were desiring her sexually, feeling bad about herself if others might see her in a negative light, and a powerful need to avoid others' negative judgments;
- the rigid prediction that she would never be able to complete graduate school and function effectively as an English teacher;
- a highly negative experience of her father (e.g., as angry, powerful, cruel, and taking pleasure in causing her pain); and
- the belief that she had no reason to live and should take her own life, given how defective she was.

In reflecting on her priorities for the therapy, Eleanor expressed a strong desire to curb her self-injury, risky sex, and suicidal behavior. In addition to utilizing MBT's strategies for addressing maladaptive behaviors (see Chapter 5), Eleanor and her therapist focused on the core rigid belief that seemed to be fueling these behaviors: the idea that Eleanor was inherently bad, worthless, and insufficient, thus deserving of punishment and disdain.

Utilizing the Mentalizing Your Certainty Toolkit, Eleanor reflected upon the "evidence" for her certainty (e.g., her shyness, lack of intelligence, social inadequacies, not having a "real job" or stable relationship), as well as its impact on her. Since Eleanor felt so certain that she was inherently flawed, she felt understandably anxious that she was going to fail at every turn, and hopeless about any possibility of change. This certainty also infused all of Eleanor's maladaptive behaviors: her self-injury and risky sex served as a form of self-punishment; her social avoidance and perfectionism were an attempt to hide her deficiencies from others; not applying to graduate school helped her to avoid the failure she knew was going to come; and her suicidality was the ultimate method of completely obliterating her badness. In turn, these behaviors seemed to keep Eleanor perpetually "stuck" in her life. She was not moving forward in her career, she was socially isolated, and she was not pursuing the committed relationship that she really wanted for herself.

As Eleanor reflected on these matters, she increasingly came to recognize that her rigid self-concept was playing a powerful role in fueling her suffering. "Looking at it in black-and-white like this, it seems really clear that my negative view of myself is a big part of why I feel so bad all the time, and why I want to engage in all of these self-destructive behaviors. But I have no idea how to see myself any differently. I would love to have better self-esteem, but that feels completely unrealistic to me, sort of like pretending that global warming isn't happening, or that there is no systemic racism. It sounds nice, but it's just not the way that things are. In my bones, I still *feel* like I am not good enough—it feels 100% true." Interestingly, despite Eleanor's continued conviction in her badness, her focus was shifting slightly. She continued to talk about her deficiencies, but she also increasingly made reference to her *belief* that she was defective. At the level of her experience, her badness was starting to become a mental state, rather than simply a "fact."

Eleanor's therapist introduced the Mentalizing Additional Perspectives Toolkit. Would Eleanor be willing to work toward seeing herself from a different perspective, in the exact moment that she was judging herself? Eleanor agreed to try. Her self-judgments came up most extensively at work, especially when she felt like she made a mistake with a student, or if she worried that her co-workers were looking down on her for her lack of knowledge. In these moments, Eleanor would reflexively think, "I am so stupid, I have no idea what I'm doing. Everybody here knows so much more than me. What is the point of me even being here, if I am so useless at this job?" With her therapist's encouragement, Eleanor started trying to "press pause" in these moments, reflecting on MBT's various mentalizing prompts in order to broaden her outlook on her self-criticisms.

Utilizing the "What am I missing?" prompt, Eleanor acknowledged that she had not been considering a range of her other experiences in her professional role, including the various times that her colleagues had given her positive feedback, as well as situations where she felt like she was really making a difference in her students' lives. Employing the "Where is my mind?" prompt, Eleanor considered how, as part of her BPD as well as her debilitating perfectionism, she could be quite strict and even cruel to herself, holding herself to rigid standards that were nearly impossible to meet: "It doesn't really feel that way, but I guess it is possible that these self-judgments are related to my diagnoses, and my tendency to be really hard on myself." And then considering the "Dismantling the certainty" prompt, Eleanor reflected on her extensive background in childcare, all of the college courses she had taken in education and child development, and the fact that many other teacher's aides at her school had no such background or training. All of these points chipped away at Eleanor's self-concept as someone without knowledge, skill, or competence.

As Eleanor worked to interrupt and reconsider her self-criticisms, she started feeling less ashamed in her work, along with a burgeoning sense of confidence and agency in her abilities as an educator. Encouraged by this progress, she started applying similar strategies to her impulses to engage in self-destructive behavior. When she felt overwhelmed by the desire to self-injure or take suicidal actions, she would direct her focus to her rigid view that there was something fundamentally wrong with her. With the help of MBT's "Challenging splitting" strategies, Eleanor reflected on factors that undermined this negative view of herself, such as her desire to help other people, her strong motivation for treatment, and her commitment to her family. Similarly, when Eleanor was gripped by the impulse to engage in risky sex, she worked to disrupt the idea that her only value was serving as a sexual object for men. Applying the "Nuance across time" techniques, she remembered her experience prior to this darker period in her life, when she longed to find a stable, loving connection with a romantic partner, with whom she could build a family. She did not quite know how to get there, but part of her still believed that this might be possible.

In these ways, Eleanor worked to broaden her perspective on her rigid negative views of herself. Over time, Eleanor's self-destructive impulses started to fall away, like dead leaves on a new branch. They arose in her less frequently, and when they did, they seemed far less compelling to her. She stopped cutting and burning herself, stopped walking into the street with her eyes closed, and stopped having risky sex with anonymous partners. As Eleanor's confidence in herself grew, she decided to finally apply to graduate school in education. To her surprise, she got in, and she proceeded to get straight A's in all of her classes. While she initially tried to write this off as a fluke ("My professors are really easy graders"), as the positive feedback continued to roll in from her professors and mentor teachers, it became more challenging for Eleanor to hold on to her view that she was unintelligent and incompetent. Her experience was starting to disturb her negative self-concept.

Despite all of this progress, there was one area of Eleanor's life that consistently threatened her emotional stability: her relationship with her father, whom she continued to see as an all-powerful monster. Eleanor felt overwhelmed with rage toward him, and at the same time panicked and vulnerable whenever she was in his presence. Eleanor reflected on the support for this experience of her father (e.g., his impatience, continued critical comments, and controlling tendencies toward her mother), as well as how it impacted her to view him in this way: "I am just a puppet on a string with him. It's humiliating—he has so much control over how I feel at any given moment." Utilizing the "Find the exceptions" prompt, Eleanor asked herself: "Are there any facts or considerations that contradict my view of my father as this omnipotent, invulnerable villain?" Eleanor observed how most people in her family seemed to shun her father, such that he spent so much of his time alone and isolated at family events. Looking at him there, he seemed sad, lonely, and even confused about how to be relating to other people. He also came across as physically weak and frail, and so *old*, compared to how she remembered him in her childhood.

Eleanor also noticed how her father would often reach out to her over text to tell her about some business accomplishment or financial venture: "It's like he wants me to be impressed with him or something. He's trying to have a relationship with me, and the only way he can think to do that is to talk about his work. I think he knows how much I hate him, and that makes him feel uncomfortable, or insecure." The therapist observed that it actually sounded like Eleanor had a lot of emotional power over her father, rather than just the other way around. Eleanor was shocked to consider this, but she could not deny that it seemed to be true.

Through utilizing all of these strategies, Eleanor gradually developed a more three-dimensional picture of her father. Sure, he was aggressive, mean, and spiteful, but he was also lonely, insecure, and somewhat clueless about what was going on in his life. "I used to feel so terrified of him. But now I just feel kind of sad for him, and sorry for him. He has driven everyone away from him, and he is all alone, but he genuinely has no idea why this has happened, or what to do to make it better. I still don't like him, but I feel for him. I know this cannot be easy."

Interestingly, as Eleanor's views of her father evolved, her own sense of self-worth seemed to follow suit. Her feelings of anxiety and self-loathing significantly improved, and she began experiencing a sense of calm, self-assuredness, and quiet dignity that she brought with her wherever she went. "All this time, I just thought that is who my father *was*—some all-powerful monster who had control over everybody. But by holding on to this rigid view of him, I was unwittingly disempowering myself, placing myself in the role of this weak, powerless victim who had no agency. I don't really understand it, but now that I am seeing him as basically just a person, I get to be a person as well. There's something liberating in that."

Armed with this newfound sense of her own value, Eleanor finally took the step of starting to date again. While the process was not easy, she is now in a stable, committed relationship, with a man who cherishes her and treats her with love and respect. To her surprise, when she finished graduate school, she was offered a job at the same school where she completed her student teaching. She currently works as a high school English teacher there. She stands in front of that classroom every day, discussing literature and helping students learn how to express themselves through the written word.

"I never thought that this would be possible for me—I just hated myself so much, and I didn't think that I had anything to offer. But when they offered me this job, I couldn't really deny it anymore: The way that people were seeing me was just so different from how I saw myself. So now when I start to judge myself, I am able to consider the possibility that maybe this is just me being hard on myself again, rather than the way that I actually am. Maybe this is just a perspective, and not a fact. I still have a long way to go, but I feel like I am finally starting to feel better about myself—more open to the idea that I am not as bad as I think I am."

Chapter Review 12.1
Introduction to the Non-mentalizing Modes

Process-related Deficits in Mentalizing

- Process-related problems in mentalizing are disruptions in "how" you relate to mental states in yourself and others.

- Mentalization-based treatment (MBT) refers to these disruptions as *non-mentalizing modes*, also dubbed "pre-" or "low" mentalizing modes. There are three different non-mentalizing modes:

  - **psychic equivalence mode,** or difficulties with certainty and rigidity in your thinking;

  - **teleological mode,** or challenges with concreteness and externalization; and

  - **pretend mode,** or trouble with disconnection and dissociation.

- These problems with reflectiveness parallel forms of thinking that children exhibit before they develop the full capacity for mentalization.

- Despite the term "non-mentalizing," these modes are not black-and-white. At any given moment, there are ways in which you are probably employing ineffective forms of thinking (e.g., rigidity, concreteness, disconnection), while simultaneously also engaging in helpful, adaptive reflectiveness about mental states in yourself and others.

The Non-mentalizing Modes in Borderline Personality Disorder

- People with borderline personality disorder (BPD) suffer from *attachment-related* disruptions in mentalizing: When your need to connect with other people gets stimulated or threatened, your "good" mentalizing can go offline.

- Then the "bad" mentalizing starts to creep in:

  - you become highly certain in your perspective *[psychic equivalence mode]*;

  - you focus excessively on external things *[teleological mode]*; or

  - you lose contact with yourself and other people *[pretend mode]*.

- When these forms of thinking take hold, you experience all of the instability in mood, self-esteem, relationships, and behavior that are endemic to BPD.

- By helping you to continue mentalizing when you are under emotional stress, MBT tries to prevent you from falling into these non-mentalizing modes, enabling you to achieve greater stability in your life.

[continued on next page]

Attachment insecurity

"Good" mentalizing goes offline

Emergence of non-mentalizing modes

Certainty   Concreteness   Disconnection

Functional challenges in mood, self-esteem,
relationships, and behavior

Chapter Review 12.2
Psychic Equivalence Mode: Excessive Certainty and Rigidity

Introduction to Psychic Equivalence Mode

- Psychic equivalence mode involves excessive certainty and rigidity in your thinking, beliefs, and viewpoints.

  - "If I think it, that makes it true."

  - You feel like you are accurately perceiving reality: *This is actually what's going on.*

  - Your thoughts do not feel like "thoughts"; you experience them as FELT FACTS.

  - When you are in psychic equivalence mode, you find it very challenging to consider alternative perspectives.

  - Sometimes you assume that other people already see things the same way that you do, while at other times, you simply believe that they *should* see things the way that you do.

- You can hold psychic equivalent beliefs about a wide range of topics: yourself; other individuals; groups of people or organizations; concrete events and occurrences in the world; and even abstract concepts or principles.

- Chronologically, these beliefs can concern the past ("I was not a good enough—that is why my partner left me"), the present ("I am still not good enough: I am boring, weak, and overly emotional . . . "), or the future ("I will never be good enough, so there is no hope for me").

- When you feel highly certain of your perspective, that perspective dominates and controls your life, leading to instability in your mood, self-esteem, relationships, and behaviors.

Rigid Beliefs about Yourself

- In borderline personality disorder (BPD), your rigid, overly certain beliefs about yourself could variously focus on:

  - *Your own characteristics or abilities:* "I am ugly, unattractive"

  - *Your psychology and internal states:* "I am too needy and emotionally sensitive"

  - *Your actions and behavior:* "What have I done? Now I have destroyed everything"

  - *Your concrete life circumstances:* "This place is so toxic, stifling, and oppressive"

  - *Negative evaluations of yourself:* "I am worthless and unlovable. I just drive people away from me"

  - *Positive evaluations of yourself:* "I am the only person at that job who actually cares about the clients"

  - *Standards or expectations for yourself:* "I should not need attention from other people. It is weak and pathetic"

  - *Experiences of self or identity:* "I need to be in a relationship to feel OK"

  - *Predictions about the future:* "I am never going to get better"

[continued on next page]

Rigid Beliefs about Other People

- In BPD, your rigid, overly certain beliefs about other individuals can focus on:

  - *Other people's characteristics or abilities:* "My co-workers have no idea how to do their jobs"

  - *Others' psychology and internal states:* "He is such a narcissist"

  - *Other individuals' actions and behavior:* "My mom never should have said that to me"

  - *Other people's concrete life circumstances:* "Everybody in this class is doing better than me"

  - *Negative evaluations of other people:* "He is the worst boss I have ever had"

  - *Positive evaluations of other people:* "She is everything I want to be"

  - *Standards or expectations for others:* "He needs to get his shit together: get a job, move out of his parents' house, and start going to therapy"

  - *Predictions about other people in the future:* "I know that she is going to break up with me"

  - *Tendency to base your own mental states on others' mental states:* "I need my partner to be happy with me, in order to feel good about myself"

Chapter Review 12.3
Mentalizing Practice Points: Mentalizing Your Certainty

When you are suffering, mentalization-based treatment (MBT) encourages you to actively wrestle with the question: "Where is the certainty?"

Rather than trying to "delete" any of your thoughts, work to recognize that these are thoughts in your mind (not necessarily facts), and then consider other ways to see the situation. You will thus be able to stand right alongside your original belief, while also acknowledging the potential validity of other viewpoints.

The first step in this process involves mentalizing your own certainty.

Mentalizing Your Certainty Toolkit
Step 1. "I am feeling certain that _____ _____."
Step 2. How certain are you that this view is correct? *(circle on the arrow below)*   0 — Completely uncertain ······························ 10 — Completely certain

Step 3. What leads you to believe this is true?		
Past or Present Behaviors/Tendencies	Personal Qualities or Characteristics	Life Circumstances

[continued on next page]

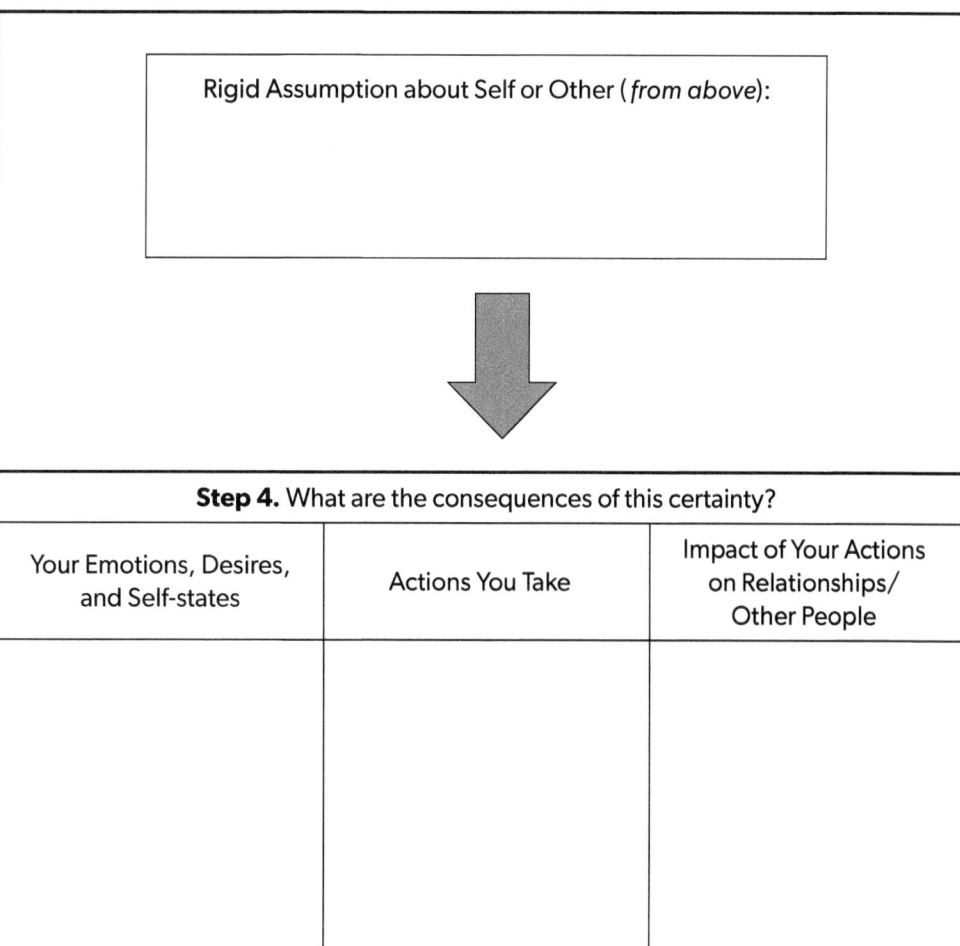

Chapter Review 12.4
Mentalizing Practice Points: Developing Greater
Curiosity and Flexibility

Once you have reflected on the support for (and consequences of) your rigid assumption, work to develop greater curiosity and flexibility around that assumption.

To that end, utilize the Mentalizing Additional Perspectives Toolkit to consider other outlooks on your original viewpoint. Then, employing the Mentalizing a Broader Perspective Toolkit, try to attain an expanded outlook on the issue in question.

Mentalizing Additional Perspectives Toolkit	
Original Rigid Assumption:	
Consider Other People's Outlooks	
Your Loved Ones' Perspective	
Close but not the Same	
Reckon with Difference	
Put Yourself in the Other Person's Shoes	
Import the Other Person's Situation	
Export Your Own Situation	

[continued on next page]

Work Toward Greater Nuance in Your Own Viewpoint	
"What am I missing?"	
Nuance across Time	
Anger and Control	
"What's my part?"	
Contextualize the Certainty	
"What else has happened?"	
"Where is my mind?"	
Patterns of Rigidity	
The MBT Formulation	
Mentalize the Consequences	

[continued on next page]

Take Issue with Your Certainty	
Dismantle the Certainty	
Find the Exceptions	
Crack the Crystal Ball	
Challenge Splitting	
Test-drive Other Perspectives	

[continued on next page]

Mentalizing a Broader Perspective Toolkit
Original Rigid Assumption:
Having considered these additional perspectives, what is your view on your original assumption now? What similarities and differences do you notice between your previous view and your current one?
Revisit your initial assumption. How certain are you now that it is correct? Has your level of certainty changed from before? *(circle on the arrow below)* **0** Completely uncertain **10** Completely certain
Even if your original belief has not changed, has your outlook on the issue broadened or expanded in any way? "I still feel strongly that _____." *[original rigid assumption]* "At the same time, I recognize that _____ _____." *[new, additional perspective]*

13

Addressing Problems with Externalization and Concreteness

Kristin sought out mentalization-based treatment (MBT) to address her difficulties with emotional dysregulation, restrictive eating, and debilitating perfectionism. A highly sensitive child, Kristin remembers experiencing emotions that were always "too big" or "too much" for every situation: desperate worry that other children would not like her, panic that she would fail in her classes, and overwhelming sadness and shame when she felt like other people were judging or rejecting her. While Kristin's father was empathic and understanding about her challenges, her mother felt impatient with Kristin's emotionality, responding by trying to talk her out of her feelings: "Why are you so upset about this? Everything is fine!" Kristin was placed on psychiatric medications from an early age, and she learned to feel ashamed of her emotions: "Everyone was trying to 'turn down the volume' of my feelings, but no matter how many meds they pumped into me, it wouldn't work. I felt like there was something intrinsically wrong with me: I was weak, defective, and too much for everyone around me."

Kristin coped with her emotions by *doing* things—taking actions that enabled her to feel like she had some control over her chaotic internal world. By the time she reached adolescence, Kristin had arrived at a perfect formula for feeling good about herself: getting straight A's, going to an Ivy League college, remaining impeccably thin, wearing designer clothes, being articulate and well-spoken, and securing the interest and attention of attractive and powerful men. When Kristin was able to meet these standards, she experienced a temporary sense of relief, calm, and self-esteem.

But the problem was that this feeling never "stuck." If Kristin ever felt like she was failing in these areas (e.g., by getting a bad grade, gaining weight, or getting rejected by a romantic partner), that same chaotic, out-of-control feeling would return. Kristin would then apply willpower to succeed in the area in question (e.g., by studying more, going shopping, doing extracurricular activities), now directing her mother's dismissive refrain toward herself: "You're fine, you're fine. Everything is fine." When these strategies could not completely eliminate her distress, Kristin would sometimes engage in more self-destructive actions (e.g., promiscuity, cutting herself with razors, restricting her food) in order to "shut off" her mind, and to regain a sense of connectedness with herself.

Armed with her high intelligence and ambition, Kristin was able to meet many of those external benchmarks for success in life. She attended that Ivy League college; she got married to an attractive, wealthy hedge fund manager; and she built a career in public relations, ultimately attaining a high-status position at a public relations firm. Yet despite all of these achievements, Kristin continued to struggle with extreme instability in her emotions and self-esteem.

At work, Kristin was continuously focused on her performance, placing a tremendous pressure on herself to always be productive and efficient, and (perhaps most importantly) to *appear* productive and efficient to her colleagues and supervisors. When her supervisors

Mentalization. Robert P. Drozek, Oxford University Press. © Oxford University Press 2025.
DOI: 10.1093/oso/9780198916857.003.0013

were giving her positive feedback about her work, she was able to feel like she was doing a good job in her role, and to feel stable in herself as a person. But if they ever failed to give her direct and explicit validation (e.g., by not responding to her e-mails, not complimenting her presentation, not giving her a promotion), she experienced intense emotional dysregulation, shame, and anger. "For me, actions speak louder than words. If they really valued me, they would SHOW that they valued me. But when it's just silent, I start to go down a rabbit hole: I'm not good enough, they *know* that I'm not good enough, and it's just a matter of time before they fire me and find someone who actually knows what they're doing."

Kristin's insecurities expressed themselves outside of work as well. Despite the fact that she was objectively attractive, she was terrified that she was gaining weight, or becoming less attractive as she got older. She coped with these feelings by checking her appearance in mirrors throughout the day, turning off Self View in Zoom meetings, skipping meals to decrease her caloric intake, and getting Botox injections, to forestall the aging process. When she noticed some imperfection in her appearance, or if she felt like her clothes were feeling too tight on her, she would talk to herself in a highly critical, unkind way: "You are so disgusting, so gross. How can you even go out of the house when you look this way? You're embarrassing yourself."

Kristin also struggled with defensiveness and interpersonal conflict in her marriage. Her husband Mark was loving but quite perfectionistic himself, and he would often give Kristin constructive feedback about how she was completing their shared chores, household responsibilities, and life tasks. Kristin felt like Mark was judging her in those moments, looking down on her and seeing her as incompetent. She would quickly become defensive—feeling enraged with him, insulting him, and telling him why he was incorrect about the matter in question. She would spend days upon days feeling resentful and victimized by Mark, leading to decreased intimacy and estrangement in their relationship. It felt clear that HE was the problem in the relationship, and that he needed to be different in order for her to feel a sense of peace and satisfaction in her life.

Kristin thus remained caught in a vicious cycle of instability: needing external things in order to feel good about herself, but in her pursuit of these things, continuously feeling like her life was not under her own control. She began to experience suicidal thinking and fantasies. "I do not really want to kill myself, but it would probably just be easier if I just never woke up in the morning. At least then I would not have to deal with all of these feelings."

EXTERNALIZATION AND CONCRETENESS IN YOUR BELIEFS ABOUT YOURSELF

As discussed at the start of Chapter 12, teleological mode involves externalization and concreteness in your thinking, beliefs, and viewpoints. The first clue that you are in teleological mode is your excessive focus on primarily external or "visible" factors in yourself or other people. Examples of external factors include:

- physical appearance;
- actions, behavioral patterns, and interpersonal approaches;
- interactions (or the lack of interaction) with specific people, groups, or animals;
- academic, professional, or social status;
- money, objects, or material possessions;
- visible events or circumstances, whether in your immediate environment or your life more broadly;
- places, settings, or geographical locations;

- chronology and time (e.g., particular times of day, specific days of the week or month, certain times of year);
- medical issues or bodily processes;
- events happening in broader society, culture, and the world; and
- relationships or affiliations with certain people, organizations, or groups.

When you are in teleological mode, you are not simply *attentive* to these external elements, the way that you might be when you are stuck at the external pole of mentalizing reviewed in Chapter 11. Rather, you end up *relying* on external factors to structure your experience of yourself and others, such that these factors hold an inordinate sway over how you feel about yourself, and how you interpret and understand other people. For this reason, MBT's motto for describing teleological mode is "The outside determines the inside." In this state, you become something like a puppet on a string: your emotions and beliefs get involuntarily controlled by the world around you, and you lack a full sense of agency in your life.

On this view, the defining feature of teleological thinking is the tendency to rigidly conflate, associate, or "link" the aforementioned external factors with mental states in yourself and others. With yourself, you might assume that you can only feel OK *[mental state]* if you get a new job *[external circumstance]*, or that you need to use drugs or alcohol *[behavior]* in order to alleviate your anxiety *[mental state]*. With other people, you may presume that your friend is angry with you *[mental state]* because they have not reached out to you recently *[another person's behavior]*, or that your co-worker is happy and fulfilled *[mental state]* because they are married, make a lot of money, and live in a fancy community *[external circumstances]*.

Sometimes you might explicitly formulate these teleological beliefs, for example if you think, "I will not be able to relax until I get a new job" or "It has been so long since she has texted me—I think she is done with me." At other times, you simply encounter the *consequences* of the teleology (e.g., quick assumptions about the meaning of others' actions; powerful emotions in response to external circumstances; intense desires to take a certain action, or for some event to transpire), with minimal awareness that you are implicitly "linking" some external and internal process. Furthermore, you can engage in teleological thinking about yourself and others at various moments in time: in past scenarios ("He spoke harshly to me, so that means he was looking down on me"), in present scenarios ("I have been unemployed for so long—I feel horrible about myself"), or in future or hypothetical scenarios ("If they do not have sex with me by the third date, they are definitely not attracted to me").

When patients and therapists are learning about MBT, one of the most common questions they ask is: "What is the difference between psychic equivalence mode and teleological mode? They seem pretty similar to me." In fact, both modes involve excessive rigidity and certainty in your thinking, but teleological mode involves a specific type of certainty—namely, certainty about the necessary *relationship* between external and internal factors. "This *[external thing]* means that *[internal thing]*." So teleology could be seen as an important "species" of psychic equivalence, one that involves you endorsing some rigid formula, along the lines of EXTERNAL = INTERNAL.

Let's consider some of the main examples of teleological thinking focused on yourself and your own experience.

- *Linking your feelings with your subsequent actions:* You might reflexively presume that, if you are feeling a particular way, you need to take some action in order to manage that feeling. For example, you could feel like you have to reach out to an ex-romantic partner whenever you feel lonely, that you need to cut yourself if you feel ashamed, or that you need to use substances when your cravings reach a certain level of intensity. You can thus get "tugged around" by your emotions, such that THEY are governing you, rather than the other way around.

- *Connecting your actions with your positive mental states:* You might also automatically associate particular behaviors with certain positive experiences *after* you take some action. For example, you could reflexively presume that you need to take some action in order to experience some positive emotion ("If I just spend all day studying, then I can feel good about myself"), or to decrease certain painful feelings ("If I eat this whole bag of chips, then I can get rid of this anxiety"). It is important to note that *avoidance* is a behavior as well, so you might feel like you need to stay away from some circumstance (e.g., a social, work, academic, family, or romantic interaction) in order to regulate your distress, and to protect yourself psychologically. All of these forms of teleology can lead to significant difficulties with compulsive behavior, impulsivity, and maladaptive interpersonal approaches. Since you are convinced that the action in question is so unequivocally *necessary*, you end up feeling compelled to do the thing, without fully reflecting on the short- and long-term consequences for yourself and other people.

- *Connecting your actions with your painful emotional states:* You also could assume that particular actions will definitely lead to painful emotions in you. For instance, you may believe that taking some action will exacerbate your distress ("I cannot go to that in-person support group . . . it will make me too anxious"), or decrease your positive emotions ("I have been in such a good mood lately. If I talk about my trauma, I am going to lose all of that"). Remember, NOT doing something counts as an action, too. So you could also presume that *refraining* from engaging in some maladaptive behavior (e.g., self-injury, criticizing someone, abusing substances, promiscuity) will generate challenging emotions in you, which will then intensify your urge to take the problematic action. "If I don't e-mail my boss giving him a piece of my mind, I am just going to keep ruminating about this all day. So I had better click 'send'. . . ." As above, this form of teleology results in various forms of addictive, compulsive behavior. Your life becomes lopsided, since you become excessively reliant on a handful of behaviors in order to regulate your emotions, while "staying away" from more adaptive behaviors that might grant you greater flexibility and fulfillment in your life.

- *Associating your visible personal characteristics with positive emotions in yourself:* In addition to connecting your feelings to your behavioral tendencies, you could also base them on your own concrete personal characteristics, such as your appearance, weight, clothing, or physical traits. For example, you might only feel confident if you are beneath a specific weight, or you only feel relaxed and comfortable if you dress a certain way in public. These processes contribute to difficulties with perfectionism and excessive self-focus. Your gaze turns primarily toward yourself, and you work tirelessly to contort yourself into an ideal that you can never fully reach. Or if you do reach the ideal (e.g., by buying the right clothes or making sure that the camera catches you at just the right angle), you feel a constant sense of pressure to *keep* meeting it, in order to maintain your sense of psychological well-being.

- *Associating your visible personal characteristics with painful emotions in yourself:* When these forms of teleology are in play, you end up experiencing more aversive emotions if you ever fail to meet your own externalized standards. For instance, you feel highly insecure if your face looks puffy, depressed if your jeans feel tight, or anxious during sexual situations, when someone else can see your body. This type of thinking can make you feel ashamed, self-conscious, and uncomfortable in your own skin, along with a constant sense of stress and anxiety that you are not measuring up.

- *Correlating external situations with positive emotions in yourself:* You could also link your emotions to various external circumstances of your life, such that you feel like you can "only feel good" if certain events and situations end up happening to you. Examples of this include basing your feelings on interpersonal relationships and interactions ("I need my partner to validate me, in order to feel emotionally safe in our relationship"); on other interpersonal relationships and interactions NOT happening ("I love hanging out with my parents, as long as they don't start talking about my childhood"); on work-related events ("I have to keep getting promoted, in order to really feel good about myself in this job"); on scenarios related to pets or animal companions ("I just need to find out that Milo is OK, and then I can focus on my work again"); on financial situations ("Once I am financially independent, I know that I will start feeling better about myself"); on issues of body, health, and appearance ("If I could lose at least ten pounds, I would be a lot less anxious in social situations"); on circumstances in your living situation ("I have to get out of this apartment, before my depression can get any better"); on conditions in your immediate environment ("As soon as the weather got nicer, my suicidality went away"); on time and chronology ("I can only feel focused and motivated when I first get up in the morning"); or on events in broader society and culture ("If we could just get this guy out of office, I could actually feel proud to live in this country again").

  In these ways, you implicitly set up "rules" for experiencing positive emotions, such that it ends up feeling like your emotional stability is significantly controlled by the world around you. This leads to a much narrower window for psychological well-being. As long as the world meets your expectations, you can feel OK, but as soon as it departs from those standards, you can get thrown into states of instability and unrest, including intense anxiety, shame, and anger. This brings us to . . .

- *Correlating external situations with painful emotions in yourself:* You might also draw connections between certain external factors with *painful* emotions in yourself. For instance, you could feel convinced that you are going to experience distress and discomfort in specific interpersonal relationships and interactions ("When my partner speaks critically to me, I immediately get angry"); when other interpersonal relationships and interactions do NOT happen ("If she leaves my text on 'read,' I feel insecure, and worried that she is upset with me"); in the context of work-related events ("If I do a bad job on that assignment, I am going to feel horrible about myself"); in scenarios related to pets or animal companions ("If anything happens to my cat, I will not have any reason to live anymore"); in financial situations ("I get so anxious whenever I get a new bill"); surrounding issues of body, health, and appearance ("This breakout is making me feel so ashamed and embarrassed"); in circumstances related to your living situation ("I need to get out of this state. My mental health has gone downhill since I moved here"); involving conditions in your immediate environment ("I feel so overwhelmed if there is too much going on around me"); surrounding time and chronology ("I always get depressed at this time of year"); and related to events in broader society and culture ("The whole world is going up in flames—I am living in a constant state of panic and dread").

When you allow your emotions to be determined by these external factors, your sense of psychological stability remains perpetually out of reach. Since you often have no direct control over these factors, you can experience distress and suffering at the drop of a hat, significantly dictated by what is happening around you at any given moment. This results in difficulties with depression, anxiety, and emotional instability, along with an overall sense of hopelessness and powerlessness in your everyday life.

- *Teleological self-esteem:* As we have discussed elsewhere (Drozek et al., 2023), many patients with personality disorders struggle with what we call *teleological self-esteem*—that is, a pattern of basing your sense of self-worth on largely visible factors, such as attractiveness; physical appearance (e.g., involving weight, clothing, or physical traits); possessions; effective behavioral performance; vocational or social standing; and interactions and relationships with specific people, organizations, or groups. With teleological self-esteem, you feel like you only have value and worth if you fulfill and actualize these visible factors, for example when you are succeeding in your career, when other people are giving you positive feedback, or when you are in a relationship with a specific person. Rather than recognizing your own inherent value as a person, you feel like self-esteem is something that has to be "earned"—you always need to be working to perfect yourself, or to attain that carrot that is going to endow you with a sense of value. This is exhausting. The good feeling just never stays put, and over time, you start to feel depressed, empty, and demoralized.

- *Teleological shame:* The underbelly of teleological self-esteem is teleological *shame*—that is, the tendency ascribe negative value to yourself when you fail to meet the aforementioned visible conditions. You thus feel badly about yourself when you look a certain way, if you do not make a specific amount of money, if you feel like you have done a poor job at some task, if you are not successful enough at work or school, or if you are not in a relationship with a particular person. Since your value perpetually rests outside of yourself, your badness is always lurking around every corner. This gives rise to difficulties with self-hatred, worthlessness, and self-disgust, as well as all of the other problems that come when you do not sufficiently value yourself: depression, anxiety, emotional instability, difficulties with motivation and concentration, problems with self-care, and relationships with people who do not treat you the way that you deserve.

Mentalizing Warm-up

With these examples of teleological mode in mind, return to Kristin's story on page 305. In what ways does Kristin struggle with concreteness and externalization in her thinking about herself? How does this concreteness affect her mood, self-esteem, relationships, and functionality?

Now it's time to apply these concepts to your own experience. Where do you observe concreteness and externalization in your beliefs about yourself? Delve into Worksheet 13.1, which helps you consider the various shapes that these processes might take in your life.

Worksheet 13.1
Teleological Mode: How Can You be Externalized in
Your Thinking about Yourself?

Teleological mode involves externalization and concreteness in your thinking, beliefs, and viewpoints. See below for examples of areas where you might experience teleological thinking. Try to provide at least three examples of your beliefs in these areas. In each category, how does this concreteness affect your emotions, self-esteem, relationships, and behavior?

(1) Linking your feelings with your subsequent actions. For example: "When I think/feel/want _____, I feel like I need to *[engage in some sort of behavior]*."

(2) Connecting your actions with your positive mental states. For example: "I need to *[engage in some sort of behavior]* in order to experience *[some positive thought, emotion, desire, or feeling about myself]*."

(3) Connecting your actions with your painful emotional states. For example: "Whenever I *[engage in some sort of behavior]*, I experience *[some painful thought, emotion, desire, or feeling about myself]*."

[continued on next page]

(4) Associating your visible personal characteristics (e.g., appearance, weight, clothing, physical traits) with positive emotions in yourself. For example: "I am only able to feel *[some positive thought, emotion, desire, or feeling about myself]* if I *[display some visible characteristic]*."

(5) Associating your visible personal characteristics (e.g., appearance, weight, clothing, physical traits) with painful emotions in yourself. For example: "Whenever I *[exhibit some visible characteristic]*, I feel *[some painful thought, emotion, desire, or feeling about myself]*."

(6) Correlating external situations with positive emotions in yourself. For example: "I need *[external event to happen]* in order to experience *[some positive thought, emotion, desire, or feeling about myself]*."

(7) Correlating external situations with painful emotions in yourself. For example: "Whenever *[external event or circumstance happens]*, I feel *[some painful thought, emotion, desire, or feeling about myself]*."

[continued on next page]

(8) Teleological self-esteem. For example: "In order to feel good about myself, I need to *[display some quality, take/not take some action, have some relationship, or experience some positive life circumstance]*."

(9) Teleological shame. For example: "Whenever I *[display some quality, take/not take some action, lack some relationship, or experience some negative life circumstance]*, I feel bad about myself."

EXTERNALIZATION AND CONCRETENESS IN YOUR BELIEFS ABOUT OTHER PEOPLE

In borderline personality disorder (BPD), you might interpret other people teleologically as well—that is, you rely extensively on visible factors in order to understand what other individuals are thinking and feeling. Your concrete, externalized beliefs about others could variously involve:

- *Connecting other people's actions with their positive mental states:* When other people behave in certain ways, you could automatically assume that this means they are FEELING some emotion, including some particular emotion toward you. For example, a romantic partner engages in physical intimacy with you, and you presume this means they want a relationship with you, or at least are considering it. Or you associate text communications with caring about someone, so you believe that, if your family member truly cares about you, they will text you regularly to check in on you. In addition, you could be very attentive to other people's explicit language when they are communicating with you. So when your boss gives you positive feedback about your work on some project, you suppose that he is seeing you in an unequivocally positive light, even though recently he raised concerns about your attendance and work performance.

  This form of teleology can lead to difficulties with rigidity and demandingness in your relationships. Since you associate a specific set of other people's actions with their positive feelings, you end up feeling like you *need* them to do certain things, in order for you to feel secure that they are valuing you. Alternatively, this teleological tendency can make you naive and overly trusting in your interactions with others. As long as other people say or do certain things (e.g., offering you attention, care, and positive feedback), you assume that they are invested in you, even when they are taking other actions potentially indicating they are feeling less positive or committed in their relationship with you.

- *Connecting other people's actions with their negative mental states:* Extensive research suggests that people with BPD have something of a "negativity bias" when reading other people's internal states, in particular interpreting others' neutral or ambiguous facial expressions as indicating more negative feelings (e.g., anger, sadness, anxiety; Meehan et al., 2017; Mitchell et al., 2014; Wrege et al., 2021). From the perspective of MBT, this amounts to a form of teleological thinking, where you reflexively "link" certain outward displays with aversive psychological processes in other individuals.

  For example, your friend does not text you back, and you presume that they are upset with you. Or your partner frowns and looks away from you, and you feel convinced that they are angry and withdrawing from you emotionally. Or your professor gives you some constructive feedback, and this feels like criticism— they are judging you negatively, and they do not think you are as smart as the other students. These forms of teleology account for much of the emotional and interpersonal instability for people with BPD. You are vigilant for these feared external cues, and when they appear, they can completely overtake your emotional life, leading to difficulties with self-consciousness, anger, defensiveness, and mistrust of other people.

- *Associating other people's visible personal characteristics with their positive emotions:* As mentioned earlier, visible personal characteristics include someone's appearance, weight, clothing, or physical traits. So this type of teleological thinking essentially involves "judging a book by its beautiful cover," specifically by assuming that certain qualities in other people point to their upbeat, euthymic subjective states. So if an individual is highly attractive, you reflexively assume that they are confident and have high self-esteem. Or if a person dresses well and appears highly "put together," you believe that they are *internally* put together: psychologically stable, healthy, and experiencing positive mood. Interestingly, this type of thinking contributes to problems with insecurity and self-devaluation. You end up "comparing your insides to other people's outsides"—arriving at an overly rosy and idealized picture of others in your mind, and feeling like you do not measure up by comparison.

- *Associating other people's visible personal characteristics with their negative emotions:* You also might associate certain visible qualities with more negative mental states in other people. For instance, you could believe that a highly attractive person is superficial and entitled, or that someone who struggles with obesity is lazy and unmotivated. This form of teleology causes you to jump to conclusions without sufficient data, drawing overly sharp distinctions between yourself and other people based on more superficial factors.

- *Correlating external situations with positive emotions in other people:* You could also place significant emphasis on other people's external circumstances, presuming that these concrete factors suggest that they are experiencing more "positive" or favorable emotions, desires, and feelings about themselves. For example, you might link other people's positive feelings to various external circumstances in their lives, such as interpersonal relationships and interactions ("Once my sister starts dating again, she is going to feel so much better about herself"); relationships and interactions NOT happening ("You need to break up with him, if you want your depression to get any better"); work-related situations ("Ever since my boyfriend got that new job, his anxiety has completely disappeared"); scenarios related to pets or animal companions ("She needs to get a dog, so that she has a reason to get out of bed in the morning"); events related to body, health, and appearance ("As soon as my father gets a clean bill of health, he will not have a care in the world"); conditions in other people's immediate environment ("She will feel so much happier if she can just get outside, and spend some time in nature"); time and chronology ("When spring comes, his mood is going to get so much better"); or occurrences in broader society and culture ("Now that Taylor Swift is back on tour, my best friend has a sense of meaning and purpose again").

  When engaging in these forms of concrete thinking, you feel convinced that the outside world holds inordinate power over other people's internal lives, in this way underestimating the importance of their own *psychological* processes in cultivating a sense of emotional well-being and fulfillment. You can thus infantilize other people, seeing them as passive pawns rather than as full, robust agents in their own life.

- *Correlating external situations with negative emotions in other people:* You also might assume that other people will always experience pain and distress when confronted with particular challenging events. Examples of this type of teleological interpretation include connecting others' negative feelings to various external circumstances in their lives, such as interpersonal relationships and interactions ("If my husband keeps being so strict with the kids, they are going to develop low self-esteem"); relationships and interactions NOT happening ("Without her to take care of him, he is just too anxious to function in his life"); work-related events ("This job is sapping her will to live"); scenarios related to pets or animal companions ("If anything ever happens to Mittens, my aunt is going to go completely downhill"); events related to body, health, and appearance ("Unless he gets on the right medications, his anxiety is just going to keep getting worse"); conditions in other people's immediate environment ("She needs to move out of this apartment, or she is going to go crazy"); time and chronology ("There is no way that these students can be motivated or focused this early in the morning"); or on events in broader society and culture ("My dad was completely fine my entire life, but ever since the pandemic started, he's been depressed and suicidal"). These forms of teleology grant the external environment significant control over other people's emotional lives, essentially "blaming" that environment for distress and instability in others. You can thus experience people largely as victims of these outside factors, leading to difficulties with anger and devaluation of the (presumed) concrete source of their suffering.

It is important to note that, in highlighting all of these forms of teleology, MBT is not denying the importance of external factors (e.g., actions, qualities, events) in understanding other people. Sometimes people give you gifts because they value you, and they want to be closer to you. Sometimes people do not respond to your texts because they are actually angry at you, and they are trying to punish you. The problem with teleological mode is not that you are focused on external things—it is that you are rigidly *equating* specific external things with particular internal processes, such that you only imagine a narrow range of mental states when people take certain actions, display certain qualities, and experience certain circumstances. "If he asks me a lot of questions about myself, then he wants to be in a relationship with me." "If she raises her voice at me, then she hates me." Under these conditions, you remain trapped in your initial, externally focused interpretations of other people, failing to mentalize a broader array of mental states in others—mental states that (when you consider them) enable you to experience a greater sense of stability, trust, and connectedness in your relationships.

Mentalizing Warm-up

Keeping in mind these examples of teleological thinking about others, return to Kristin's story on page 305. How does Kristin struggle with concreteness and externalization in her interpretations of other people? Consider the ways in which this concreteness affects her mood, self-esteem, relationships, and functionality.

But what about you: Where do you observe concreteness and externalization in your beliefs about others? Work on completing Worksheet 13.2, which walks you through the various shapes these processes could take in your everyday life and experience.

Worksheet 13.2
Teleological Mode: How Can You be Externalized in Your Thinking about Other People?

Teleological mode involves externalization and concreteness in your thinking, beliefs, and viewpoints. See below for examples of areas where you might experience teleological thinking. Try to provide at least three examples of your beliefs in these areas. In each category, how does this concreteness affect your emotions, self-esteem, relationships, and behavior?

(1) Connecting other people's actions with their positive mental states. For example: "When *[another person takes/does not take some action]*, they are experiencing *[some positive feeling about you, themself, or something else]*."

(2) Connecting other people's actions with their negative mental states. For example: "When *[another person takes/does not take some action]*, they are experiencing *[some negative feeling about you, themself, or something else]*."

(3) Associating other people's visible personal characteristics (e.g., appearance, weight, clothing, physical traits) with their positive emotions. For example: "When *[another person exhibits/does not exhibit some visible characteristic]*, they are experiencing *[some positive feeling about you, themself, or something else]*."

[continued on next page]

(4) Associating other people's visible personal characteristics (e.g., appearance, weight, clothing, physical traits) with their negative emotions. For example: "When *[another person exhibits/does not exhibit some visible characteristic]*, they are experiencing *[some negative feeling about you, themself, or something else]*."

(5) Correlating external situations with positive emotions in other people. For example: "When *[external events happen/do not happen to another person]*, they are experiencing *[some positive feeling about you, themself, or something else]*."

(6) Correlating external situations with negative emotions in other people. For example: "When *[external events happen/do not happen to another person]*, they are experiencing *[some negative feeling about you, themself, or something else]*."

MENTALIZING PRACTICE POINTS: DISRUPTING THE EXTERNALIZATION

In BPD, teleological mode is notoriously difficult to treat. When you are engaged in teleological thinking, you usually feel utterly convinced that both your problems and your solutions reside entirely outside of you. You feel like you are suffering *because* you look a certain way, you have done a bad job on some task, you are not successful enough, you do not have the right relationships, or other people are treating you in a way that is clearly problematic. And if those external factors are the problem, then the solution is simple: Get the good thing, avoid the bad thing, and then you will feel better.

When you are able to effectively manage the external environment in this way, you usually *do* end up feeling better, at least for a little while. This just reinforces the idea that the outside world is the locus for change, and so you just need to try harder to control it, or to control yourself. Accordingly, it can be difficult to feel motivated to address your teleological thinking. Why work on changing your psychology when you can just focus on getting more "quick fixes"?

From the perspective of MBT, there is significant reason to try to address your difficulties with externalization and concreteness. While your teleological pursuits can offer you some short-term relief in the moment, these emotions never stay put, and you have to continuously work to "keep the good feelings around." This gives rise to an almost constant sense of pressure, anxiety, and over time, emotional exhaustion. And then, when the external world inevitably does not comply with your efforts, you end up experiencing the range of painful emotions than anyone with BPD knows all too well: sadness, anger, shame, and hopelessness. So MBT suggests that, in order to achieve any durable emotional stability and fulfillment, you need to address the teleological thinking that undergirds this roller coaster of emotions. But how do you do this?

In MBT, the therapeutic approach for teleological mode can be summed up by the dictum:

Disrupt the externalization.

From a big picture perspective, this prescription involves two broad steps, which parallel the strategies for psychic equivalence mode introduced in Chapter 12:

(1) *Make the externalization mental.* When you are in teleological mode, the problem is that you are rigidly "equating" some outside thing with some internal process. Someone disagrees with you about some topic in current events *[external factor]*, and you automatically assume that they do not respect you *[mental state]*. Often you are not even aware of the two things you are linking together, or even that you are doing this linking in the first place! So the first step in treating teleological mode involves recognizing that you are engaged in this psychological process, and that this psychological TENDENCY in you is a key driver of your suffering.

(2) *Reflect on the teleological equation.* Once you understand that you are conflating some external factor with another internal process, you can start to consider the teleological association itself. Are there any additional ways to see this presumed connection? Could *other* mental states be unfolding alongside the external factor? For instance, you might consider other mental states that the person could be experiencing when they are disagreeing with you, including an emotion of excitement around intellectual engagement, or a sense of care and affection for you as a person. When reflecting in these ways, you broaden your range of perspectives about the scenario, thus introducing greater flexibility and curiosity about the necessary connection between the outside and the inside.

As you learn how to apply these mentalizing strategies in your life, you start to feel less controlled and dominated by the outside world. You gain access to an experience of peace, stability, and connectedness to yourself. By disrupting the externalization, you create space for a reliable *inner* world, which is able to persist independently of what you look like, how people are treating you, and how well you feel like you are "performing" in your various roles and relationships.

This is all admittedly quite abstract, so let's drill down on the specific mentalizing strategies that can help you along these lines. Like the techniques for psychic equivalence mode, these strategies are progressive and build on each other, so there is value in applying them in a step-by-step fashion.

Step 1: Articulate the teleological belief you want to address. In order to address your teleological thinking, you first need to be aware of how you are thinking teleologically! Employing the Teleological Equation Toolkit below, start by identifying the specific external factor on which you are focused at the moment: your own behavior, visible characteristics, or circumstances, or another person's actions, physical characteristics, or circumstances.

The Teleological Equation Toolkit

External Factor on which You are Focused *(Action, visible characteristic, or circumstance involving you or another person)*

Related Internal Factors			
Thoughts	Emotions	Desires	Feelings about the Self

Articulate the Teleological Equation:

"I feel certain that

_____

[external factor from above]

means that

_____."

[internal factor(s) from above]

Then reflect on the internal states you are associating with the external factor in question, which are essentially thoughts, emotions, desires, or feelings about the self. Finally, synthesizing all of these reflections, "put words on" the teleological equation likely in play. For example, you might be assuming that your employee failing to follow your directions *[external factor]* means that she does not respect you *[internal factor]*, or that you are not good enough *[internal factor]* because you are not in a relationship *[external factor]*.

Let's consider these examples in turn, utilizing the Teleological Equation Toolkit.

The Teleological Equation Toolkit
External Factor on which You are Focused   *(Action, visible characteristic, or circumstance involving you or another person)*   My employee did not follow my directions on that project.

Related Internal Factors			
Thoughts	Emotions	Desires	Feelings about the Self
She does not respect me. She just thinks that I will let her do whatever she wants.	She is angry at me for assigning her that project in the first place.	She wants to get away with doing a little work as possible, without me noticing.	She walks around with a sense of superiority: She feels like she is better than me, and that she is above the rules.

Articulate the Teleological Equation:

"I feel certain that

my employee not following my directions
_____
[external factor from above]

means that

she thinks she is better than me,
and she doesn't respect me
_____ ,"
[internal factor(s) from above]

In this toolkit, the patient started by identifying the external factor that was bothering him, namely his employee not following his directions on a particular project. He then proceeded to itemize his employee's potential internal states that he was linking with her behavior (e.g., her anger, superiority, desire to avoid work, and her lack of respect for him), ultimately arriving at a succinct statement of his teleological assumption: "I feel certain that my employee not following my directions means that she thinks she is better than me, and she doesn't respect me."

Now consider a Teleological Equation Toolkit focused on one patient's concrete belief about herself.

The Teleological Equation Toolkit

External Factor on which You are Focused *(Action, visible characteristic, or circumstance involving you or another person)* I am 35 years old and still not in a relationship.

Related Internal Factors			
Thoughts	Emotions	Desires	Feelings about the Self
I am constantly comparing myself to other people my age, thinking, "What is wrong with me that I am the only one who does not have somebody?"	I feel lonely, depressed, and worried that I will never find someone.	I want to be in a relationship so bad. I feel a bit desperate, even willing to date losers so that I do not have to be alone.	I feel worthless and unlovable, like there is something inherently wrong with me. I also feel embarrassed and ashamed, especially when I am at family events.

Articulate the Teleological Equation: "I feel certain that not being in a relationship *[external factor from above]* means that I am worthless and unlovable, like there is something inherently wrong with me   ," *[internal factor(s) from above]*

In this toolkit, the patient pinpointed the external factor that was causing her distress ("I am 35 years old and still not in a relationship"), then reflecting on the internal processes she connected with this fact: negative thoughts about herself, loneliness and depression, the desperate desire to have a relationship, and a sense of worthlessness and defectiveness. Bringing all of these ideas together, the patient gave voice to the teleological equation potentially at play in this experience: "I feel certain that not being in a relationship means that I am worthless and unlovable, like there is something inherently wrong with me."

In both of these examples, the patients employed the Teleological Equation Toolkit to sift through a range of complex and emotionally messy experiences, ultimately defining a bite-sized teleological belief that was serving a key role in fueling their suffering. Once you have your hands on such a belief, you now have a clear point of focus for implementing MBT's additional strategies for teleological mode. Before proceeding, feel free to try out the Teleological Equation Toolkit yourself, on some situation where you are feeling highly focused on (and distressed about) a concrete, visible factor involving yourself or other people.

Step 2: Try to make the teleology feel more "mental." The next step in addressing teleological mode involves appreciating how the externalization actually involves mental processes unfolding inside of you. This might sound overly obvious: Of course you are aware that your thoughts are in your head—where else would they be? However, as we discussed regarding psychic equivalence mode in Chapter 12, you can cognitively "know" that something is a thought while still 100% *feeling* like it is a fact. So in order to disrupt your externalization, you have to start making the teleological feel *psychological*.

The Mentalizing the Teleology Toolkit presents a handful of strategies that gently nudge you in that direction, without directly challenging your teleological belief. Start by trying to visualize the teleological equation you have already identified in Step 1 above, namely by writing down the external factor in the box on the left and describing your attendant mental states in the circle on the right. As reflected in the image, these objects are visually distinct from each other, and yet you are seeing them as "equal" in some way. By envisioning these two different factors in a clear spatial relationship to each other, you begin to recognize that *you* are identifying them with each other in your mind, but these factors are not one and the same thing.

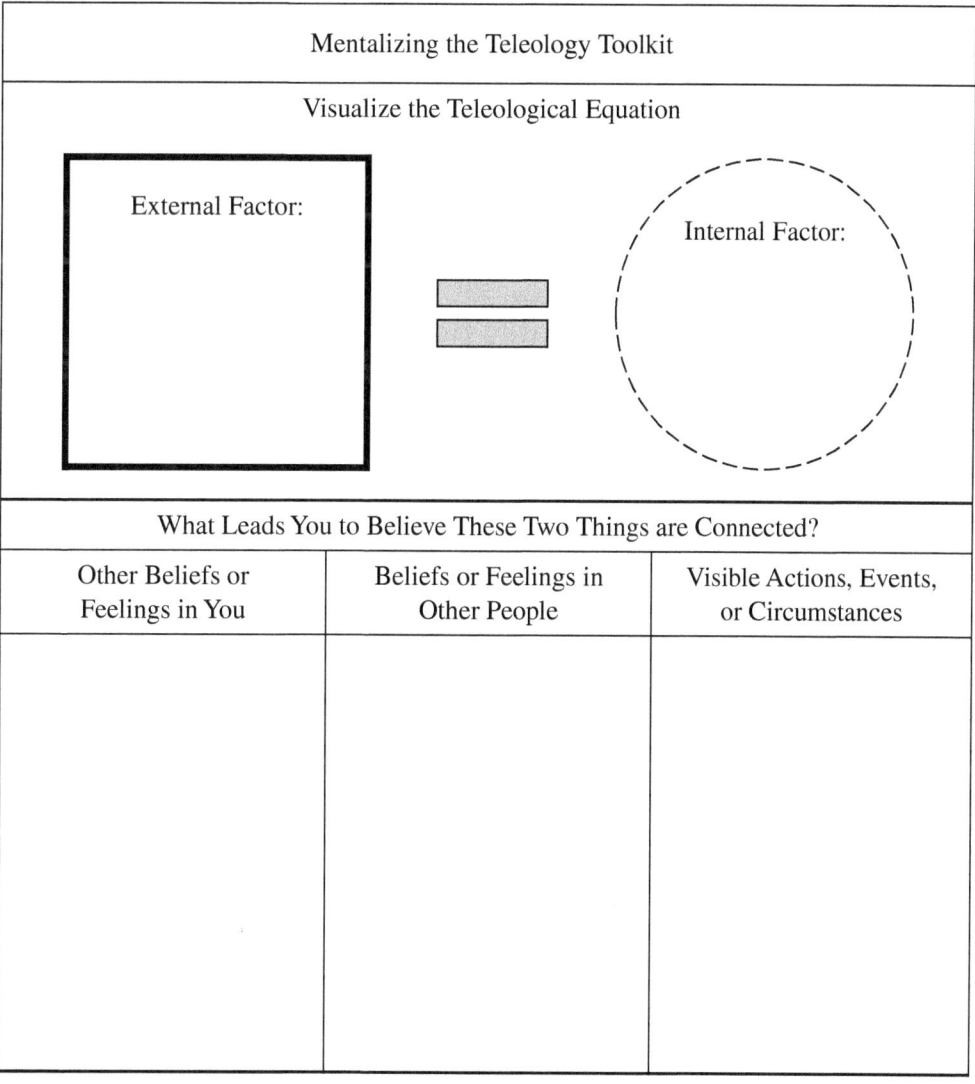

What are the Consequences of Your Teleological Belief?		
Your Emotions, Desires, and Self-states	Actions You Take	Impact of Your Actions on Relationships/ Other People

Contextualize Your Suffering
Ask yourself the question:
"Is it possible that I am suffering not because
_____,
[external factor from above]
but because I am assuming that
_____
[external factor from above]
means that
_____?"
[internal factor(s) from above]

Next take a step back from the teleological equation itself, and ask yourself the question: "What leads you to believe these two things are connected?" This is where you reflect on potential "support" for your externalized belief, usually falling into the categories of other beliefs or feelings you have ("When *I* respect my boss, I always do exactly what they say"), beliefs or feelings in other people ("Our co-workers all agree that she has no respect for authority"), or more "objective" actions, events, or circumstances in yourself, other people, or the world more broadly ("Since she started here, she has never really gone along with our rules or policies"; "All of my other employees follow my instructions without any trouble").

Interestingly, when considering these matters, you might struggle to fully explain why you believe what you do, in the same way that you cannot really explain why you believe that water is wet. It just *feels* true, almost by definition. Do not put too much pressure on yourself here. Rather, simply notice how you feel so convinced that these external and internal things are connected (e.g., your employee's action and her lack of respect for you, your relationship status and your worthlessness), without any incontrovertible "evidence" for that conviction. Whatever the outcome of these inquiries (e.g., if you arrive at support for your teleological view, or if you fail to find support for it), in the process of asking yourself "What makes me believe this?," you are relating to the teleology *as a belief state*, and thus ushering it into the realm of psychology rather than fact.

Next work to examine the consequences of you holding this teleological belief. When you feel so certain that these external and internal factors are linked, how does that impact you and other people? Such consequences include internal processes unfolding inside of you, such as your emotions, desires, and feelings about yourself (e.g., anger toward your employee, desire to retaliate against her, shame and embarrassment that she is looking down on you); actions that you take in the situation (e.g., giving your employee the silent treatment, not calling on her in staff meetings, talking harshly to her in her performance review); and the impact of your actions on other people (e.g., your employee feeling insecure about her job and less motivated to do her work, other staff feeling awkward in meetings).

Once again, as you reflect on these matters, you are implicitly relating to the teleology as a mental state in you: It is your concrete *belief* that leads you to feel these ways and take these actions, thus impacting the people in your life. This further underscores that you are contending with a psychological process in yourself, which is potentially amenable to treatment. And since the aforementioned consequences of the teleology are usually more "problematic" in nature (e.g., actions that cause trouble for yourself and other people, painful emotions in yourself and others), you start to recognize that this belief could be playing a pivotal role in fueling your difficulties.

Along similar lines, you can utilize these reflections on your teleological thinking to further contextualize the suffering that you are experiencing in the situation. Specifically, try wrestling with the question: "Is it possible that I am suffering not due to this external thing, but because I am ASSUMING that this external thing is linked with a very specific mental state?" For instance, continuing with the example of your employee not following your directions, you might ask yourself: "Is it possible that I am suffering right now not because my employee did not follow my directions, but because I am assuming that her not following my directions means she does not respect me?"

By reflecting in these ways, you are entertaining the possibility that the source of your suffering is not the outside world, but your manner of *relating* to that world. This is ultimately good news. If the problem exists outside of you, then you have very little control over it. External things just tend to do what they do, whether we like it or not. But if the problem is located fundamentally INSIDE of you (i.e., that is, in your manner of interpreting concrete and visible factors), then you can actually do something about it—namely, by utilizing the principles of mentalizing to shift your psychological relationship to external reality. This opens up the door for the possibility of change, and ultimately to a feeling of hope that there might be a way out of this mess.

See here for a completed version of the Mentalizing the Teleology Toolkit, focusing on the patient's belief that she is worthless and unlovable because she is not in a romantic relationship.

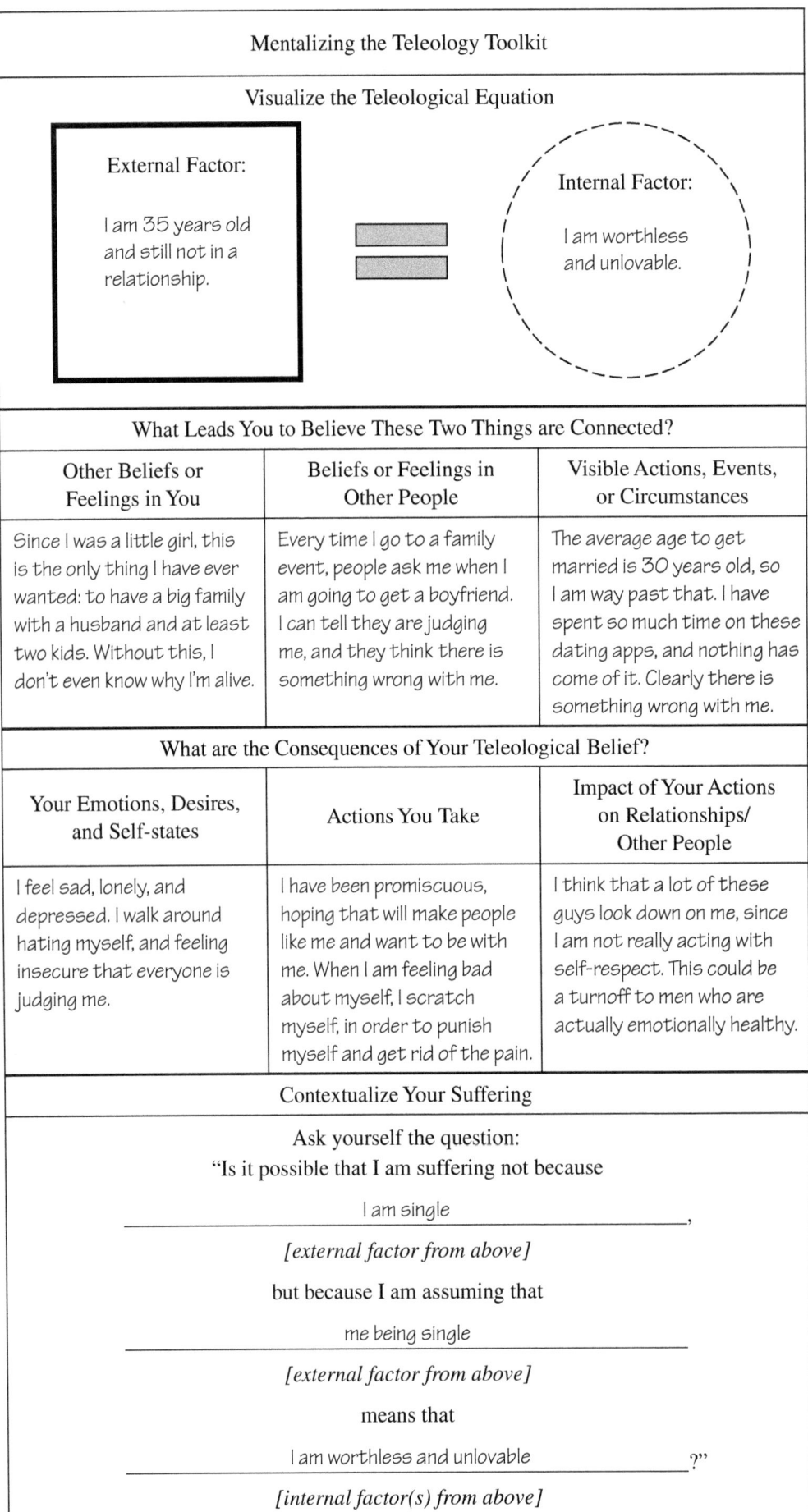

Mentalizing the Teleology Toolkit

Visualize the Teleological Equation

External Factor:

I am 35 years old and still not in a relationship.

=

Internal Factor:

I am worthless and unlovable.

What Leads You to Believe These Two Things are Connected?

Other Beliefs or Feelings in You	Beliefs or Feelings in Other People	Visible Actions, Events, or Circumstances
Since I was a little girl, this is the only thing I have ever wanted: to have a big family with a husband and at least two kids. Without this, I don't even know why I'm alive.	Every time I go to a family event, people ask me when I am going to get a boyfriend. I can tell they are judging me, and they think there is something wrong with me.	The average age to get married is 30 years old, so I am way past that. I have spent so much time on these dating apps, and nothing has come of it. Clearly there is something wrong with me.

What are the Consequences of Your Teleological Belief?

Your Emotions, Desires, and Self-states	Actions You Take	Impact of Your Actions on Relationships/ Other People
I feel sad, lonely, and depressed. I walk around hating myself, and feeling insecure that everyone is judging me.	I have been promiscuous, hoping that will make people like me and want to be with me. When I am feeling bad about myself, I scratch myself, in order to punish myself and get rid of the pain.	I think that a lot of these guys look down on me, since I am not really acting with self-respect. This could be a turnoff to men who are actually emotionally healthy.

Contextualize Your Suffering

Ask yourself the question:
"Is it possible that I am suffering not because

_____I am single_____ ,

[external factor from above]

but because I am assuming that

_____me being single_____

[external factor from above]

means that

_____I am worthless and unlovable_____ ?"

[internal factor(s) from above]

Step 3: Challenge the teleological equation. Once the teleology is feeling more like a *belief* in you, the next step is challenging and disrupting the belief in question. Utilizing the Challenging the Teleology Toolkit, first restate the teleological equation that you want to address, along the following lines:

- "My partner has not been initiating sex with me" *[external factor]* = "They are less excited about me, and they are pulling away from me emotionally" *[internal factor]*
- "If I ever lose my job" *[external factor]* = "I will have no reason to live anymore" *[internal factor]*
- "She is so stylish, poised, and well put together" *[external factor]* = "She must be confident and comfortable with herself" *[internal factor]*
- "I talked way too much at that dinner party" *[external factor]* = "I feel completely embarrassed" *[internal factor]*

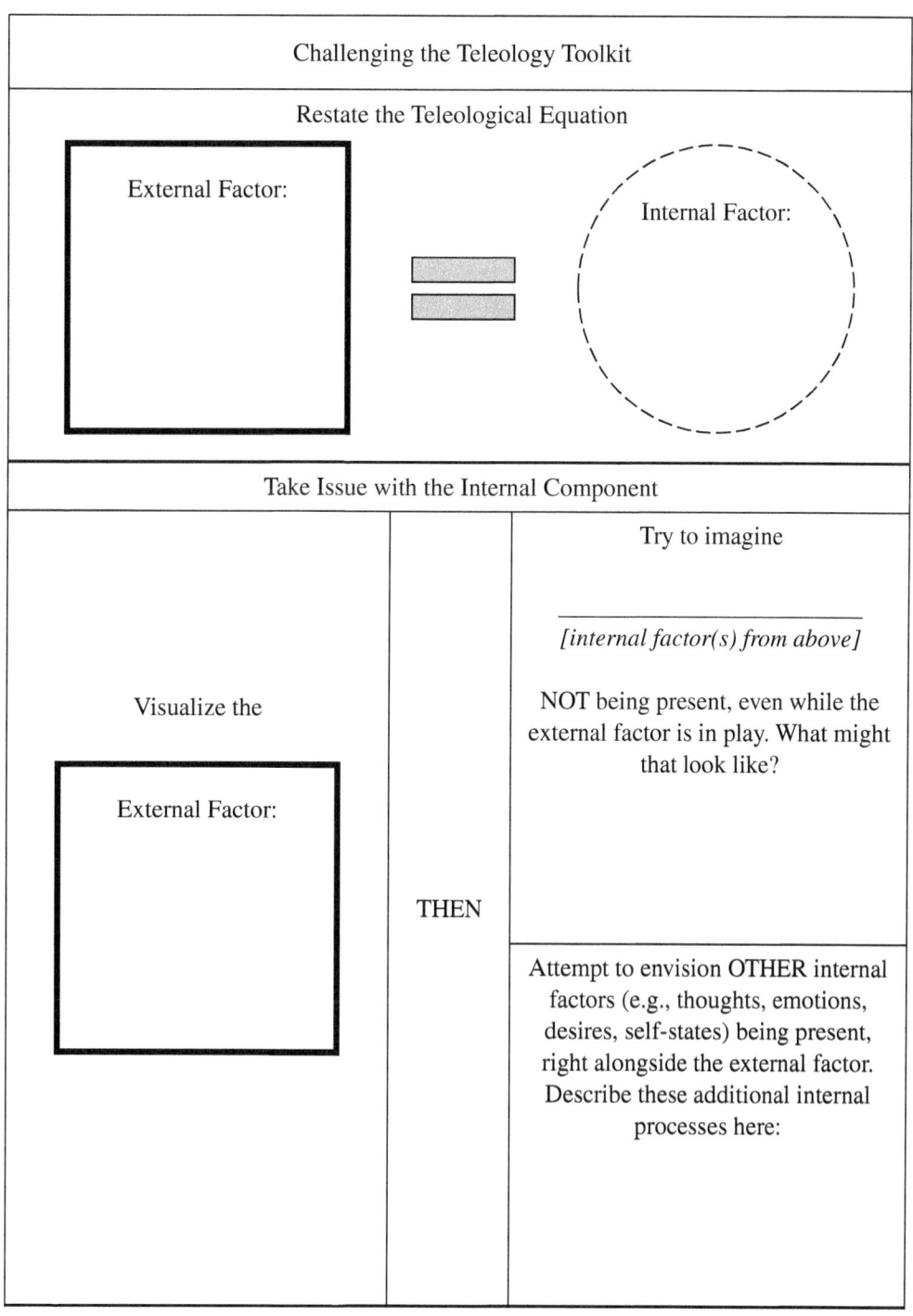

Take Issue with the External Component		
Envision the external factor NOT being present. 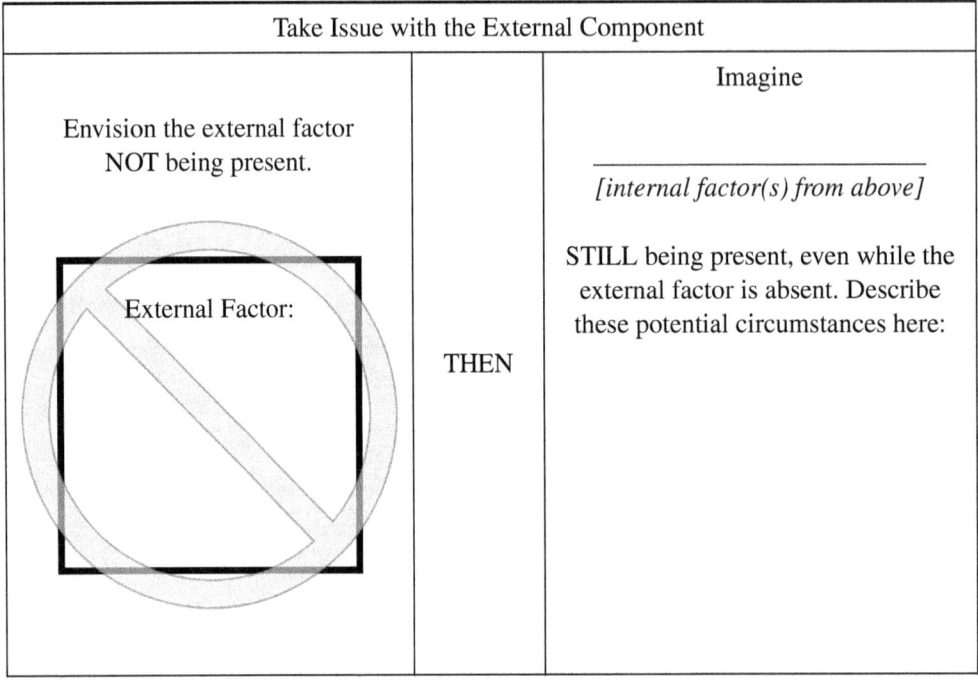	THEN	Imagine ——————————— *[internal factor(s) from above]* STILL being present, even while the external factor is absent. Describe these potential circumstances here:

You can work to challenge the teleological linkage in two primary ways: taking issue with the internal component in the equation, and taking issue with the external component. To challenge the internal component, visualize the external factor being present, and then try to imagine the internal factor being absent. For example, in order to challenge the teleological belief that your employee not following your directions means she does not respect you, envision your employee acting that way while still having full emotional respect for you as a boss, and as a person. Or to disrupt the belief that you are worthless and unlovable for not being in a romantic relationship, observe the fact that you are not in such a relationship, and imagine the possibility that you could still have unconditional, inherent worth as a person.

Just to be clear on this one: I am not suggesting that you should attempt to *believe* or convince yourself that the internal factor is absent (e.g., that your employee actually respects you, or that you are a worthwhile person). That is a tall order, if not an impossible one, especially since when you are in teleological mode, you truly believe that the external and internal factors are definitively linked. In MBT, we simply invite you to IMAGINE other possibilities about the teleology, in the exact same moment that you are feeling convinced of your concrete view. In particular, try practicing what we call *authentic* imagination—that is, fully and wholeheartedly considering the potential reality of the idea in question.

So rather than simply cognitively acknowledging "Sure, it's possible that my employee respects me," take a moment to imagine that your employee *actually, truly* respects you as a boss, even though it does not feel that way to you at the time. This technique is entirely consistent with MBT's "addition not subtraction" therapeutic approach: Even as you are feeling certain of your externalized belief, genuinely consider that some other psychological reality might also be true, in such a way that you are not prioritizing or elevating any particular viewpoint over another.

Going one step further, work to articulate OTHER potential mental states that could conceivably be present, right alongside the external factor in question. So when your employee is not following your directions, you might reflect on her feelings of stress and sadness related to her ongoing divorce, her strong opinions about how the project should be completed, and her desire to have more time for her other work projects—all mental states that your employee could potentially be experiencing, in addition to any feelings of disrespect or superiority toward you.

If you are feeling particularly stuck in your thinking here, feel free to unlock your imagination by switching up some of the incidental details of the situation in question. This could involve some of the following mentalizing strategies:

- *Consider the person's feelings at other moments in time:* how your employee used to feel about you, or how you could imagine her feeling about you in the future; what you used to feel about being single, or what you could imagine feeling in the future (or in some other hypothetical scenario)
- *Contemplate another person's feelings in relation to the external factor:* what might motivate another employee to complete a project in their own way; how other people could feel when they are not dating anyone
- *Reflect on how you would mentalize another person in similar circumstances:* how you might interpret an employee you like who does not follow their boss's directions; how you view your good friends who are single
- *Ponder how another person would mentalize the individual in question:* what another colleague might hypothesize about your employee's motives and emotions, or what your employee might say about her *own* motives and emotions; your loved one's perspective on your value and worth, even though you are not in a relationship

For instance, when you are thinking about the fact that you are not in a relationship, you could imagine a world in which you felt largely content with that fact, or a sense of security and self-love that is independent of your relationship status. You could observe that many people feel content and confident when they are not in a relationship, and that *you* tend to feel accepting and supportive of your close friends who are single. You also might note your friends' and family members' views of you: namely as being worthwhile and lovable as a person, even though you are not with anyone.

Finally, to take issue with the external component in the teleological equation, imagine the visible factor NOT being present, and yet the internal component in that equation continues to exist. So here you would visualize your employee following your directions in completing the project, at the same time envisioning her thinking she is better than you, and not respecting you. Or you could picture yourself finally being in a relationship while continuing to feel worthless and unlovable. Really try to *see* these things, in a way that feels true and authentic to you, at an emotional level.

All of these strategies represent ways to challenge and disrupt your teleological thinking. By affirming the external factor and negating the internal factor, and then by negating the external factor and affirming the internal factor, you are imagining scenarios in which "the outside" and "the inside" are not as rigidly linked. As you consider these other possibilities, you start to feel less overwhelmed by the concrete issues, and more curious about the range of potential mental states unfolding in relation to them.

See here for a completed version of the Challenging the Teleology Toolkit, applied to the teleological belief we have been following, that the patient is worthless and unlovable because she is not in a relationship.

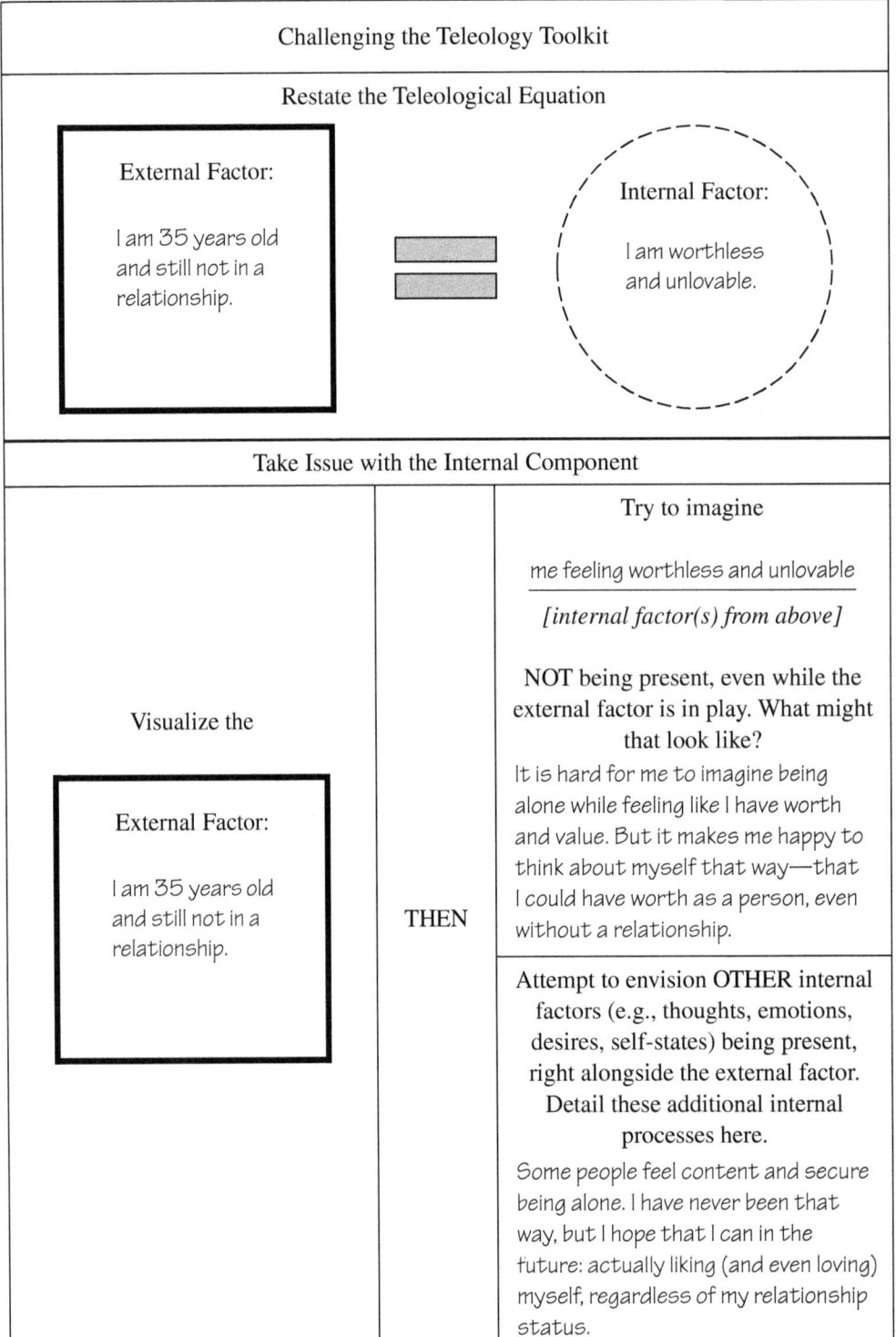

Challenging the Teleology Toolkit

Restate the Teleological Equation

External Factor:

I am 35 years old and still not in a relationship.

=

Internal Factor:

I am worthless and unlovable.

Take Issue with the Internal Component

Visualize the

External Factor:

I am 35 years old and still not in a relationship.

THEN

Try to imagine

me feeling worthless and unlovable
_____
[internal factor(s) from above]

NOT being present, even while the external factor is in play. What might that look like?

It is hard for me to imagine being alone while feeling like I have worth and value. But it makes me happy to think about myself that way—that I could have worth as a person, even without a relationship.

Attempt to envision OTHER internal factors (e.g., thoughts, emotions, desires, self-states) being present, right alongside the external factor. Detail these additional internal processes here.

Some people feel content and secure being alone. I have never been that way, but I hope that I can in the future: actually liking (and even loving) myself, regardless of my relationship status.

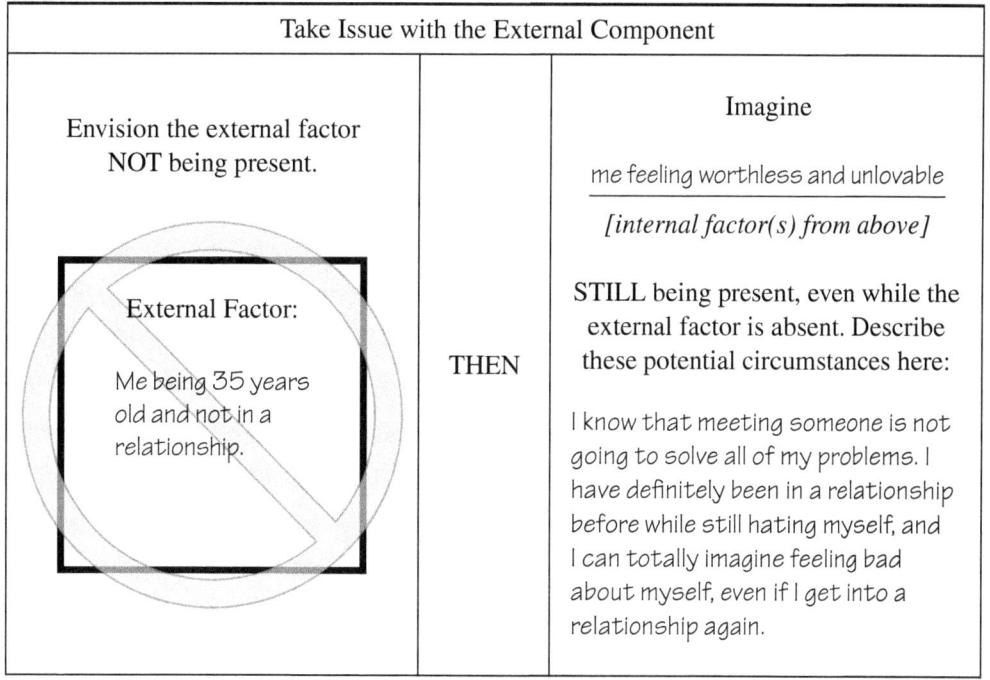

Step 4: Revisit and reconsider the teleological equation. Having "imaginatively disrupted" your teleological thinking, you can now revisit your original concrete assumption. Employing the "More than Meets the Eye" Toolkit below, ask yourself: What is your view on the teleological equation now? Are you still 100% certain that the internal factor is present? What other mental states can you also imagine alongside the external factor, either now or in the future? By reflecting in these ways, you work toward attaining a broader perspective on the teleology, one that includes mental states you did not originally associate with the visible thing in question.

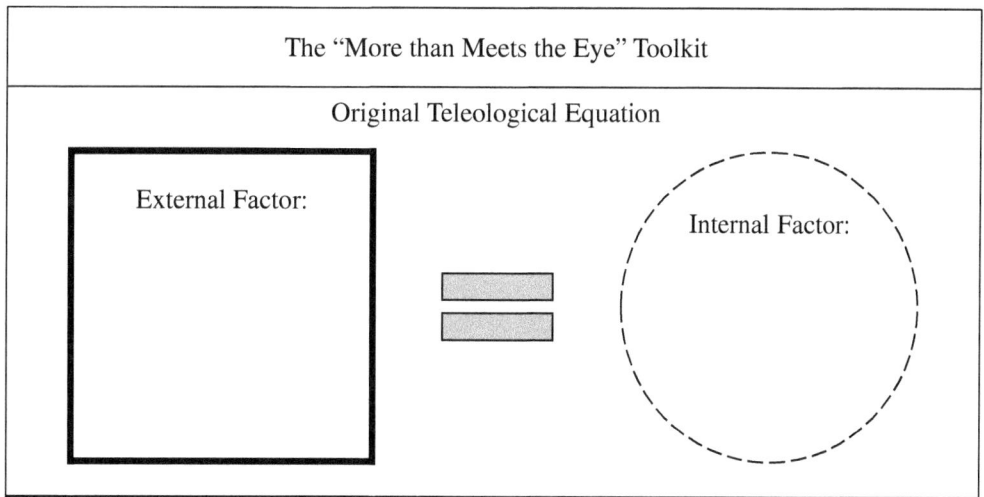

What other mental states can you also imagine alongside the external factor, either now or in the future? "Expand" the teleological equation by describing these below.

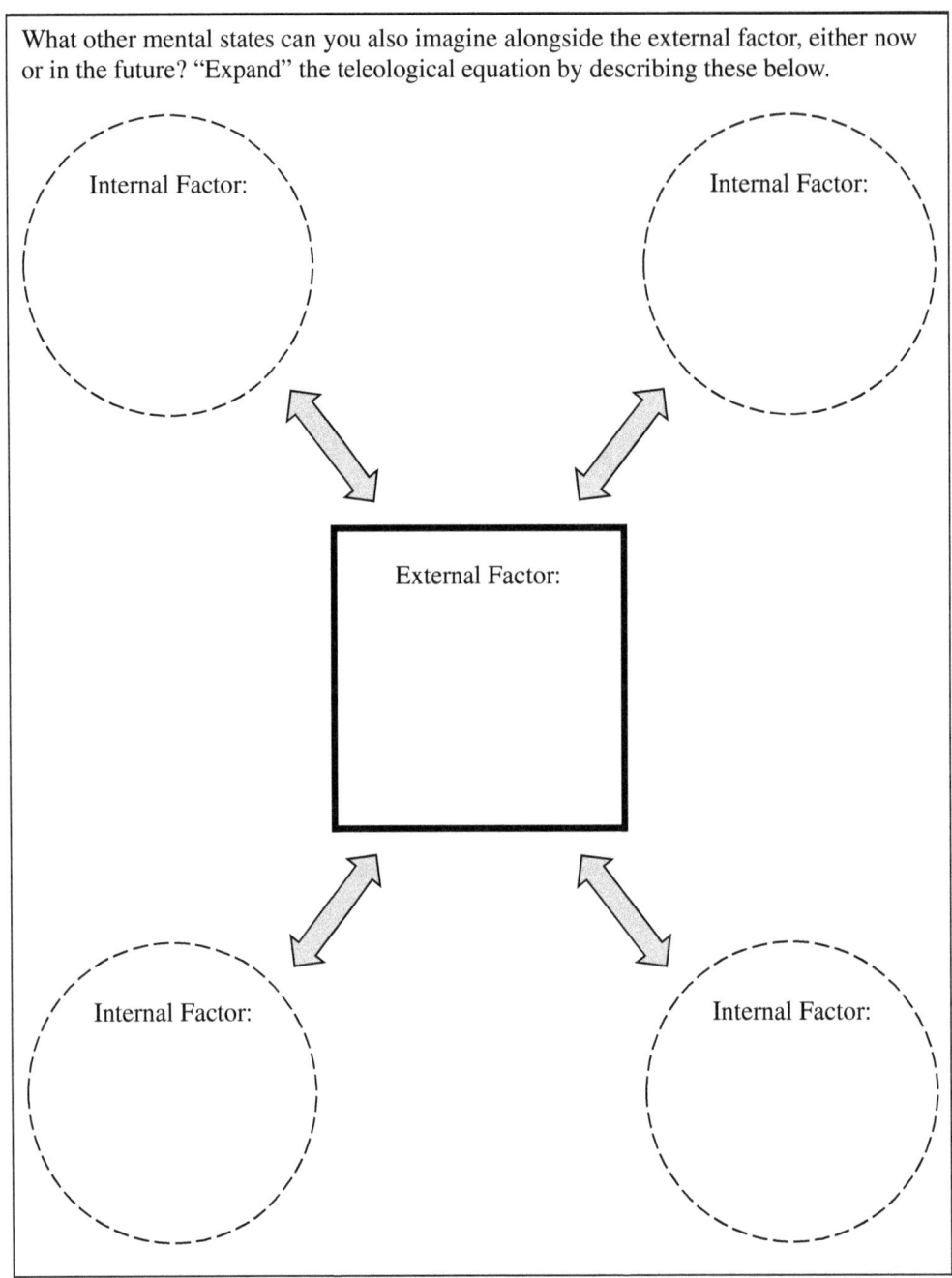

For example, concerning the belief that your employee not following your directions means that she does not respect you, you might observe that you still believe that the employee struggles with entitlement and superiority. However, upon reflection, you wonder if perhaps you have been taking her behavior a little personally. You are also aware that your employee could be experiencing a range of other mental states that might explain why she has not been prioritizing your preferences: her stress and sadness related to her ongoing divorce; her strong opinions about how the project should be completed; and her desire to have more time for her other work projects, which you know she really values.

Once you identify a broader array of mental states that could be present, expand the teleological equation by itemizing these in the various "internal factor" circles on the toolkit. This allows you to appreciate, in a clear visual way, the range of psychological possibilities that are potentially relevant to the external factor at issue. See here for a completed version of the "More than Meets the Eye" Toolkit, applied to the patient's belief that she is worthless and unlovable because she is not in a romantic relationship.

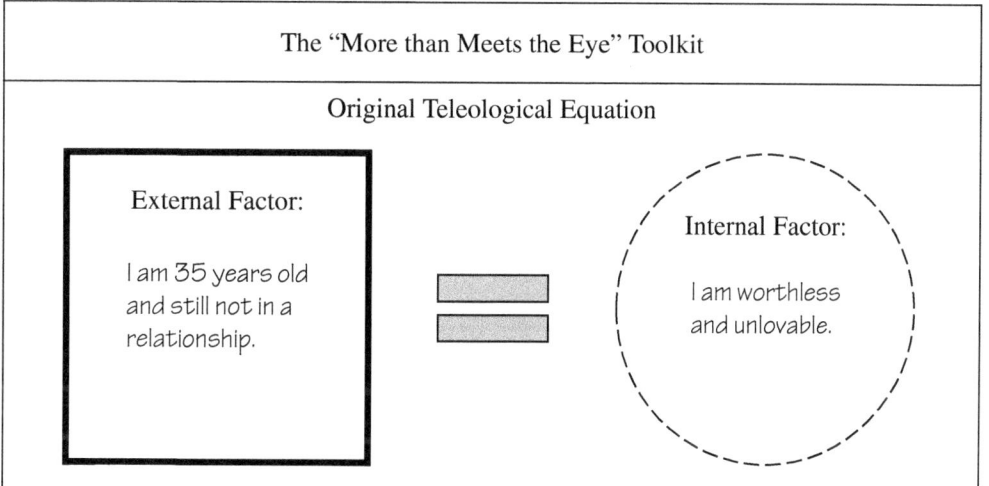

The "More than Meets the Eye" Toolkit

Original Teleological Equation

External Factor:

I am 35 years old and still not in a relationship.

Internal Factor:

I am worthless and unlovable.

Having challenged the rigid connection between the two above elements, what is your view on the teleological equation now? Are you still 100% certain that the internal factor is present? If you are seeing things any differently, what leads you to reevaluate your view?

I still feel really horrible about myself for not being in a relationship. I am not 100% certain that this means I am worthless, but I definitely FEEL worthless. Weirdly, I do not judge other people when they are single, so it is possible that I have a double standard here. I also do not want to feel this way, so I am hoping that over time, I can learn how to be a little kinder to myself in this department.

What other mental states can you also imagine alongside the external factor, either now or in the future? "Expand" the teleological equation by describing these below.

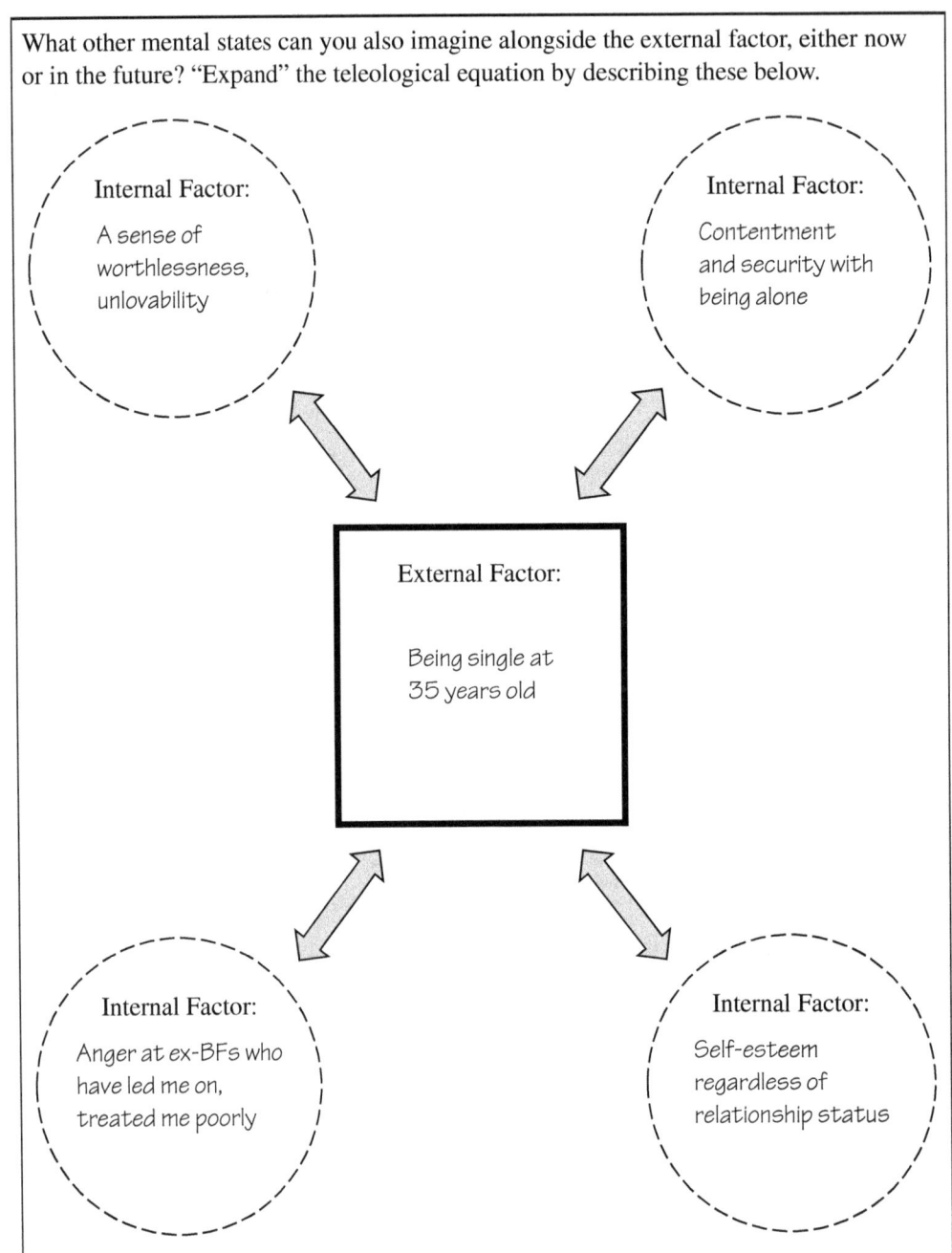

Internal Factor:

A sense of worthlessness, unlovability

Internal Factor:

Contentment and security with being alone

External Factor:

Being single at 35 years old

Internal Factor:

Anger at ex-BFs who have led me on, treated me poorly

Internal Factor:

Self-esteem regardless of relationship status

In this toolkit, the patient started by summarizing her original teleological belief ("I am worthless and unlovable because I am 35 years old and still not in a relationship"), then reevaluating this view based on her efforts to disrupt the teleological linkage. The patient's new perspective was more flexible on multiple fronts. She explicitly framed the teleology as a psychological process ("I definitely FEEL worthless"); she expressed some level of doubt about the teleological equation ("I am not 100% certain that this means I am worthless"); she recognized a discrepancy between her view of herself and her view of others ("I do not judge other people when they are single, so it is possible that I have a double standard here"); she expressed a desire to see herself differently ("I also do not want to feel this way"); and she acknowledged the possibility of evolving her self-concept in the future ("I am hoping that over time, I can learn how to be a little kinder to myself in this department"). The patient also worked to expand the teleological equation beyond this initial linking of "being single" and "worthlessness," ultimately considering several other mental states (e.g., contentment, anger at ex-boyfriends, self-esteem) she could imagine experiencing in that external circumstance of not being in a relationship.

This patient's reflections illustrate our overarching approach to treating teleological mode in MBT: starting to question the concrete thinking, and then broadening the range of mental states potentially associated with the external factor. As you learn how to do this, you feel less controlled by outside things, and more grounded in the *internal* experiences of yourself and other people.

Mentalizing Cool-down

Now that you have learned about how MBT treats concrete and externalized thinking, return to Kristin's story on page 305. What might it look like for Kristin to apply these strategies in her life, in order to address her challenges with perfectionism, emotional dysregulation, and suicidality?

RETURNING TO KRISTIN

At the outset of MBT, Kristin and her therapist worked together to develop her MBT formulation, which itemized her challenges in mentalizing. In particular, Kristin's difficulties with externalization and concrete thinking (AKA teleological mode) included:

- A pattern of basing her self-esteem primarily on external factors: appearance, attractiveness, academic and professional achievement, productivity and efficiency, social performance, positive feedback from others, and sexual attention from men
- Experiencing emotional stability when she met these visible standards, and emotional dysregulation/self-hatred when she failed to meet them
- Relying on concrete behaviors in order to regulate her distress: self-injury and suicidality, promiscuity, body-related compulsions (e.g., restriction, mirror checking, avoidance, Botox), engaging in dismissive and critical self-talk ("You're fine, everything is fine"; "You're disgusting")
- At work, presuming that her colleagues and supervisors valued her when they were giving her explicit validation, and assuming that they were viewing her negatively in the absence of that validation
- In her marriage, feeling convinced that her husband's constructive feedback meant that he was judging her and looking down on her
- In those moments, feeling compelled to take immediate action (e.g., arguing, defending herself, insulting her husband) in order to manage her emotions

Given her high levels of stress and anxiety in the workplace, Kristin and her therapist decided to prioritize her difficulties with externalization in interactions with her colleagues. Utilizing the Teleological Equation Toolkit, Kristin identified the equation: "If my boss and co-workers do not give me positive feedback about a project, that means they are judging me." Kristin's therapist worked with her to explore the psychological dimensions of this assumption: What led her to feel like these two factors were connected? Kristin was initially taken aback by this question, since it seemed so obvious: "If they thought I had done a good job, of course they would say something about it. Why would they just be quiet if they were impressed with my work?"

Ultimately, Kristin was able to articulate her "reasons" for holding this belief. Whenever she was impressed with someone, she always made sure to communicate this to them explicitly. She had also literally *seen* her supervisors compliment other employees, if they really admired her colleagues' work. Plus she was not the only one to feel this way, since she felt like most people agree that there is a basic connection between "giving positive feedback" and "seeing something positively."

Kristin also reflected on the negative consequences of this teleological belief, including significant feelings of anxiety, shame, and irritability, as well as a pattern of reassurance-seeking at work, sometimes even "showing off" her knowledge and accomplishments. This potentially led her co-workers and supervisors to *see* her as more insecure, and to feel overwhelmed and frustrated by having to manage her intense emotions.

With her therapist's encouragement, Kristin worked to challenge this linking of "lack of positive feedback" with "negative judgment." She had the opportunity to do this when, after presenting on her work in a staff meeting one day, her supervisor had a more "neutral" expression on his face, and he did not mention anything about her presentation. Employing the Challenging the Teleology Toolkit, Kristin started by considering that perhaps her supervisor was *not* judging her presentation in a negative light. This was difficult to imagine, but it felt sort of liberating—the idea that his radio silence did not necessarily mean that something bad was going on. But what else could be going on in his head? He might be distracted with other things, especially all of his other responsibilities at the firm. He had been wanting to move another project forward, but she knew that he was feeling worried that it was not going well. Kristin shared in session, "I guess it is also possible that he appreciated my presentation but just didn't say anything about it. I find that hard to believe, but we really haven't seen each other much since that meeting, so it's not out of the question."

As Kristin reflected in these ways, she experienced her colleagues and supervisors as far less threatening. *Maybe* they were judging her, but also they could be feeling a broader array of positive and neutral feelings toward her, including warmth, respect, positive regard for her work, and appreciation for her as a person. She started feeling less anxious and on edge in the workplace, and more confident about the work she was doing there.

Despite these improvements in mentalizing others, Kristin continued to interpret *herself* teleologically, namely by basing her self-esteem and emotions primarily on external factors. "Even though I am not as convinced that other people are judging me, I still feel like I need them to like me, and to be impressed with me, in order to feel OK. I guess if I were to put words on the teleological equation here, it would be something like, 'I feel certain that I am only worthwhile if I am attractive, thin, professionally successful, continuously efficient and productive, and seen in a positive light by others'."

Aided by the Mentalizing the Teleology Toolkit, Kristin applied these ideas to broaden her perspective on her myriad anxieties and insecurities. She tried reckoning with the question: "Is it possible that I am suffering so much not because I do not have these external things, but because I am assuming that I am only worthwhile IF I have these external things?" Interestingly, this made her feel far less hopeless about the issues in question. Based on her past experience, she felt like she could never sufficiently meet her own external standards, which led her to feel hopeless and demoralized. But if the problem was her standards *themselves*, that introduced the possibility of change. "I may never be thin enough, and I may be getting less attractive as I get older. But if the reason why I feel so stressed out and ashamed is because I am basing my self-esteem on those things, then maybe I can actually do something about that."

Kristin thus devoted herself to challenging and disrupting these concrete linkages. When she was judging herself for not being productive and efficient enough at work, she worked to "press pause," and to imagine any instances where she has been productive and efficient, and yet NOT felt worthwhile and good about herself. "That happens all of the time, actually. Even when I have a really good day and get a lot accomplished, I still feel like I haven't done enough, and there is something wrong with me as a person. Sort of like nothing is ever enough for me. Now that I think about it, it is kind of a shitty deal: I set up all of these conditions for my value, and yet I never end up feeling very good about myself."

Kristin also worked to apply these strategies whenever she was feeling insecure about her weight and appearance. She envisioned what she saw as the worst case scenario along these lines: her getting wrinkles and gaining a lot of weight as she got older, such that other people saw her as "old" and no longer found her attractive. Following the Challenging the Teleology Toolkit, Kristin tried to imagine the possibility that she could have intrinsic worth and value, even if these external conditions were to transpire. "I can't really picture what that would look like for me—it's like trying to imagine a square circle, or an invisible color. For everybody else in my life, I would be so offended by the idea that their value is based on how they look. With my friends, family, and even my husband, I love them for who they are— unconditionally, regardless of their appearance. I do really like the idea of this: that somehow I could have a sense of peace no matter how I looked, and that I wouldn't have to keep doing all of this stuff in order to feel good about myself."

As Kristin reflected more flexibly about these issues of self-esteem, she started to feel less overwhelmed and controlled by all of the external factors in her life. She felt calmer and more comfortable at work, putting less pressure on herself to do everything perfectly, all the time. While she still did not like how she looked, she felt more accepting of her appearance, and less focused on all of these minor "imperfections" that would previously dominate her thinking. Kristin also started experiencing an increased sense of agency surrounding her body-focused behaviors. She discontinued her mirror-checking, stopped receiving Botox injections, and took the leap of enabling Self View in Zoom meetings. She also stopped restricting her food, and she began consistently following a food and exercise plan, as recommended by her dietitian.

Heartened by this progress, Kristin shifted her focus onto her challenges with reactivity and defensiveness in her relationship with her husband Mark. She formulated the teleological equation: "Whenever he criticizes me, I need to attack him back, or else I am going to feel horrible about myself." With this pattern on her radar, Kristin worked to "reflect rather than reflex" in those moments when Mark would give her constructive feedback about their shared household tasks. She acknowledged that, even when she did insult and criticize him for the feedback, she still ended up experiencing negative feelings about herself, now compounded with guilt and shame for her aggressive outbursts. In an effort to further disrupt the teleological equation, Kristin envisioned what it might feel like to NOT criticize and insult her husband. Could she ever imagine not criticizing him, without feeling intense shame and worthlessness?

"If this were to happen today, I don't think it would be possible. Even if I were to hold my tongue and not respond, I would still believe he was talking down to me, so I would feel really bad about myself. In order to not feel worthless and ashamed in the moment, I would have to have a much stronger sense of self—some sense of self-worth independent of what he thinks of me, or how he is treating me. I'm not there yet, but I do want to work toward it, especially since I don't want to keep being so aggressive toward him."

Utilizing the Expanding the Teleology Toolkit, Kristin worked to reflect more broadly on Mark's mental states when he was disagreeing with how she completed some household chore. Other than potentially looking down on her (her teleological assumption), what might he be feeling in those moments? She knew that Mark was highly perfectionistic, just like she was. He could get quite anxious around household matters, especially when things seemed messy or disorganized. In light of this, Kristin wondered if perhaps Mark was simply wanting the house to be cleaner in order to manage his own anxiety, without necessarily looking down on her and seeing her as incompetent. Kristin shared in her therapy appointments, "The more that I sit with this, I think that I have been kind of taking things personally with him. This is just who he is, and it doesn't really have much to do with me, even if it might feel that way in the moment."

Kristin's experience of these discussions with Mark gradually began to shift. She felt less victimized and controlled by him, and also less reliant on criticizing him in order to manage her own feelings of shame. Instead, she worked to communicate her emotions and desires in a more open and flexible way, without needing to "change his mind" and his manner of seeing her. "I have just been trying to pay more attention to what I am feeling in these discussions, and also not just jump to quick conclusions about what Mark is feeling. As long as I keep those things on my radar, I feel like I have a lot more self-control over what I do next. Sometimes I go along with what Mark wants me to do, and other times, I decide to keep doing what I was doing. But in the end, 'what I do' seems less important than how I am thinking about it."

After several years in treatment, Kristin experienced significant improvements in her overall level of stability and self-esteem. While she remained quite ambitious and high-achieving, she felt far less anxious, irritable, and pressured as she moved throughout her days, and more accepting of all of the messiness and "imperfections" (e.g., in work, appearance, and her relationships) that are just part of everyday life. As she became less reliant on visible behaviors (e.g., perfectionism, self-injury, defensiveness, self-criticism) to manage and suppress her feelings, Kristin actually started *feeling* her feelings, even if they were painful and initially upsetting to her. Her depression improved, along with her hopelessness and suicidality.

"I used to hate my emotions, but even more, I used to hate myself for having emotions in the first place. Something was only real if I could see it, so I just did whatever I could to change myself on the outside. I am learning that there is more to me than meets the eye, and more to other people too. There is something scary about that, but also kind of comforting. It makes me feel more centered in myself—just knowing that there is some part of me that is real, alive, and even *good*, no matter what is going on around me."

Chapter Review 13.1
Teleological Mode: Concreteness and Externalization

Introduction to Teleological Mode

- Teleological mode involves excessive concreteness and externalization, such that you rely extensively on external factors in order to understand yourself and other people.

- These external factors can include physical appearance; bodily processes; money; material possessions; actions; interpersonal interactions; academic, professional, or social status; places; time; relationships with certain people, organizations, or groups; and events and circumstances, in your own life or in the broader world.

- With teleology, you become highly certain that some external thing is connected (or "linked") to an internal state.

  - "The outside determines the inside."

  - "This *[external thing]* means that *[internal thing]*."

- Since both non-mentalizing modes involve excessive certainty, teleology can be seen as an important "species" of psychic equivalence mode, one that involves you endorsing some rigid formula, along the lines of EXTERNAL = INTERNAL.

- When in teleological mode, you remain trapped in your initial, externally focused interpretations of other people, failing to mentalize a broader array of mental states in others.

- You become something like a puppet on a string: your emotions and beliefs get involuntarily controlled by the world around you, and you lack of full sense of agency in your life.

Concrete Beliefs about Yourself

- In borderline personality disorder (BPD), your teleological thinking can variously involve:

  - *Linking your feelings with your subsequent actions:* "If I feel lonely, then I have to reach out to my ex."

  - *Connecting your actions with your positive mental states:* "If I just spend all day studying, then I can feel good about myself."

  - *Connecting your actions with your painful emotional states:* "I cannot go to that in-person support group . . . it will make me too anxious."

  - *Associating your visible personal characteristics with positive emotions in yourself:* "I can only feel confident if I am beneath a specific weight."

  - *Associating your visible personal characteristics with painful emotions in yourself:* "I feel so anxious whenever I have a breakout. . . . I don't want anyone to be able to see me."

  - *Correlating external situations with positive emotions in yourself:* "I need my partner to validate me, in order to feel emotionally safe in our relationship."

[continued on next page]

- *Correlating external situations with painful emotions in yourself:* "I feel so overwhelmed if there is too much going on around me."
- *Teleological self-esteem:* "I feel like I only have value when I am in a romantic relationship, and when other people are giving me positive feedback."
- *Teleological shame:* "I feel horrible about myself because I have not lived up to my potential: I am not successful enough, I do not make enough money, and I still do not own my own home."

Concrete Beliefs about Other People

- In BPD, your teleological beliefs about other individuals can focus on:
  - *Connecting other people's actions with their positive mental states:* "They just texted me out of the blue, so they definitely are interested in me."
  - *Connecting other people's actions with their negative mental states:* "I can tell that he is angry with me, since he frowned and looked away from me as soon as I walked into the room."
  - *Associating other people's visible personal characteristics with their positive emotions:* "She seems so confident and self-assured: she's beautiful, thin, and always has the right outfit for every occasion."
  - *Associating other people's visible personal characteristics with their negative emotions:* "He had bedhead, and his shirt was wrinkled. . . . Clearly, he did not care about this date."
  - *Correlating external situations with positive emotions in other people:* "You need to quit that job, if you want your depression to get any better."
  - *Correlating external situations with negative emotions in other people:* "Without a relationship, she is just too anxious to function in her life."

Chapter Review 13.2
Mentalizing Practice Points: Mentalizing the Teleology

In mentalization-based treatment (MBT), the therapeutic approach for addressing teleological mode can be summed up by the dictum: "Disrupt the externalization."

This involves recognizing that you are engaged in a psychological process, and that this psychological TENDENCY in you is a key driver of your suffering. Once the teleology feels more mental, you can challenge your beliefs about how the "outside" and the "inside" are definitively linked.

The first step in this process involves identifying the teleological belief that you want to address.

The Teleological Equation Toolkit			
External Factor on which You are Focused *(Action, visible characteristic, or circumstance involving you or another person)*			
Related Internal Factors			
Thoughts	Emotions	Desires	Feelings about the Self

Articulate the Teleological Equation:

"I feel certain that

_____

[external factor from above]

means that

_____."

[internal factor(s) from above]

[continued on next page]

With this equation in hand, follow these steps to reflect on the psychological dimensions of the teleological experience.

Mentalizing the Teleology Toolkit

Visualize the Teleological Equation

External Factor:

=

Internal Factor:

What Leads You to Believe These Two Things are Connected?

Other Beliefs or Feelings in You	Beliefs or Feelings in Other People	Visible Actions, Events, or Circumstances

What are the Consequences of Your Teleological Belief?

Your Emotions, Desires, and Self-states	Actions You Take	Impact of Your Actions on Relationships/Other People

[continued on next page]

Contextualize Your Suffering
Ask yourself the question:
"Is it possible that I am suffering not because
_____ ,
[external factor from above]
but because I am assuming that
_____
[external factor from above]
means that
_____ ?"
[internal factor(s) from above]

Chapter Review 13.3
Mentalizing Practice Points: Challenging the Teleology

Once the teleology feels more like a *belief* in you, the next step is challenging and disrupting the belief in question. Utilizing the following toolkit, try "taking issue" with both components in the teleological equation.

Challenging the Teleology Toolkit

Restate the Teleological Equation

External Factor: ▭ ▭ = Internal Factor:

Take Issue with the Internal Component

Visualize the External Factor:	THEN	Try to imagine _____ *[internal factor(s) from above]* NOT being present, even while the external factor is in play. What might that look like?
		Attempt to envision OTHER internal factors (e.g., thoughts, emotions, desires, self-states) being present, right alongside the external factor. Describe these additional internal processes here:

[continued on next page]

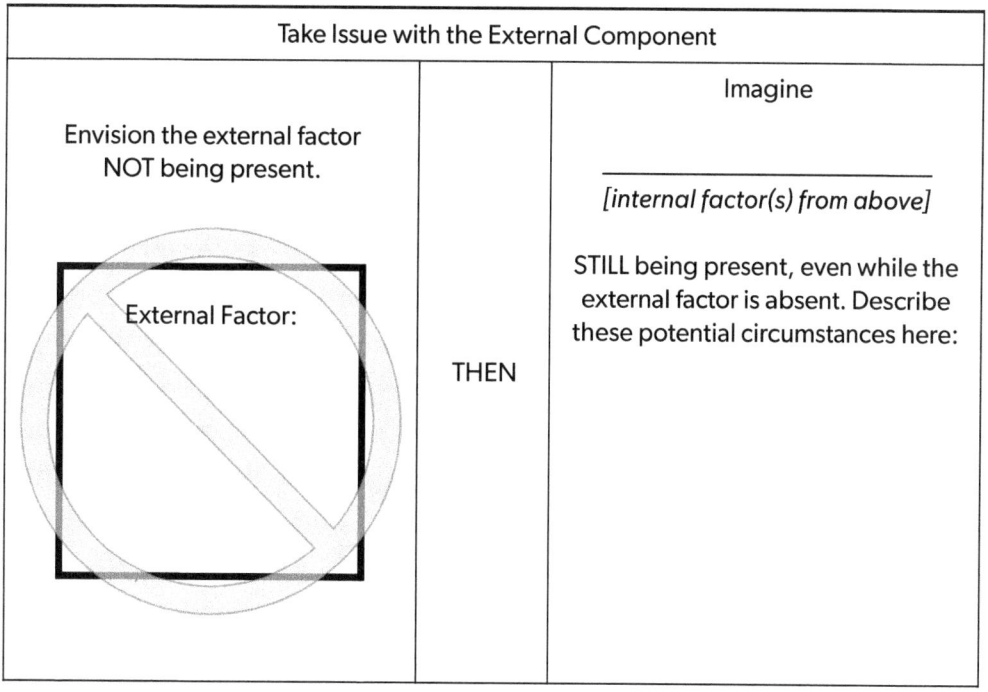

Now that you have "imaginatively disrupted" your teleological thinking, revisit your original concrete assumption. Work toward attaining a broader perspective on the teleology—one that includes mental states you did not originally associate with the visible thing in question.

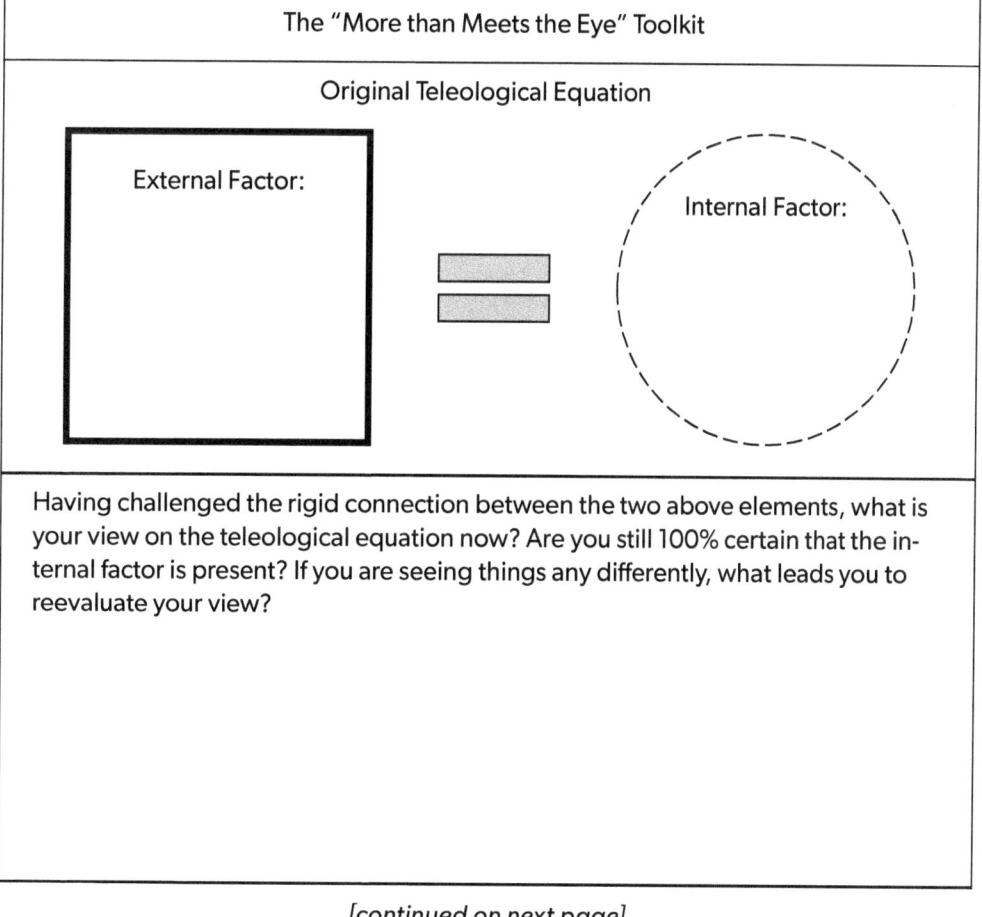

[continued on next page]

What other mental states can you also imagine alongside the external factor, either now or in the future? "Expand" the teleological equation by describing these below.

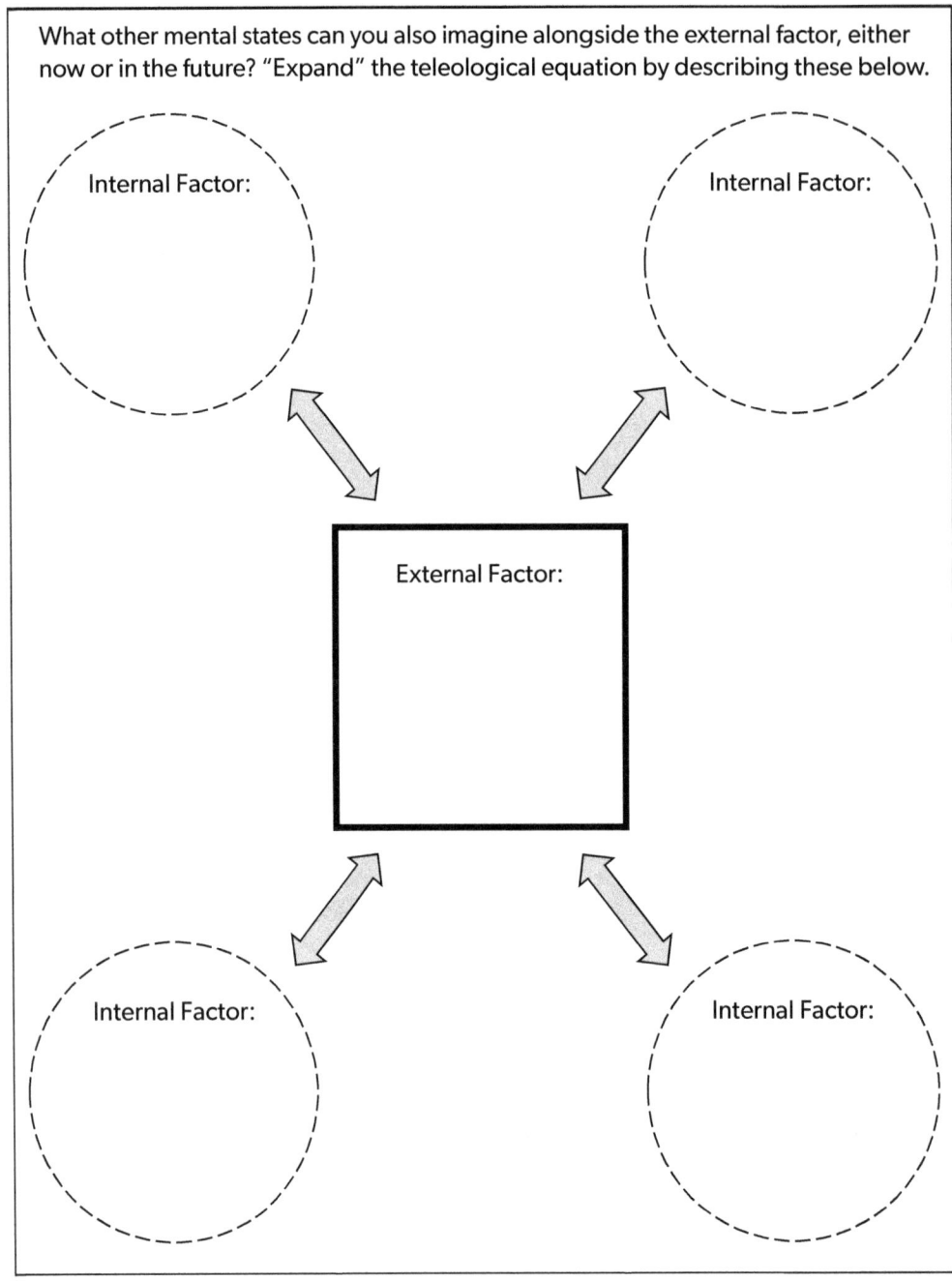

14

Addressing Problems with Disconnection and Dissociation

For as long as he could remember, Paul struggled with suicidal thinking, sensitivity to rejection, and disconnection from his emotions. A college philosophy professor, Paul grew up in a family of highly successful academics, who valued intelligence and abstract thinking above all else. Throughout his childhood, there were no discussions of emotions, desires, or interactions with his peers. Around the dinner table, his family lived on a steady diet of science, literature, and philosophy, with a side of politics thrown in for good measure. He knew that his parents loved him, but he never felt *seen* by them as a full person.

While Paul always excelled academically, he struggled with nearly constant, unbearable feelings of emptiness. For reasons he never understood, he felt dead inside—a dull, aching sense of numbness that followed him around wherever he went. Intellectually, he knew that he must be struggling with some challenging emotions, but he just could not find them in himself, or feel them in any deep way. He always felt like he was a thousand miles away from himself, on the outside looking in.

The only thing that gave Paul any relief was thinking about suicide. When the Internet came out, he immediately began researching suicide methods online. He fantasized about these methods in excruciating detail: gathering the implements, writing the notes, carrying out his plan, his family discovering his body, and what people would say about him at his funeral. When picturing these things, he would then be able to cry—a full-throated sobbing that finally enabled him to get connected to his body, and to feel like he was real. There were no thoughts in these tears, just an experience of being overwhelmed and flooded with pure, unthinking emotion.

All of this changed in graduate school, when Paul met his wife Sonia. Paul had never been in a romantic relationship before, and he was enamored. They spent all of their time together: going for walks, having sex multiple times per day, spending long afternoons at the library, discussing their research, travelling to conferences, and attending classical music concerts. For the first time in his life, Paul felt like he was truly important to someone, and that he was not alone. His mood improved, and he felt more connected to himself, at least as long as Sonia was around.

The problem, from Paul's perspective, was that Sonia was not always around. When Sonia took time away from their dynamic—to run errands, take care of work obligations, or visit with her family and friends—Paul felt abandoned by her, becoming despondent and resentful at her for leaving him. He withdrew from her emotionally, giving her the silent treatment in the hopes that she would ask what was wrong, apologize, and try to connect with him again. When Sonia did not pursue him in this way, Paul became critical of her, accusing her of not caring enough about him and making his depression worse.

These challenges only intensified when Paul and Sonia starting having children, and Sonia's energy was significantly focused on them and their needs. They spent less alone time together, the frequency of their sexual intimacy dramatically decreased, and Sonia

Mentalization. Robert P. Drozek, Oxford University Press. © Oxford University Press 2025.
DOI: 10.1093/oso/9780198916857.003.0014

seemed far less emotionally present with him—less attuned to how Paul was feeling, and less concerned when he was struggling. While Paul loved the children, he also felt resentful of them for taking up so much of Sonia's time and attention. Those old feelings of emptiness crept back in, along with the desire to end things. Rather than partnering with Sonia to take care of the children, Paul would isolate in his office and research suicide methods online. Sonia confronted him about his separateness, but Paul was defensive and dismissive of her concerns: "I'm around as much as you are! You're just emotionally enmeshed with the kids, and you can't handle the fact that I actually have boundaries."

Paul and Sonia gradually became more estranged and distant from each other. Paul started writing suicide notes to Sonia and the children, and he "rehearsed" tying the noose that he would one day use to hang himself. When Sonia found the notes and noose in Paul's office, she was horrified, and Paul agreed to finally seek out treatment for his difficulties. He found a therapist who specialized in mentalization-based treatment (MBT).

Paul had no experience engaging in any type of therapy. In his therapy sessions, Paul presented as highly intellectual and "in his head"—speaking in a monotone with minimal emotional expression, even when he was discussing topics (e.g., his marital problems and suicidal gestures) that many people would find emotionally painful. Paul spent most of his time describing external circumstances in his life: his academic responsibilities, his various medications, and the different activities that Sonia would do with the children. When the therapist inquired about Paul's emotional challenges, Paul responded in an abstract and intellectualized fashion, sharing his theories about what he was going through, influenced by various psychological concepts and jargon he had picked up online.

"I think that the problem is that I have an anxious attachment style, while Sonia has a more secure attachment style. There has been codependency and enmeshment on my part, likely driven by narcissistic abuse and neglect from my parents, who were never able to meet my emotional needs. I also suspect there might be some trauma bonding in play, but that is kind of a new concept for me, so I have to learn more about that." When the therapist invited Paul to elaborate more on these abstractions ("Could you share about what you are getting at when you say that you have 'anxious attachment'?"), Paul responded by simply restating the same terms: "You know, anxious attachment: where the person struggles to feel secure in their relationships, and experiences fears of abandonment and low self-esteem."

The therapist thus felt quite distant from Paul and his challenges, as if there was a tremendous gulf between what Paul was saying and how he was actually struggling. Paul also did not seem that interested in what the therapist *herself* was thinking and feeling in their interactions. He spoke in monologues, talking for minutes on end about his intellectual formulations and explanations about himself and other people. If the therapist tried to interrupt him to further explore what he was saying, he appeared irritated with her. Sighing audibly, he would briefly respond to her question and then immediately return to spooling out his previous line of thought. Regardless of what Paul was explicitly *saying*, he seemed fundamentally adrift: separated from his own emotions, and disconnected from other people's minds, including the mind of the therapist who was trying to help him.

DISCONNECTION FROM MENTAL STATES IN YOURSELF

As mentioned in Chapter 12, pretend mode involves difficulties with disconnection and dissociation: disconnection from your own emotions and desires, and detachment from other people's mental states as well. At the outset, I want to make one thing clear: The term "pretend mode" does not imply dishonesty, or any intentional misrepresentation of facts. Rather, the "pretend" in pretend mode derives from the notion of pretend play in childhood, where the child is entirely absorbed in a world of their own creation and imagination, and (in the moment) less attentive to their own emotions, other people's emotions, or the world around them (Bateman et al., 2023). As they play, the child can talk and talk and talk: "And then this happened, and then that happened, and then he said this. But she had never been to the place before, so everybody took a break and looked around at the scenery. And they were like, 'Woah'. . . ." In these moments, most children are *not* asking themselves "What emotions am I experiencing right now in my life?" or "What are the people around me feeling?"

According to MBT's theory of borderline personality disorder (BPD), pretend mode develops due to deficits in parental mirroring. As we reviewed in Chapter 4, when caregivers fail to adequately mentalize the child's emotions, the child internalizes images or "representations" of the caregiver, but those representations do not reflect the child's primary feeling states. As development unfolds, this leads to a sense of vacancy and emptiness in the sense of self. You might possess language to describe yourself and others, but that language does not map onto your actual emotions and desires. This could be seen as the tagline for pretend mode: "Words without feelings." And if you cannot fully access and experience your own feelings, you lack the robust emotional foundation for empathizing and resonating with other people's emotions.

When you are struggling with pretend mode, these difficulties do not necessarily manifest themselves across the board, in all relationships and circumstances. While you could potentially experience more "global" problems with pretend mode (e.g., complete disconnection from your own emotions, or utter inability to empathize with others), you most likely encounter what we call *context-dependent* difficulties with pretend mode—that is, the tendency to "disconnect" from yourself and other people under certain emotional or interpersonal conditions. For instance, you might start to dissociate when you are under stress, or you could find it difficult to empathize with others when you feel like they are criticizing you.

Accordingly, as we are reviewing the different examples of pretend mode in this chapter, try to be curious about the specific factors that tend to "trigger" you falling into pretend mode. Examples include particular internal states (e.g., some emotion, desire, or feeling about yourself), interpersonal scenarios (e.g., certain relationships or types of relationships, specific interactions or experiences with select individuals), or events and circumstances that are not directly "about" other people (e.g., involving work, academics, finances, possessions, health and body, living situation, time of day/year, or your immediate environment).

In yourself, pretend mode can present itself in a variety of ways:

- *Lack of interest in or curiosity about your own mental states:* At times, you might feel little to no curiosity about the topic of what you are feeling. The question "What is happening inside of me?" is simply not that compelling to you. If someone (e.g., your therapist, your partner) asks you about your emotional states, you could feel a sense of apathy, indifference, or even irritation, as if the issue is completely inconsequential or irrelevant. Who cares? Why does that matter, given everything else that is going on? Importantly, without that basic level of curiosity or interest, no mentalization is possible. And as we have discussed throughout this book, when mentalization is offline, you are vulnerable to all of the forms of instability that are central to BPD. From that perspective, this "lack of curiosity about mental states" could be seen as one of the most counterproductive and even dangerous attitudes you can hold in the treatment of BPD.
- *Detachment from your own emotions and desires:* In Chapter 9, we reviewed your difficulties with content-mentalizing, where you find it challenging to identify and "put words on" your internal states. With pretend mode, you might cognitively "know" what you are feeling, but you struggle to actually *feel* the thing. For example, you feel largely neutral or unbothered when discussing emotionally charged topics (e.g., falling in love, past traumatic experiences), failing to access and inhabit the emotions you suspect have to be in there somewhere. Or people

might tell you that your non-verbal displays (e.g., tone of voice, facial expressions) do not properly match the content of what you are talking about: You may smile when talking about your self-injury, or appear emotionally "flat" when discussing your recent promotion.

These experiences are consistent with research linking BPD with decreased emotional awareness and alexithymia, or difficulties identifying and expressing emotional states (Derks et al., 2017). This disconnection from your emotions can lead you to feel separate from yourself as a person—from who you are, what you want, and what you deserve in your life. And when you are disconnected from yourself, people feel less emotionally connected to you. They can neglect you and ignore you, on some level sensing that you are not fully *there* in a meaningful way. In the worst case scenario, when you fail to appreciate your own needs and rights in your relationships, you are at risk for abuse, mistreatment, and exploitation from others.

- *Chronic feelings of emptiness:* As we discussed in Chapter 1, "chronic feelings of emptiness" are one of the nine diagnostic criteria for BPD. These feelings can be understood in various ways, but research suggests that this experience involves "a feeling of disconnection from both self and others" (Miller et al., 2021). This understanding situates emptiness squarely in the realm of pretend mode. Framed another way, emptiness is the feeling that comes when you cannot feel your feelings. This can manifest as a sense of numbness, nothingness, purposelessness, dissatisfaction, restlessness, unfulfillment, or feeling "dead inside." Something is missing, but you do not know what it is. You might then try to cope with these feelings through impulsive behaviors, hurting yourself, or distracting yourself by filling up your life with productive activities (Miller et al., 2020; Miller et al., 2021).

- *Dissociative symptoms:* Jumping forward to criterion nine for BPD, "severe dissociative symptoms" can also be present in pretend mode. From a technical perspective, the American Psychiatric Association (2022) defines dissociation as "discontinuity in the normal integration of consciousness, memory, identity, emotion, perception, body representation, motor control, and behavior" (p. 329). Talk about a mouthful! Put more simply, dissociation is essentially losing contact with your own experience. This can include feeling separate from your emotions, disconnecting from your body, feeling like you are seeing yourself from the outside, getting lost in daydreams or fantasy, zoning out and "losing time," memory problems, and losing contact with who you are as a person. In addition to causing stress and anxiety for you, these difficulties can significantly impact your ability to function in your life. You might feel less connected to your loved ones, struggle to concentrate at work, or try to feel more connected to yourself by engaging in risky behaviors like abusing substances, self-injury, or promiscuity.

- *Overreliance on intellectualization, abstractions, and jargon about yourself:* Pretend mode often involves you being more "in your head" than "in your heart." You could be prone to extensively sharing your ideas about yourself, without fully accessing and inhabiting your own emotions and desires. Examples include talking in generalities rather than specifics ("I am the sort of person who . . . "; "My problem is that I tend to . . . "); explaining rather than describing your experiences ("This links back to my childhood . . . "; "I think that I became this way because . . . "); communicating in a highly vague fashion ("I have been through a lot of things in my life, which have really impacted me"; "This week was really difficult, mostly due to challenges in my relationships"); focusing on what you presume you "should" be thinking and feeling ("I need to maintain a positive attitude"; "I should not be so upset about this . . . "; "If I were more focused on achieving my goals, I could finally move forward in my life"); and employing "jargon" and technical psychological concepts to describe your internal experiences (e.g., "I'm feeling manic," "I have a lot of intrusive thoughts," "Do you know about complex trauma?", "My depression was getting so bad," "My attachment style is . . . ," "I'm very codependent," "I'm an empath").

While there is nothing inherently wrong with this sort of language, it is one step removed from your actual lived experience. This means that, if you rely on it too much, it can inadvertently cut you off from your felt emotions and desires. In your relationships, other people might understand your ideas about yourself, but they are not seeing you *feel things* while you are engaging in this way, and so they may feel more distant and alienated from you.

- *Disconnection from certain objective facts about your life:* Throughout this book, we have considered ways in which you might ignore or "miss" specific emotions and desires in yourself and other people. Interestingly, something similar can happen with external reality: You can ignore, minimize, or "miss" seemingly important objective factors about yourself and your life situation. These may be factors that lead you to experience painful emotions whenever you think about them, for example some physical quality of yours that you dislike, your past actions that make you feel embarrassed or ashamed, or an area of your life where you feel like you are not measuring up. Or if you are seeing yourself in a more negative light, these factors could be more "positive" things about you, such as your talents, interpersonal strengths, past successful actions, physical traits that you actually *do* find attractive, or more pleasant events or circumstances in your life. In other cases, these factors might be more emotionally "neutral" (e.g., some obligation or plan, some past action or interaction, a current situation or event in your life), but you are simply not thinking about them, despite the fact that they are relevant and meaningful to you. They are not on your radar.

These forms of disconnection can lead you to develop a highly incomplete picture of yourself, which is divorced from external reality. You are then unable to take steps to modify your maladaptive behaviors, improve your circumstances, or address your challenging emotions around the parts of reality from which you are disconnected. For example, if you fail to appreciate your pattern of "chasing" romantic partners who are less invested in you, there is nothing to stop you from continuing that. If you try to ignore your significant difficulties in your work situation, those problems will just continue. You can thus remain trapped in a "pretend mode sense of self," lacking the key information about yourself that is necessary to spur change.

Mentalizing Warm-up

Having learned more about pretend mode, revisit Paul's story on page 347. What examples of disconnection and dissociation can you observe in Paul's experience of himself? How do these challenges impact his mood, self-esteem, relationships, and functionality?

Utilizing Worksheet 14.1, apply these ideas about pretend mode to your own life. In what ways have you experienced disconnection and dissociation from your internal experience?

Worksheet 14.1
Pretend Mode: How do You Experience Disconnection from Yourself?

(1) What does it look like when you experience a lack of curiosity about your own mental states? Are there any circumstances where you are less likely to be interested in what you are feeling?

(2) Detail any examples when you have experienced a sense of detachment from your own emotions and desires. What conditions have triggered this detachment in you?

(3) If you have been more detached from your feelings, how has that impacted your mood, self-esteem, relationships, and behavior?

(4) In what ways have you experienced feelings of emptiness in your life? What circumstances tend to elicit these feelings in you?

[continued on next page]

(5) How have your feelings of emptiness impacted your mood, self-esteem, relationships, and behavior?

(6) See below for a list of dissociative symptoms often associated with trauma and borderline personality disorder (BPD). Circle any of these that you have experienced in your life.

Feeling separate from your emotions	Disconnecting from your body
Feeling like you are seeing yourself from the outside	Losing contact with who you are as a person
Memory problems	Zoning out and "losing time"
Getting lost in daydreams or fantasy	Other dissociative symptoms:

(7) What events or situations are likely to instigate these difficulties? Describe any ways in which these forms of dissociation have affected your mood, self-esteem, relationships, and behavior.

(8) *Intellectualization* includes talking or thinking in generalities ("I tend to . . . "), explanation-giving, using psychological jargon, focusing on "shoulds" or ideals, or communicating in a vague or confusing manner. Recount any examples where you have engaged in intellectualization about yourself, as well as the negative consequences this has had in your life and relationships.

[continued on next page]

(9) How have you been disconnected from any objective facts about yourself and your life? Such facts could include your physical characteristics, past or present actions, relationships, or life circumstances. Outline any examples of this disconnection, as well as how this has negatively affected your everyday functioning.

DISCONNECTION FROM MENTAL STATES IN OTHER PEOPLE

When you are in pretend mode, you can become disconnected from *other* individuals' mental states as well. That is, you might cognitively recognize what others are feeling and wanting (i.e., engaging in the "content-mentalizing" reviewed in Chapter 9), but you remain somewhat detached, separated, and disengaged from these emotions and desires. In MBT, we call this "pretend mode with other people."

Before we proceed, a word of warning. We will be talking about your difficulties taking other people in, and responding to them in an empathic and compassionate way—the so-called "problems in empathy." While these problems are highly common in BPD and other personality disorders (Burghart & Mier, 2022; Ohse et al., 2024; Salgado et al., 2020; Urbonaviciute & Hepper, 2020), reflecting on them can sometimes bring up strong feelings for people, including guilt, shame, and self-judgment. *"If I struggle with empathy, that means I do not care about people. And if I do not care about people, that makes me a bad person. That has always been my biggest fear."* This kind of thinking is only reinforced in popular culture and social media (e.g., TikTok, Reddit), which is overrun with portrayals of people with BPD as aggressive, self-centered, and low-functioning, thus perpetuating stigma and unfair stereotypes.

As you make your way through this section, do your best to avoid going down these unhelpful roads. *All of us* struggle with deficits in empathy, which then influence how we treat the people we love. This is a human problem, not just a personality disorder problem. And these problems do not mean that we are not *also* kind, thoughtful, and responsive to other people's needs. As mentioned earlier in the chapter, if you have BPD, you most likely experience *context-dependent* disconnectedness from yourself and others. This means that your ability to connect and resonate with others likely goes "up and down," sort of like the bars on a cell phone, but depending on what you are feeling and what is going on around you. So rather than criticize yourself for these challenges, simply ask yourself: "How might these difficulties show themselves in my life? When are they most likely to arise, and when are they less likely to appear?" This approach enables you to reflect on these issues in a more nuanced and self-accepting manner, without drawing any grand conclusions about yourself as a person.

In BPD, common forms of disconnectedness from other people include:

- *Lack of interest in or curiosity about other people's mental states:* You might find yourself feeling somewhat indifferent or apathetic about the question of "What is this other person feeling?" This may arise with particular people, for example someone against whom you have anger or resentment, or you could experience this toward people more generally: not really being curious about or invested in understanding what they are going through. Without this curiosity, you remain trapped in your "own little world." Your perspective becomes THE perspective, and since you are not *seeking out* the experiences of others, you are less likely to encounter information that could expand and disrupt your automatic feelings and assumptions.
- *Overreliance on intellectualization, abstractions, and jargon about other people:* As mentioned earlier in the chapter, pretend mode often involves getting "stuck in your head," rather than feeling your feelings. An analogous process can happen in your relationships with other people, where you relate to others in an overly intellectual fashion, finding it more challenging to identify, resonate, and empathize with their emotions and desires.

Examples include talking in generalities rather than specifics about others ("My mother is just a very critical person"; "He really struggles with anxiety, which has never been treated"; "In all of her relationships, she tends to put other people in front of herself"); explaining rather than describing other people's experiences ("He reacted like that because of his history of childhood trauma . . . "; "She is just seeing me through the lens of her past abusive relationships . . . "; "I blame this all on her alcoholic father . . . "); talking about others in a highly vague fashion ("She is a really sensitive person, which has created a lot of stress for her"; "He has made so much progress, but he has a long way to go"); focusing on what you think other people "should" be thinking and feeling ("She needs to work through her unresolved issues of grief and loss"; "He has no right to be angry at me"; "They are way too focused on . . . "); and employing "jargon" and technical psychological concepts to describe other people's experiences ("He's a narcissist, and he was just grooming and love bombing me"; "She just gets into toxic relationships, over and over again"; "They won't stop gaslighting me"; "His favorite defense mechanism is projection").

At first listen, these sorts of communications *sound* insightful, but they are not actually focusing on the other person's emotions and desires. When engaging in these forms of intellectualization and abstraction, you can struggle to fully connect and empathize with others, and other people are less likely to feel like you are *seeing* them as full, emotionally complex individuals.

- *Monologues and self-focused communications:* When interacting with other people, you might find yourself falling into what could be called *self-focused* communications: engaging in monologues, or talking for prolonged periods of time without interruption; speaking extensively about yourself, your experiences, and your ideas about things; not asking other people questions; neglecting to listen when others speak, and to explicitly "reflect back" what they are saying; not answering others' questions or addressing their concerns; interrupting others; turning conversation topics back to you and your life ("That reminds me of when I . . . "); arguing with other individuals, or dismissing and criticizing their views; or even mumbling and talking with a low voice volume, such that other people cannot easily hear you.

  When communicating in these ways, there is a stark imbalance of "Self over Other" (Chapter 11), such that you end up occupying an inordinate amount of space in the interpersonal interaction, and the other person is "smaller" and less prominent. It is like you are the star of a one-person show, and the other person is the lone audience member in the back row, rather than being up there on the stage with you. From the perspective of mentalizing, this means that other people's *mental states* are less prominent in the interchange, and so you are less able to recognize and empathize with what others are going through. Other people can thus feel less connected to you, and you can feel more isolated and alone in your relationships, since you are deprived of the vital experience of relating to others in a truly dynamic, reciprocal way.

- *Disconnection from certain objective facts about other people:* At times, you might not be sufficiently engaged with external reality: ignoring, minimizing, or "missing" objective factors about the people around you. These factors include others' actions, interpersonal patterns, appearance, or life circumstances (e.g., concerning work, school, finances, possessions, medical issues, living situation)—either in the past or in the present. We see this form of dissociation especially in tendencies toward idealization and devaluation (discussed in Chapter 12), where you focus less on external things that undermine or contradict your rigid view of the other person. For example, if you feel really excited about a new romantic partner, you might not want to think about your ambiguous relationship status, and the fact that they were a bit cagey when you asked about what was happening between the two of you: "Let's just see where things go." Or if you feel quite angry at a close friend for not prioritizing your relationship, you could be less attentive to the times when they have been highly supportive, consistent, and devoted to you.

When disconnected in these ways, you are working with an incomplete picture of the other individual, one that fails to reflect the full reality of who they are as a person. This ends up affecting how you feel and behave in your relationships. You continue relating to the other person in an overly idealizing or devaluing manner, and you remain disconnected from the specific feelings (e.g., anxiety, sadness, shame, love, desires for closeness) that you *would* experience, if you were acknowledging the objective factors in question.

- *Deficits in empathy for other people:* "Empathy" can be defined as the ability to resonate with, care about, and be motivated by other people's mental states. The psychoanalyst Heinz Kohut (1984) described empathy as *vicarious introspection*, or "the capacity to think and feel oneself into the inner life of another person" (p. 82). Empathy is a complex construct in BPD. While some studies suggest that individuals with BPD are actually *more* empathically attuned to others, most research finds that people diagnosed with BPD can suffer from notable impairments and disruptions in the ability to empathize with other people (Salgado et al., 2020). Research on empathy suggests that empathic deficits fall into two main categories: passive deficits and active deficits (Decety & Meyer, 2008; Jones et al., 2010; Rhee et al., 2013, 2016, 2021). *Passive* empathic deficits involve not fully "keeping other people in mind": not being attentive to other people's feelings, not experiencing robust concern or compassion for others, and failing to resonate with and feel motivated by other individuals' emotions, needs, and rights. Under these conditions, you can struggle with self-centeredness, self-involvement, entitlement, or a pattern of "using" others to satisfy your own desires and preferences (e.g., for emotional support, attention, or financial assistance). People feel neglected and taken advantage of by you, as if you are not fully invested in them as independent, worthwhile individuals.

  On the other hand, *active* empathic deficits involve actually experiencing desires and wishes that undermine other people's dignity or well-being. You might cognitively understand what others are feeling, and you still want to do or say something to make them experience some form of emotional or physical pain. People can end up feeling hurt, mistreated, and victimized by you, since you are not treating them with the respect that they deserve. This can lead to significant disruptions in relationships, including conflicts, frequent break-ups, estrangement, and alienation from others.

  See below for examples of the different "types" of empathic deficits that we see in BPD. Bear in mind that, for each category of difficulty, you could experience either active or passive empathic deficits, or perhaps a bit of both, depending on your unique personality traits and relationship with the people in question.

  - *Person-specific empathic deficits:* While you might be highly empathic to many people, your ability to empathize could get "turned down" or even "shut off" with particular individuals in your life: your parents, siblings, boss, or former friends. For example, when describing these challenges, you might reflect: "I can often take my boyfriend for granted—using him for emotional support whenever I am upset, but not thinking about his emotions and needs, or even how all of my difficulties are impacting hm. I also forget to ask him about how his day is going, instead just launching into whatever is happening with me" *[passive empathic deficits]*. Or you could observe: "I feel intense hatred for my mother, for never really being a parent to me. I want her to know how much she has fucked me up, and to feel all the pain that I have felt in my life: the shame, desperation, and hopelessness. I try to punish and hurt her by not talking to her, not answering her texts, and reaching out to my dad instead of her" *[active empathic deficits]*.

- *Group-specific empathic deficits:* At times, you might find it challenging to empathize with people who possess particular personal qualities (e.g., personality traits, identity, or demographic characteristics), who have certain group affiliations (e.g., with political parties, companies, or religions), or who serve in a defined vocational or cultural role (e.g., as a boss, teacher, law enforcement officer, therapist). For instance, you could reflect: "I really want nothing to do with people from the opposing political party. Given what they support, I tend to see them as 'less than human,' and I don't really care if anything bad happens to them in their lives" *[passive empathic deficits]*. You might notice: "I tend to struggle with people I see as overly self-centered and entitled. I immediately shut them out, but then I try to make underhanded comments to make them feel bad about themselves for being so selfish" *[mix of active and passive empathic deficits]*. Or you could recognize: "I have a lot of problems with people in positions of power, especially my bosses. I get worried that they are talking down to me, so I always want to argue with them, dismiss what they say, and knock them off their pedestal" *[active empathic deficits]*.

- *Interaction-specific empathic deficits:* You could also experience decreased empathy when you are engaged in particular kinds of interpersonal interchanges and dynamics with others, largely independent of the particular person involved. For example, you could note: "When other people give me constructive feedback, I get immediately defensive—telling others why they are wrong, criticizing them, and trying to make them feel bad for attacking me" *[active empathic deficits]*. Or you may acknowledge: "If I have to complete a project or assignment, I only focus on myself, my performance, and trying to do things perfectly. I never think about connecting with the other people involved (e.g., my boss, my co-workers, the clients), or trying to understand what *they* want and need in the situation" *[passive empathic deficits]*.

- *Constrained or "biased" empathy:* In much the same way that you can have "mentalizing blind spots" (i.e., specific mental states you can "miss" in yourself and other people; see Chapter 9), you can also have *empathic* blind spots, or particular feelings in others that are less likely to motivate you, or that might even inspire your aggression or ire. When reflecting on these challenges, you can explicitly highlight the empathic "bias" in play: "While I can easily be motivated by other people's sadness and anxiety, I find it much more challenging to identify with and care about their feelings of anger and frustration, especially when those feelings are directed toward me" *[passive empathic deficits]*. Or you can simply acknowledge the particular mental states with which you struggle to empathize: "When I see other people crave attention or recognition, I immediately feel disgusted with them, and I want to punish them for feeling that way" *[active empathic deficits]*.

- *Emotion-dependent empathic deficits:* Your ability to empathize with other people could be significantly dependent on what *you* happen to be feeling at the time. For example, you might be quite kind and compassionate when you are feeling calm and confident in yourself, but you become self-focused and irritable when you feel overwhelmed. By and large, these sorts of empathic deficits tend to be triggered by your emotions ("If I feel stressed out, I can get tunnel vision: just putting my head down and not thinking of anyone but myself, until I feel better again" *[passive empathic deficits]*); your desires ("When I want someone to see me in a positive light, I can sometimes lie and misrepresent myself. I don't really think about how they would feel if they knew I was lying, or their rights to have an honest relationship with me" *[passive empathic deficits]*); and your feelings about yourself ("When I feel ashamed in my relationship with my girlfriend, I get angry with her and try to make her feel bad—the same way that I am feeling about myself" *[active empathic deficits]*).

- *Situational empathic deficits:* You also could find it harder to empathize with other people in the context of certain objective life circumstances, for example involving work, academics, finances, possessions, health and body, living situation, time of day or year, or your immediate environment. For example, you might become more self-absorbed when there is instability in your living situation *[passive empathic deficits]*, more impatient and irritable with other people when you are feeling physical discomfort *[active empathic deficits]*, or envious and resentful toward people you see as "successful" when your own career is not moving forward *[active empathic deficits]*.

- *Global lack of empathy:* In some cases, you may experience more categorical or "across the board" problems with empathy—that is, struggling to empathize with others under a broad array of conditions, independently of what you are experiencing internally or externally. Here you might observe, "I tend to think about myself most of the time: what I am feeling, what I want, and how to make myself feel better. I am rarely focused on what other people are going through, or what they might need from me" *[passive empathic deficits]*. Or you could notice, "I walk around with a sense of hatred and spite everywhere that I go. When good things happen to other people, I feel jealous and resentful of them, and when bad things happen to people, I sometimes feel a secret sense of pleasure and satisfaction. If I can't have a good life, I don't want anyone else to have one either" *[active empathic deficits]*.

Mentalizing Warm-up

Keeping these examples of pretend mode in mind, return to Paul's story on page 347. Where do you observe disconnection and dissociation in Paul's experience of other people? How do these challenges impact his mood, self-esteem, relationships, and functionality?

Employing Worksheets 14.2, 14.3, and 14.4, try relating these ideas about pretend mode to your own life. In what ways do you experience disconnection from others, and challenges with empathy in your relationships with others?

Worksheet 14.2
Pretend Mode: How do You Experience Disconnection
from Other People?

(1) What does it look like when you feel a lack of interest in or curiosity about other people's mental states? Are there any circumstances where you are less likely to be curious about what others are feeling?

(2) *Intellectualization* includes talking or thinking in generalities ("They tend to . . . "), explanation-giving, using psychological jargon, focusing on "shoulds" or ideals, or communicating in a vague or confusing manner. Detail any examples where you engage in intellectualization about other people, as well as the negative consequences this has had on your life and relationships.

(3) See below for examples of self-focused communication. Circle any of these that you have experienced in your life.

Monologues, or talking for extended periods of time without interruption	Turning conversation topics back to you and your life
Speaking extensively about yourself, your experiences, and your own ideas	Neglecting to listen to others, and to "reflect back" what they are saying
Not answering others' questions or addressing their concerns	Arguing with others, or dismissing and criticizing their views
Not asking other people questions	Mumbling, talking in a low voice volume
Interrupting others	Other forms of self-focused communication:

[continued on next page]

(4) What events or situations are likely to instigate these difficulties? Describe any ways in which this type of communication has affected your mood, behavior, and relationships, including how other people feel about you.

(5) How have you been disconnected from objective facts about other people? Such "facts" include others' actions, interpersonal patterns, appearance, or life circumstances—either in the past or in the present. Detail any examples of this disconnection, as well as negative consequences this has had on your life and relationships.

Worksheet 14.3
Pretend Mode: How do You Experience Empathic Deficits
with Other People?

"Empathy" is the ability to resonate with, care about, and be motivated by other people's mental states. Problems with empathy fall into two main categories: passive deficits and active deficits.

Passive empathic deficits involve not being fully attentive and responsive to other people's emotions and desires, leading to self-centeredness, entitlement, and "using" others. *Active* empathic deficits involve actually experiencing desires and wishes that undermine other people's dignity or well-being, resulting in anger, argumentativeness, aggression, or actions intended to cause others emotional or physical pain.

Utilizing the table below, map out your various problems in empathy, including how they have impacted yourself and other people. Do your best to provide specific examples of these challenges, drawing from your life and relationships.

Deficits in Empathy	
Person-specific Empathic Deficits	
Passive Deficits	Active Deficits
"When I interact with [specific person], I am not attentive to or motivated by their [emotions, desires, feelings about themself]."	"When I interact with [specific person], I want them to feel [some painful emotion, desire, physical state, feeling about themself]."
How have these deficits affected your emotions and behavior?	

[continued on next page]

When you have felt/acted in these ways, how has that impacted others' emotions, desires, and feelings about you?	

Group-specific Empathic Deficits	
Passive Deficits	Active Deficits
"When I interact with *[people from specific groups]*, I am not attentive to or motivated by their *[emotions, desires, feelings about themself]*."	"When I interact with *[people from specific groups]*, I want them to feel *[some painful emotion, desire, physical state, feeling about themself]*."

How have these deficits affected your emotions and behavior?	

When you have felt/acted in these ways, how has that impacted others' emotions, desires, and feelings about you?	

[continued on next page]

Interaction-specific Empathic Deficits	
Passive Deficits	Active Deficits
"When I experience *[some particular interpersonal interaction]*, I am not attentive to or motivated by the other person's *[emotions, desires, feelings about themself]*."	"When I experience *[some particular interpersonal interaction]*, I want the other person to feel *[some painful emotion, desire, physical state, feeling about themself]*."
How have these deficits affected your emotions and behavior?	
When you have felt/acted in these ways, how has that impacted others' emotions, desires, and feelings about you?	

Worksheet 14.4
Pretend Mode: Additional Problems with Empathy

Utilizing the table below, continue detailing your empathic deficits, including how they have impacted yourself and other people. Do your best to provide specific examples of these challenges, drawing from your life and relationships.

Additional Deficits in Empathy	
Constrained or "Biased" Empathy	
Passive Deficits	Active Deficits
"When other people experience [specific emotions, desires, and feelings about themselves], I feel less attentive to them, and less compassionate toward them."	"When other people experience [particular emotions, desires, and feelings about themselves], I want them to feel [some painful emotion, desire, physical state, feeling about themself]."
How have these deficits affected your emotions and behavior?	
When you have felt/acted in these ways, how has that impacted others' emotions, desires, and feelings about you?	

[continued on next page]

Emotion-dependent Empathic Deficits	
Passive Deficits	Active Deficits
"When I experience *[specific emotions, desires, feelings about myself]*, I feel less attentive to other people, and less compassionate toward them."	"When I experience *[specific emotions, desires, feelings about myself]*, I want other people to feel *[some painful emotion, desire, physical state, feeling about themself]*."
How have these deficits affected your emotions and behavior?	
When you have felt/acted in these ways, how has that impacted others' emotions, desires, and feelings about you?	

[continued on next page]

Situational Empathic Deficits	
Passive Deficits	Active Deficits
"When I experience *[some external event or situation]*, I feel less attentive to other people, and less compassionate toward them."	"When I experience *[some external event or situation]*, I want other people to feel *[some painful emotion, desire, physical state, feeling about themself]*."
How have these deficits affected your emotions and behavior?	
When you have felt/acted in these ways, how has that impacted others' emotions, desires, and feelings about you?	

[continued on next page]

Global Lack of Empathy	
Passive Deficits	Active Deficits
Describe any ways in which you experience "across the board" forms of self-focus, selfishness, entitlement, use of others, and lack of attentiveness to others' feelings and needs.	Describe any ways you experience "across the board" desires to cause other people emotional or physical pain, or to undermine others' dignity or well-being.
How have these deficits affected your emotions and behavior?	
When you have felt/acted in these ways, how has that impacted others' emotions, desires, and feelings about you?	

MENTALIZING PRACTICE POINTS: GETTING CONNECTED

According to MBT, pretend mode is one of the most significant barriers to progress in the treatment of BPD and other personality disorders (Bateman & Fonagy, 2016; Bateman et al., 2023; Drozek et al., 2023). This is because, when you are in pretend mode, you *sound* like you are connected to yourself and other people. You have a wealth of insights and formulations about yourself, your challenges, and other people's challenges, as well as what led these difficulties to develop in the first place. You think extensively about the "healthy" or "rational" way to see things, and you share your ideas about what you SHOULD be doing in order to move yourself forward. You can even deftly wield concepts drawn from psychology, mental health, and different modalities of therapy, at a level that matches some clinicians! And yet, even in the face of all of this intellectual understanding, the problems in your life can persist outside of sessions. You continue to struggle with extreme emotional pain, negative feelings about yourself, unstable relationships, and an inability to successfully follow through on all of your best intentions. This just makes you feel worse about yourself: You know what you "should" be doing, but you are just not able to make yourself do it.

MBT suggests that the problem here is that you are not authentically connected to your own experiences, or to the experiences of other people. You thus end up "flip-flopping" between intense emotionality and stark disconnection, and never the twain shall meet. However impressive your insights in therapy, you never learn how to *inhabit* your emotions while also reflecting on them, or to empathize with other people without being overwhelmed by their feelings.

This is the overarching aim of MBT's therapeutic strategies for pretend mode:

Getting connected.

Specifically, in treating pretend mode, MBT helps you to

(a) *Get connected to yourself*—to access, inhabit, and experience your emotions and desires in a deep way, less encumbered by intellect and reason; and to
(b) *Get connected to others*—to feel curious about, empathize with, and genuinely care about other people and what they are going through.

Once you are actually "in" yourself and other people in these ways, then the work of treatment can begin. In many cases, your emotions are highly painful and overwhelming, so when you are finally *feeling* them, you can utilize the strategies for psychic equivalence mode and teleological mode to target the areas of stuckness that are making you suffer in the first place (Chapters 12 and 13). This opens up the door for you to begin feeling better, as you move toward a position of greater flexibility in curiosity in your thinking.

Similarly, once you are more curious and empathically engaged in your relationships, your relationships start to move forward, often in new and exciting ways. Other people feel seen and understood by you, and like you genuinely care about them for who they are. You experience a growing sense of connectedness, vulnerability, and mutual trust with the people who matter to you. Interestingly, this then positively impacts *your* mood and self-esteem. As you find yourself more interested in how you can contribute to others' experiences, you feel less overwhelmed by your own emotional challenges. Your mood improves, and you experience an increased sense of meaning, purpose, and direction in your life. Paradoxically, by working to get more connected to other people, you end up feeling more connected to yourself.

In this chapter, we will be specifically focusing on MBT's strategies for helping you to disrupt your own experience of pretend mode, when you are stuck in it—to "pop your own bubble," so to speak. This is consistent with the approach of this entire book, which shows you how to self-apply MBT's therapeutic techniques. That said, perhaps more so than any other problem in mentalizing, it can be extremely challenging to get yourself out of pretend mode without help from other people. You might struggle to even identify *when* you are disconnected from yourself and others ("You don't know what you don't know"), or you feel confused about *how* to get connected again. So when working on these issues, consider seeking out support and guidance from a therapist, especially someone who has experience treating problems of disconnectedness and dissociation.

If you are already seeing an MBT therapist, buckle up! As far as therapeutic techniques go, MBT's interventions for pretend mode tend to be more challenging, provocative, and even confrontational. Examples include your therapist interrupting you, insisting that you provide specific examples from your life, asking you to reflect on hypothetical situations, explicitly "calling out" your disconnectedness, making a joke, saying something strange or bizarre, directly contradicting your viewpoint, communicating their own emotional experience, or calling attention to something about yourself or other people that you might prefer to ignore (see Drozek et al., 2023). In different ways, all of these strategies "wake you up" into accessing your own emotions, or considering the emotions of other people, including the therapist. Once you have found your way back to reality, you and your therapist can resume working on the challenges that brought you to treatment in the first place.

Before we lay out MBT's specific strategies for pretend mode, I should clarify the specific focus of our discussion. We have discussed how pretend mode sometimes includes dissociative symptoms, where you can become disconnected from emotions, memories, time, external reality, and even your own body. In this book, given our focus on mentalization, we will focus specifically on *mentalizing* strategies to address these forms of disconnection, which will enable you to increasingly access emotions and desires in yourself and other people. However, we will not be reviewing more behavioral strategies for treating dissociation (e.g., utilizing "ice dives," breathing exercises, balance boards, smelling salts, spicy foods, and so on), which are often highly effective at helping you connect to your physical experience and external environment. For more information about these approaches, try googling "anti-dissociation skills" online, or explore some of the excellent books out there that teach behavioral strategies to address dissociative symptoms (Boon et al. 2011; Linehan, 2015a; Marich, 2023; Reutter, 2019; Shielke et al., 2022). These strategies are entirely consistent with MBT, and can be seamlessly integrated with the techniques we will be reviewing in this chapter.

So now let's consider MBT's techniques for helping you get more connected to yourself and other people.

"Press pause" on your intellect. As we have discussed, when you rely too heavily on intellect and reason, you can inadvertently distance yourself from your emotions, and other people's emotions. So the first step in treating pretend mode is "pressing pause" on all of the forms of intellectualization that we reviewed earlier in the chapter: analyzing, rationalizing, thinking and communicating in generalities and abstractions, trying to "explain" people's experiences, utilizing jargon, and focusing on "shoulds" and ideals. When you are doing these things in an interpersonal interaction with another person (e.g., your therapist, a loved one), the best strategy is to literally *cease talking*, since that will stop the intellectualization dead in its tracks. Once you have "interrupted" the intellectual activity, you can utilize the other mentalizing practice points outlined below, especially "Getting connected with yourself" and "Cultivating empathy for other people."

Double down on stopping "pretend mode" problem behaviors. In Chapter 5, you worked to identify your problem behaviors, understood as actions you take that can interfere with your health, well-being, and stability in your life. In some cases, these problem behaviors can significantly contribute to pretend mode—that is, they can have the effect of disconnecting you from your emotions, or of making it more challenging for you to empathize with others. For example, you might feel more separate from yourself when you criticize yourself, play video games all day long, use cannabis gummies regularly, or engage in promiscuous sexual behavior. Or you could struggle to identify and emotionally resonate with other people when you are criticizing them, lying to them, or talking extensively about yourself without asking others questions about themselves.

In cases like this, it is important to do everything that you can to not engage in these "dissociative behaviors," prior to tackling your pretend mode. Otherwise you will be working at cross purposes with yourself: utilizing MBT's strategies for pretend mode to get connected to yourself and others, while simultaneously taking actions that separate you from yourself and others. That is a roadmap for going nowhere! So actively try to avoid engaging in these behaviors, by utilizing the crisis plan you developed in Chapter 5, and also by relying heavily on all of the mentalizing practice points reviewed in this book—MBT's principles that have been shown to be highly effective for addressing behavioral challenges in BPD.

Get connected to your own emotions and desires. When you are in pretend mode, you struggle to feel fully connected to your own emotional states. To begin addressing this problem, first employ MBT's techniques for identifying and "putting words on" your internal experience, reviewed in Chapter 9. You cannot access something if you do not know what that "something" is! Once you have discerned what you are probably feeling, utilize the Getting Connected to Yourself Toolkit on the next page, which compiles a handful of strategies to help you access and experience your emotions and desires.

Start by identifying the feeling from which you feel disconnected: sadness, anger, hurt, desire for attention, shame, and so on. Then using the "Connectedness Meter" in Step 2, draw an arrow to rate your level of connectedness to the feeling, with 0 being "completely disconnected" and 10 being "completely connected." This image is based on the Volume Unit Meter, a device used to measure the level of audio signals. And when you are in pretend mode, this is what we are trying to do: to "pump up the volume" on your emotions! **Remember to only use this toolkit when you are struggling to feel your feelings, and NOT when you are experiencing more intense emotions or urges.**

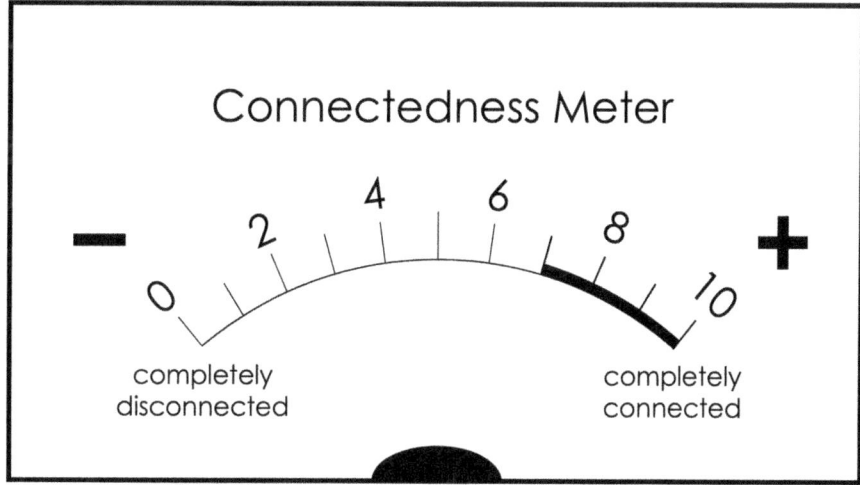

If you have determined that you are disconnected from the emotion listed in Step 1, feel free to utilize any of the remaining strategies in the toolkit, in whatever order you find most helpful. **Once you start feeling your feelings, stop using the toolkit at that stage, especially if you are feeling distressed or overwhelmed.** The whole point of MBT's techniques for pretend mode is to help you connect to yourself again. When that happens, you can resume living your life, or utilize the other mentalizing practice points in the book, which are best suited to times when you are already accessing your emotions.

Getting Connected to Yourself Toolkit

Step 1. Identify the feeling state.
(emotion, desire, or feeling about the self)

Step 2. Assess your level of connectedness.

How connected to the feeling state do you feel right now? Draw an arrow on the Connectedness Meter below.

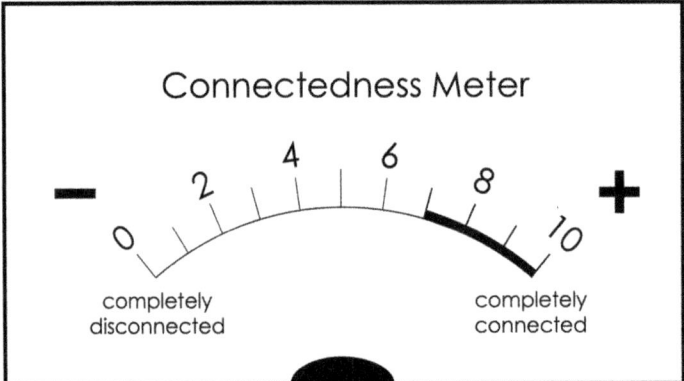

If you feel quite disconnected from the feeling, utilize the strategies below to access it more deeply. As soon as you start accessing the feeling, stop using the toolkit, to avoid becoming too distressed or overwhelmed.

Validate the Feeling State.

"It is understandable that I am feeling _____ because of . . ."

My History and Background	My Other Mental States Related to the Emotion	Factors in the External Situation	How Others Feel under Similar Circumstances

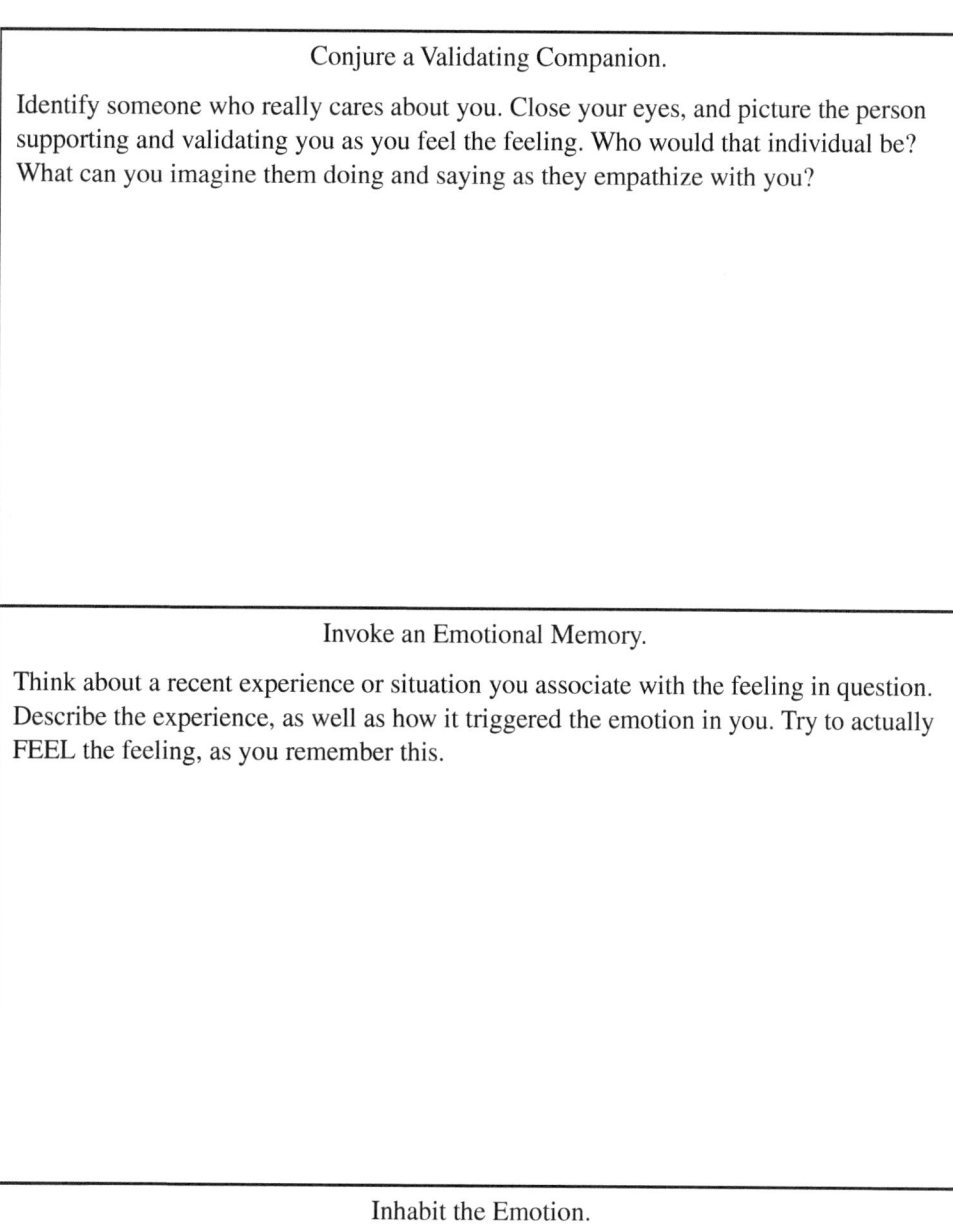

Conjure a Validating Companion.

Identify someone who really cares about you. Close your eyes, and picture the person supporting and validating you as you feel the feeling. Who would that individual be? What can you imagine them doing and saying as they empathize with you?

Invoke an Emotional Memory.

Think about a recent experience or situation you associate with the feeling in question. Describe the experience, as well as how it triggered the emotion in you. Try to actually FEEL the feeling, as you remember this.

Inhabit the Emotion.

Close your eyes, and actively work to ACCESS, INHABIT, and EXPERIENCE the feeling. Find the feeling in your body, and try to surrender to it, at an emotional level.

Do NOT dismiss or invalidate the emotion. Simply experience it, without taking any action on it.

Validate the feeling state. One core strategy for starting to access your emotions is explicitly validating them, or "getting in touch with" how your feelings are reasonable, understandable, and legitimate. When you have BPD, you can often be highly invalidating of your emotions—focusing on why you *shouldn't* feel a certain way, or even criticizing yourself for having a particular feeling, which can have the effect of blocking or inhibiting your internal experience. In contrast, by validating your affective states, you open up the door to feeling your emotions more deeply.

In general, you can validate your emotions by considering how they are reasonable in light of other factors outside of them: your history and background ("It makes sense that I am afraid and panicked right now, given my history of abuse and neglect in childhood"); other mental states connected to the emotion ("I base a lot of my self-esteem on my appearance, so it is reasonable that I want him to validate me"); aspects of the external situation leading to the emotion ("I have every right to be angry about this. My boss was not following protocol, and it created a ton of unnecessary work for me"); or how other people might feel under similar circumstances ("I think that most people would feel hurt by her comment—it was cruel and unkind").

Conjure a validating companion. In MBT's view, emotions are inherently relational—that is, you learn what you are feeling through your relationships with people who care about you (Chapter 4), and your emotions are significantly impacted by your interactions with the people around you (Chapter 10). So when you are disconnected from a particular emotion, you can get an "assist" in accessing the emotion by identifying someone who really cares about you, with whom you feel safe and connected. This could be a parent, therapist, or close friend—essentially anyone who really "gets" you. Close your eyes, so that you enter into a space where you can envision the person supporting and validating you as you feel the feeling. What do you imagine them doing and saying as they empathize with you? For example, you might picture your partner holding you and comforting you as you feel sad about a challenging medical issue. Or you could visualize yourself talking to your grandmother about feeling anxious about your upcoming job interview, with her saying to you: "No matter what happens, we love you, and you're going to be OK." Interestingly, while you might struggle to feel your feelings on your own, by imaginatively "entering into" these supportive interactions with others, you are often able to connect more fully with the emotions in question.

Invoke an emotional memory. You can also draw on your own experience in order to access your emotions. Pinpoint some situation or moment in time you associate with the feeling state you are trying to inhabit. This could be a scenario in the past where you actually felt the feeling (e.g., some stressful or upsetting circumstance), or it could be some state of affairs that, when you think about it now, really triggers the emotion in you. Remember as many details of the situation as you can, especially focusing on the aspects of the event that you find emotionally salient and intense. For example, if you are trying to experience your feelings of anger toward your past romantic partner, you could recall some of the unkind things they said to you, as well as any actions they took (e.g., infidelity, dishonesty, not following through on plans) that caused you pain and suffering. Or if you want to reconnect with your desire for closeness with your best friend, you might recollect all of the times when you have felt intellectually stimulated by them, gone on adventures together, and shared in a vulnerable way about your challenges. As you review the details of these memories, try to actually FEEL your emotions associated with them, in an authentic and visceral way. By remaining grounded in the reality of your emotionally charged experiences, you can move yourself closer to feelings that seem more distant and "far away" in your internal world.

Inhabit the emotion. The final strategy for connecting to yourself involves actively working to experience and access the emotion itself, or what MBT calls "inhabiting the emotion." To prevent any external distractions, close your eyes, and try to find the feeling in your body. Where is it located in your physical experience? Are there any bodily sensations connected to it? This could be a pounding in your chest, a sense of pressure behind your eyes, or a pit in your stomach. As you connect to these sensations, try to surrender to the affective state associated with them (e.g., sadness, pride, a desire to assert yourself), at a deep emotional level. Although no rule can be laid down, this is usually best achieved without using words or language. Whereas content-mentalizing involves identifying and labeling your inner states (Chapter 9), inhabiting the emotion involves simply *experiencing* your feelings, as directly and fully as possible. It is thus essential that you avoid doing anything to suppress or distance yourself from the affective state: judging it, criticizing it, analyzing it, or engaging in any external behaviors that might intentionally or unintentionally divert your attention away from the feeling.

Readers familiar with dialectical behavior therapy (DBT) might notice some similarities between these strategies and the Mindfulness of Current Emotion (MoCE) skill from DBT (e.g., trying not to judge or suppress the emotion, attending to physical sensations; Linehan, 2015a). The aim of MoCE is to acknowledge and notice your feeling states, without trying to either block or intensify them. The MoCE skill—which parallels the self-focused content-mentalizing strategies reviewed in Chapter 9—is especially useful when you are experiencing emotional dysregulation, since this more neutral "observing" process can enable the emotions to pass without taking over your experience and behavior (Hollander, 2017). In contrast, MBT's Inhabit the Emotion technique is most helpful when you are *disconnected* from yourself, since it intentionally tries to amplify your feeling states, in order to get you over the hump into accessing your emotions again.

When you are seeking to inhabit your emotions, do your best to refrain from taking action on them, at least in the moment of utilizing the strategy. In BPD, you might blur the distinction between "feeling your feelings" and ACTING on your feelings, such that you feel compelled to indulge in certain behaviors (e.g., self-injury, reassurance-seeking, substance use) when you are experiencing painful emotions, in order to make yourself feel better. This is the problem of teleological mode discussed in Chapter 13. However, by *accessing* your emotions without *acting on* your emotions, you can shift out of pretend mode while preventing yourself from inadvertently dropping into teleological mode. This enables you to "reflect rather than reflex" on what is going on inside you, and to finally start feeling your feelings, rather than being controlled or overwhelmed by them.

To illustrate the above strategies in action, review an example of the Getting Connected to Yourself Toolkit, completed by a patient trying to access her feelings of hurt toward her best friend, who had been pulling away from the patient following an intense argument.

Getting Connected to Yourself Toolkit

Step 1. Identify the feeling state.
(emotion, desire, or feeling about the self)

Feeling hurt by my best friend

Step 2. Assess your level of connectedness.

How connected to the feeling state do you feel right now? Draw an arrow on the Connectedness Meter below.

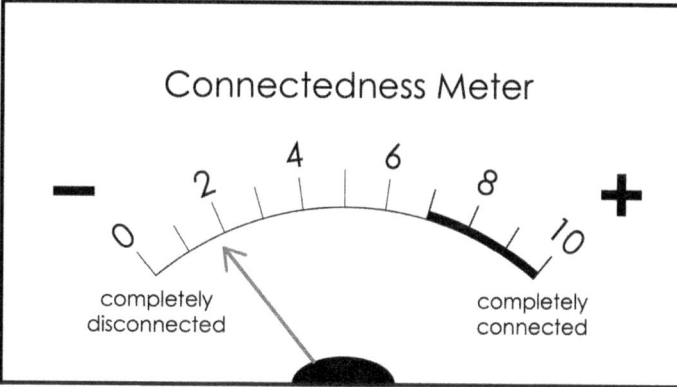

If you feel quite disconnected from the feeling, utilize the strategies below to access it more deeply. As soon as you start accessing the feeling, stop using the toolkit, to avoid becoming too distressed or overwhelmed.

Validate the Feeling State. "It is understandable that I am feeling ___hurt___ because of . . ."			
My History and Background	My Other Mental States Related to the Emotion	Factors in the External Situation	How Others Feel Under Similar Circumstances
I was bullied a lot in childhood, so I understand why I am so sensitive to feeling left out and rejected by her.	I really love her, and I want to be close to her. So I get why I feel hurt by her acting so cold toward me. It seems like she doesn't care about me anymore.	She has been MIA for the past few weeks, with no explanation. It makes sense that I feel hurt, given how much time we were spending together before that.	I think that a lot of people would feel hurt by her at this point, especially with her calling me "needy" and stopping inviting me to things.

Conjure a Validating Companion.

Identify someone who really cares about you. Close your eyes, and picture the person supporting and validating you as you feel the feeling. Who would that individual be? What can you imagine them doing and saying as they empathize with you?

I am thinking of my dad here—he is my biggest champion, and he is always there for me. I can imagine myself talking with him about this, and feeling really sad and hurt as I tell him about the situation. He would just lift me up, give me a huge hug, and say, "You're my girl, and we're gonna get through this."

Invoke an Emotional Memory.

Think about a recent experience or situation you associate with the feeling in question. Describe the experience, as well as how it triggered the emotion in you. Try to actually FEEL the feeling, as you remember this.

Probably the worst moment was when she called me "needy," after we got into that argument on our road trip together. She knows that is my biggest fear—being a burden on people—so I feel like she was really trying to hurt me. She seemed so cold, almost like a different person. I felt humiliated and sad, like I wanted to hide so she couldn't see me. I DO feel the hurt as I remember this right now.

Inhabit the Emotion.

Close your eyes, and actively work to ACCESS, INHABIT, and EXPERIENCE the feeling. Find the feeling in your body, and try to surrender to it, at an emotional level.

Do NOT dismiss or invalidate the emotion. Simply experience it, without taking any action on it.

Cultivate empathy for other people. In Chapter 9, you learned a range of strategies for recognizing other people's emotions and desires. But what if you "know" what another person is feeling, but you do not really care about it? This is the problem that we discussed in Chapter 11: having cognitive empathy without emotional empathy, where you might struggle to empathically resonate with others (Salgado et al., 2020). To work on this issue, utilize the Getting Connected to Other People Toolkit below, which reviews several different strategies to cultivate a greater sense of empathy for other people. Start by describing the person's internal states, whether those be emotions, desires, or feelings about themself. From there, feel free to try out the various techniques contained in the toolkit, or just pick and choose the particular approaches that feel relevant to your challenges.

Getting Connected to Other People Toolkit			
Other Person:			
Describe the Other Person's Feeling States. *(emotion, desire, or feeling about the self)*			
Try to Identify with the Other Person. What similarities do you notice between yourself and the other person? These could be present across various domains.			
Internal States/Personality	Behaviors/ Interpersonal Patterns	Current External Circumstances	History and Background

Import the Other Person's Situation. What would it be like for you if similar circumstances were happening in your own life?			
Your Emotions	Your Desires	Your Feelings about Yourself	Your Perspective on the Situation

Validate the Other Person's Feeling State. "It is understandable that the other person is feeling _____ because of . . ."			
Their History and Background	Their Other Mental States Connected to the Emotion	Factors in the External Situation	How Others Feel under Similar Circumstances

"What's my part?" Reflect on your own contributions to your challenges with the person, especially how you have engaged with them in maladaptive ways.			
Active Empathic Deficits	Passive Empathic Deficits	Your Problematic Actions/ Interpersonal Approaches	Positive Actions You have NOT Taken

Test-drive a More Empathic Perspective.			
If you were relating to the other person in a more empathic manner, how would your experience with them be different? Consider this question in several domains.			
Your Focus and Curiosity	Your Emotions and Desires	Your Actions/ Interpersonal Approaches	Impact on the Other Person

Try to Care about the Other Person.

Close your eyes, and actively work to empathize with the other individual. Try to feel what they are feeling—to resonate with them at a deep level.

Do NOT dismiss or invalidate what they are going through. Do your best to simply CARE about the person, and to allow their experience to matter to you.

Try to identify with the other person. By and large, it is easiest to empathize with other people when you feel a kinship with them—when you feel like they are like you, and you are like them. So one step toward greater empathy is working to *identify* with the other person, namely by wondering: What similarities do you notice between yourself and the other individual? These could be in general or in the situation under discussion, across several different domains: internal states and personality ("We both have struggled extensively with depression"); behaviors and interpersonal patterns ("I tend to be a people-pleaser, and she really has no backbone either, just doing what other people want"); current external circumstances ("Both of us live alone, and neither of us has been in a relationship for a really long time"); and history and background ("He grew up in an alcoholic family, and so did I. That might be why we are both so sensitive"). When focusing on the similarities rather than differences between yourself and other people, the barriers that separate you start to weaken and dissolve. You find it easier to resonate with others at an emotional level, and to care about what they are going through in their lives.

Import the other individual's situation. A similar strategy involves imaginatively "importing" the other person's situation into your own life. We discussed this technique in Chapter 12, as an aid to broadening your perspective when you are seeing someone in a negative light. It can also be useful when you are struggling to empathize with another person. Ask yourself the question: What would it be like for you if similar circumstances were happening in your own life? Consider the impact of this on your emotions, desires, feelings about yourself, or your broader perspective on the situation.

For example, if you were finding it challenging to empathize with your mother, you might reflect on what it would feel like for you if you were to encounter her life challenges: social isolation, significant financial stress, lack of daily structure, and your kids not communicating with you. You could acknowledge that you would probably feel depressed, lonely, and hurt by your children *[emotions]*; you would long for a greater connection with your kids, as well as a more fulfilling life *[desires]*; you might feel embarrassed and ashamed about the state of your relationships and finances *[feelings about yourself]*; and you would likely feel like you had been unfairly treated in the situation, and that other people should be more understanding of your difficulties *[perspective on the scenario]*. Rather than asking yourself to directly empathize with the other individual, by "bringing the other person's situation to you," you are simply reflecting on your *own* feelings in analogous circumstances. This helps you to better understand the other person, and also to resonate and connect with them at an emotional level—an essential condition for cultivating empathy.

Validate the person's feeling state. As mentioned earlier, when you explicitly validate your own emotions, you are able to access and experience those emotions more fully. Similarly, if you want to deepen your ability to empathize with another person, try reflecting on how it is *reasonable and understandable* that they are feeling what they are feeling. You can validate another individual's emotions by considering how the emotions are justified, in light of other factors outside of them: the person's history and background ("She has a long history of abusive relationships, so I understand why she is suspicious of him"); other mental states connected to the emotion ("He has been so depressed ever since the break-up. This makes sense, given how much he loved her"); aspects of the external situation leading to the emotion ("I get why she is feeling overwhelmed—she has had so many losses in such a brief period of time"); or how other people might feel under similar circumstances ("I see where he is coming from: Anyone would want to escape from such intense feelings of shame"). When you focus on the *validity* of another's feelings, it is often much easier to be motivated by these feelings, and to care about what the person is going through.

"What's my part?" In BPD, one of the biggest barriers to empathizing with other people is feeling like they have done something wrong or problematic in their interactions with you. Why would you want to empathize with someone who has mistreated and victimized you? However, when you examine your own problematic tendencies in the scenario in question, you recognize that you—just like the other person—have often played some role in perpetuating the challenges in the relationship. You can interrogate "your part" by mentalizing a variety of factors, including your active empathic deficits ("I secretly hope that they will break up, so that he will suffer in the same way that I have suffered"); your passive empathic deficits ("I've just been so caught up in my own shit—I have never really thought much about how my inpatient admissions have impacted my parents"); your problematic actions and interpersonal approaches ("I think that I've been pretty argumentative lately—just telling her why her perspective is wrong, rather than actively trying to understand where she is coming from"); or positive actions that you have failed to take ("I never really offered to help when my brother was out of work and struggling with those medical issues"). By reflecting in these ways, you realize how *you* have often impacted the other party in the dynamic, opening up the door for you to further empathize with their feelings, needs, and desires.

Test-drive a more empathic perspective. Another way to move toward empathizing with others is imagining what empathy would *look like* in those relationships. If you were relating to the other person in a more empathic manner, how would your experience with them be different? For example, consider what you would be focusing on and curious about in the situation ("I would be more focused on how she has been feeling lately, especially her difficulties with depression and social isolation. I would be curious if there is anything I can do to help her feel better"); the emotions and desires you would experience ("I would probably feel concerned about how anxious he has been at his job. I would want him to succeed there—to feel fulfilled by what he is doing, and for his co-workers to see him in a positive light"); the actions you would take ("I would try harder to stay sober; I know how upset she gets when I relapse"), or the interpersonal approaches you would use ("I would take the time to ask my parents about their day, and find out more about the challenges they are experiencing in their life"); and how all of these changes would impact the other person ("He might feel more relaxed and content, since he wouldn't have to be worried about me all of the time").

By envisioning these more empathic experiences, you are imaginatively expanding your empathic repertoire—"test-driving the empathy car" before you decide to buy it! Over time, you find yourself naturally caring more about other people, genuinely wanting to contribute to their experience, and automatically engaging in the compassionate behaviors that make a positive impact on their experience.

Try to care about the other person. "Try to empathize" might sound like a strange prescription. How can you make yourself care about someone from whom you feel separate and disengaged? However, in much the same way that you can work to connect to your own emotions, you can seek to authentically resonate and connect with other people's feelings. To start, make sure to refrain from dismissing or invalidating the other person's experience, whether internally (e.g., by mentally focusing on their wrongs and deficiencies) or behaviorally (e.g., by criticizing or arguing with them). Such approaches will only lead you to feel more frustrated and upset with the individual, making it that much harder to experience concern for them.

Now close your eyes, and actively work to empathize with the person. Try to feel what they are feeling—to resonate with them at a deep level. If you do not naturally feel a sense of compassion for the person, do not "pretend" that you really care about them, or criticize yourself for any problems with empathy that you notice in yourself. Rather, simply think about the individual's various emotions and desires identified throughout this toolkit, and do your best to CARE about the person—to allow their experience to matter to you in a real way.

To elucidate these principles, review an example of the Getting Connected to Other People Toolkit, completed by a patient experiencing jealousy and anger toward her boyfriend for going out to a bachelor party rather than spending time with her for their regular date night.

Getting Connected to Other People Toolkit

Other Person: My boyfriend Mike

Describe the Other Person's Feeling States. *(emotion, desire, or feeling about the self)* Desire to hang out with his friends for the bachelor party

Try to Identify with the Other Person.

What similarities do you notice between yourself and the other person? These could be present across various domains, in the situation or in general.

Internal States/Personality	Behaviors/ Interpersonal Patterns	Current External Circumstances	History and Background
We both struggle with social anxiety and low self-esteem. And we feel really insecure about what our friends think of us.	Both of us are pretty conflict-avoidant—I think this is why he waited to bring up the bachelor party until the very last minute.	Our daily routines are nearly identical: We go from home to work, and then right back to home again. We usually only see friends every now and then.	Our parents are emotionally stunted, so we are used to indirect communication. We also both grew up in working class families, so we are pretty down-to-earth and low maintenance.

Import the Other Person's Situation.			
What would it be like for you if similar circumstances were happening in your own life?			
Your Emotions	Your Desires	Your Feelings about Yourself	Your Perspective on the Situation
I would be pissed off if he gave me trouble about going to Kim's bachelorette party. I would also feel hurt, like he didn't care about something that was important to me.	I would want to support my friend—to be there for her for this important milestone. I would want Mike to WANT me to go to the party, so that I could invest in my friendships.	I would feel confident in myself, and secure that I needed to go to the bachelorette party. I would feel embarrassed and ashamed if I skipped it—definitely not something you do as a friend.	If Mike was telling me I shouldn't go to the party, I would feel strongly that he was being selfish, and that I needed to be there to support Kim, regardless of what he thought.

Validate the Other Person's Feeling State.			
"It is understandable that the other person is feeling _a desire to hang out with his friends_ because of . . ."			
Their History and Background	Their Other Mental States Connected to the Emotion	Factors in the External Situation	How Others Feel Under Similar Circumstances
Mike and Justin grew up together, and they have known each other forever. Justin is probably the closest thing to a "best friend" that Mike has.	Mike values his relationship with Justin, and he wants to maintain their friendship. Mike would feel really guilty if he blew off the bachelor party, especially since he is in the wedding party.	Justin doesn't have many friends, so he is relying on Mike to be there. And apparently they scheduled the party based on Mike's schedule, so he can't really back out at this point.	Most people would feel obligated to go to an event like this, given how close Mike and Justin are to each other. I know that I would be that way with Kim, which is why I feel a little guilty that I gave Mike such a hard time about everything.

"What's my part?"			
Reflect on your own contributions to your challenges with the person, especially how you have engaged with them in maladaptive ways.			
Active Empathic Deficits	Passive Empathic Deficits	Your Problematic Actions/ Interpersonal Approaches	Positive Actions You Have NOT Taken
I definitely wanted to make Mike feel guilty for going to the party—to punish him, hurt his feelings, and make him regret blowing me off.	I was not really thinking about Mike's desire to support his friend, or his recent feelings of disconnection in his friendships. I was so focused on my own insecurities that I basically ignored Mike's feelings.	I have been really critical of him, accusing him of not caring about me because he would not cancel his plans. I also withdrew from him and stopped talking to him, in order to pressure him to do what I wanted.	I feel guilty about this, but I have not given him any reassurance or encouragement about this decision. I have not told him to make the decision that he thinks is best, and that I will back him up no matter what.
Test-drive a More Empathic Perspective.			
If you were relating to the other person in a more empathic manner, how would your experience with them be different? Consider this question in several domains.			
Your Focus and Curiosity	Your Emotions and Desires	Your Actions/ Interpersonal Approaches	Impact on the Other Person
I would be more focused on Mike's emotions and desires, rather than just thinking about myself and what I want. I would feel more curious about what he is going through, as well as how important this all is for Justin and his fiancé.	I would feel genuinely excited for Mike to have the opportunity to celebrate his friend. I would want Mike to go to the party, and to have a good time. I would also probably believe he is doing this for Justin, not just to go to a strip club.	I would be kind, loving, and supportive of Mike surrounding this party. When he reminded me about it, I would have just suggested rescheduling our date night, without making a big deal about it.	If I had responded in this way, Mike would have felt much more comfortable and relaxed around this whole thing. He would probably feel more connected to me, maybe even grateful that I was putting his needs first, ahead of my own.
Try to Care about the Other Person.			
Close your eyes, and actively work to empathize with the other individual. Try to feel what they are feeling—to resonate with them at a deep level. Do NOT dismiss or invalidate what they are going through. Do your best to simply CARE about the person, and to allow their experience to matter to you.			

Get connected to reality. As discussed earlier in the chapter, pretend mode often manifests itself as disconnection from certain objective facts (e.g., behaviors, circumstances, qualities or characteristics) about yourself or other people. For example, if you really look up to someone, you might pay less attention to their more problematic tendencies. Or if you are seeing yourself in a highly negative light, you could overlook your positive qualities, and all of the things you have done to help other people.

To address these forms of disconnection, try following the Getting Connected to Reality Toolkit below. Start by specifying the person on whom you would like to focus, either yourself or someone else in your life. Then proceed to describe the "facts" about the person that you have been ignoring or minimizing. This could variously be information that (a) generates distress in you; (b) you want to avoid considering; (c) contradicts your beliefs about the person, especially when those beliefs are overly positive or overly negative (i.e., the idealization or devaluation associated with BPD; see Chapters 1 and 12); or (d) you have not been keeping in mind—it has not been on your radar.

Examples include the person's history or background ("My boyfriend told me that he was not texting with his ex, but I found out that this had been happening for several months"; "I said so many embarrassing things at that party—I cannot bear to think about it"); the person's current actions, interpersonal approach, or manner of communicating ("I call myself an 'artist,' but if I really think about it, I have not really spent any time on my art in the past year"; "I say that she is a horrible person, but I cannot deny that she can be extremely kind and self-sacrificing in her other relationships"); the person's objective characteristics ("I know that she has end-stage cancer, but I just try to pretend that everything is fine whenever I see her"; "I am kind of in denial about how much weight I have gained—I won't even look at myself in the mirror"); or the person's external circumstances ("I have not been thinking about the fact that I am about to be evicted from my apartment, and I need to find another place to live"; "Technically he is unemployed, but I like to think about him as an 'entrepreneur' ").

Getting Connected to Reality Toolkit
Working to Get Connected to Facts about (*circle one*) Yourself   OR   Another Person:
Describe facts/objective factors that • generate distress in you • you want to avoid considering • contradict your (e.g., overly positive or overly negative) beliefs about the person • have not been on your radar

History and Background	

Actions, Interpersonal Approach, or Manner of Communicating	
Objective Characteristics	
External Circumstances	

Try to really FOCUS on these objective factors, to "take in" the fact that they are real. When you do this, what do you feel?		
Emotions	Desires	Feelings about Yourself

Work to actually FEEL, access, and inhabit these feeling states—in your body, and deep in your heart.

When you are hunting out these facts, you know that you are on the right track when they make you feel upset or distressed in some way. You find yourself not *wanting* to think about the topic, so it just "bounces off" your mind. Accordingly, once you have identified the objective factors that you have been downplaying, try to really FOCUS on them, to "take in" the fact that they are real. When you do this, what do you feel? In particular, consider the emotions, desires, and feelings about yourself that arise in you. For example, when you focus on your parents' history of interfering with your treatment, you end up feeling sad, anxious, and angry *[emotions]*; you want to criticize them and withdraw from them *[desires]*; and you feel humiliated that they still do not trust your ability to manage your own life *[self-states]*. Once these feelings are within the plane of your experience, work to actually FEEL, access, and inhabit them—in your body, and deep in your heart.

To illustrate this process, see here for a completed version of the Getting Connected to Reality Toolkit, from a patient who had a long history of idealizing his girlfriend, even as she was treating him in problematic ways.

Getting Connected to Reality Toolkit	
Working to Get Connected to Facts about *(circle one)* Yourself OR Another Person: *My girlfriend Gina*	
Describe facts/objective factors that • generate distress in you • you want to avoid considering • contradict your (e.g., overly positive or overly negative) beliefs about the person • have not been on your radar	
History and Background	She cheated on me at the start of the relationship. She recently downloaded a dating app, but she said that it was an accident.
Actions, Interpersonal Approach, or Manner of Communicating	She smokes pot every day, which I don't like. She sometimes makes fun of me in front of my friends, saying that I am socially awkward and have a weird laugh.
Objective Characteristics	Not applicable.
External Circumstances	She has not been working for a long time due to her fibromyalgia, so she does not really have any money to contribute to our expenses.

Try to really FOCUS on these objective factors, to "take in" the fact that they are real. When you do this, what do you feel?		
Emotions	Desires	Feelings about Yourself
Worried that she is possibly taking advantage of me. A bit angry that she makes fun of me in front of my friends, since I would never do that to her.	I kind of want to ask her about when she is going to start looking for work again. I want to stand up for myself more, but I don't think that would go over very well.	When I actually think about this stuff, I feel embarrassed and ashamed that I let her treat me this way. If other people knew about all of this, they would tell me to run for the hills!
Work to actually FEEL, access, and inhabit these feeling states—in your body, and deep in your heart.		

See here for a second version of the toolkit, completed by a patient who was judging herself as being worthless and unlovable, after her girlfriend broke up with her following a six-year relationship.

Getting Connected to Reality Toolkit	
Working to Get Connected to Facts about *(circle one)* (Yourself) OR Another Person:	
Describe facts/objective factors that • generate distress in you • you want to avoid considering • contradict your (e.g., overly positive or overly negative) beliefs about the person • have not been on your radar	
History and Background	I have had a several long-term romantic relationships, so I guess some people like me. Also Janet and I stayed together for a long time, until she decided that she didn't want to have kids.

Actions, Interpersonal Approach, or Manner of Communicating	I tend to be pretty nice. Everybody tells me that I always put other people in front of myself: asking them questions, validating their feelings, and supporting them when they are struggling. I do this with my mom, my friends, and until recently, Janet.
Objective Characteristics	My friends and exes have always said that I am "hot." I don't see myself that way, but if I am being honest, I probably am more objectively attractive than a lot of people.
External Circumstances	This is one area where I actually feel good about myself. I make a lot of money, I own my own home, and I have really close relationships with my friends and family. So at least I have these things going for me.

Try to really FOCUS on these objective factors, to "take in" the fact that they are real. When you do this, what do you feel?

Emotions	Desires	Feelings about Yourself
I feel calmer and less anxious when I think about my positive traits. I also feel more hopeful, like I actually might have a future in some other relationship.	I am not ready for a relationship right now, but I definitely want to be in one someday, and I want to have kids. This makes me a little less upset that things didn't work out with Janet.	When I remember what I brought to my relationships in the past, I feel more confident in myself. I feel a greater sense of self-esteem, like I actually might have something to offer to someone.

Work to actually FEEL, access, and inhabit these feeling states—in your body, and deep in your heart.

As you can see in the above toolkits, both patients are considering aspects of reality that they had been minimizing in their thinking (e.g., a romantic partner's problematic tendencies in one case, the patient's own positive traits in the other), and then "using" those facts as a tool to help them access their emotions. These strategies underscore a core principle in MBT's treatment of pretend mode: By getting connected to reality, you get more connected to *yourself*, and to your complex feelings about your life.

Mentalizing Cool-down

With these strategies in mind, return to Paul's story on page 347. What would it look like for Paul to utilize these principles in his life, in order to address his tendencies toward intellectualization, emotional disconnection, and problems with empathy?

RETURNING TO PAUL

In developing Paul's MBT formulation, Paul and his therapist itemized his various challenges with disconnection from himself and other people:

- A pervasive experience of emptiness and emotional numbness, along with a sense of feeling "dead inside"
- Difficulties with dissociation: feeling like he was not real, seeing himself from the outside, and disconnection from his body
- Decreased curiosity about his own mental states, and the thoughts and feelings of other people
- Significant tendencies toward intellectualization, abstraction, and use of psychological jargon about himself and others: "anxious attachment," "codependency," "enmeshment," "narcissistic abuse," "trauma bonding"
- Challenges accessing and inhabiting his emotions (e.g., feeling separate from his feelings, speaking in a monotone with minimal emotional expression)
- Disconnection from objective facts about his own life, especially his behaviors of isolating from and neglecting his family
- Significant problems with empathy in his relationship with Sonia
  - Active empathic deficits, in the form of wanting to punish Sonia and make her feel guilty. These impulses arose whenever Paul felt resentful and hurt by Sonia *[emotion-dependent deficits]*, if Sonia was insufficiently attentive to him *[interaction-specific deficits]*, and when Sonia was focused on her other activities and obligations *[interaction-specific deficits]*.
  - Passive empathic deficits, in terms of Paul neglecting to consistently consider and care about Sonia's needs and experiences. Here Paul often displayed more "biased" empathy, such that he was highly attuned to Sonia's feelings about *him*, but less motivated by Sonia's feelings about other aspects of her life (e.g., her work, their children, her relationships with her friends and family).
- When Paul was overwhelmed by his depression and suicidal thinking, he exhibited "passive" problems with empathy: not considering his children's needs and desires for connectedness with him; neglecting to recognize how his avoidance and isolation was impacting Sonia and their children; and failing to appreciate the impact of his planned suicide on his family *[emotion-dependent empathic deficits]*.
- In therapy sessions, a pattern of monologues and self-focused communication, with decreased interest in his therapist's perspective and feelings.

As a first step in addressing these challenges, Paul and his therapist started by utilizing MBT's content-focused therapeutic strategies, in order to help Paul identify and "put words on" emotions and desires in himself and other people (see Chapter 9). With the help of the Content-mentalizing Toolkit and the Mentalizing from the Outside In Toolkit, Paul acknowledged his diverse feelings about himself and his relationships:

- His powerful desires for Sonia to nurture and take care of him, so that he could feel soothed and regulated in himself
- His emotions of hurt, insecurity, and resentment when Sonia would occupy herself with other things, along with the impulse to punish Sonia for (from his perspective) neglecting him. He felt panicked and even terrified that Sonia was pulling away from him—that she would ultimately get sick of him and abandon him, and that his life would return to the time before he met Sonia, when he felt fundamentally empty and alone.
- His deep feelings of love for Sonia and his children, in addition to anger and resentment at the children for taking up so much of Sonia's time and emotional energy
- His sense of hopelessness and helplessness about the state of his life, and his desire to commit suicide to permanently end his emotional suffering

Paul's therapist also encouraged him to reflect on *Sonia's* emotions about all of these matters ("When you withdraw from Sonia and refuse to engage with her, what do you think that makes her feel?"; "Do you have a sense of how that impacted her, when she found the noose in your office?"), and Paul was able to hypothesize about a range of Sonia's emotions surrounding their recent troubles, including her sadness about Paul's withdrawal from her; her anxiety and stress about having to manage her various responsibilities (e.g., in work, parenting, and family relationships); her desire for Paul to be more engaged in their family life, and to help her take care of their children; and her abiding sense of love for Paul, along with her terror that he would kill himself and she would lose him.

Even as Paul learned how to recognize and articulate all of these internal states in himself and others, he found it difficult to fully *experience* those states in a deep and authentic way. He remained quite "in his head" when he spoke about his own problems, and he continued to struggle with dismissiveness and indifference in his interactions with Sonia and their children. In order to address these issues, Paul and his therapist worked to implement MBT's therapeutic strategies for pretend mode. To start, Paul's therapist encouraged him to "press pause" on all of the intellectual maneuvers that Paul was enacting in the therapy: analyzing himself and Sonia, talking in generalities and abstractions, deploying lots of psychological jargon, focusing on what he and other people "should" be doing and thinking, and trying to explain "why" he developed his psychiatric challenges.

Paul was initially taken aback by these recommendations: "I am realizing that so much of what I do, every moment of every day, is some form of thinking, or trying to analyze myself and other people. So when you suggest that I 'press pause' on my intellectualization, it's highly disorienting, like you're telling me to drive with my eyes closed. If I'm not trying to figure things out, what would my life even look like? And what am I supposed to do instead? I literally have no idea."

Paul and his therapist also explored the role of his suicidal behavior (e.g., fantasizing about killing himself, researching suicide methods, writing suicide notes, rehearsing his plans) in his emotional life. Paul recognized that he would often start to experience some painful emotion (e.g., hurt, anger, loneliness, insecurity), but then as soon as he engaged in those behaviors, he would experience an immediate relief, as if he was temporarily "shutting off" his mind. In light of this, Paul's therapist wondered if, in order for Paul to start accessing his emotions, he might need to refrain from holding on to suicide as an "out" from his emotional experience. Paul agreed to double down on this. "I have used suicide for so long as a method for managing my emotions. Without it, I am terrified that I am not going to be able to function, or to get anything done."

Relying less extensively on his intellectualization and suicidality, Paul began to actively work to access and experience his internal states. So when he suspected that he was feeling hurt that Sonia was spending all of her time working and taking care of their children, he tried to follow the Getting Connected to Yourself Toolkit, first assessing his level of connectedness to the emotion. He noticed that his experience of the feeling state was more cognitive than emotional: "I am aware that I probably feel hurt by her, since that is the sort of thing I have felt in the past. But I am not actually *feeling* the emotion—it still seems really far away from me."

Paul thus proceeded to validate his sense of hurt. "I understand why I feel so hurt about all of this. I grew up feeling emotionally neglected by my parents all of the time, so I am really sensitive to being ignored and rejected by other people *[history and background]*. I also want to feel connected to her, so I get afraid whenever it seems like she is pulling away from me *[other mental states connected to the emotion]*. Also objectively speaking, we have not been spending much time together, and we have not had sex in several months, so I get why I am feeling hurt and insecure *[factors in external situation]*. I know that this happens a lot when couples have little kids—the man ends up feeling like his wife is neglecting him, and this can lead to hurt feelings *[how others feel under similar circumstances]*."

Paul felt a bit more stuck when he attempted to imagine a loved one who could validate his emotions. "The only person in my life who ever validates me is Sonia, so how can I imagine her validating me when she is the person causing me pain?" He proceeded in spite of this, imagining them lying in their bed together as he conveyed how upset he was by them growing apart from each other, and how scared he was that she was going to get fed up with him and leave him. He envisioned Sonia holding him, stroking his head, and telling him how she understood why he was feeling afraid. They had been together for a long time, and they were so important to each other—the emotional foundation for each other's lives.

As Paul pictured this, he felt something shift inside of him: a feeling of physical pain in his stomach, as if something sharp was puncturing a barrier in him. It was not quite an emotion, but it definitely *hurt*, and he did not like it, which perhaps was a sign that he was making some progress. To capitalize on this, Paul progressed to the "invoke an emotional memory" section of the toolkit. Paul remembered an experience when he was in first grade, when he had an assignment to memorize and learn how to spell words on a gigantic word list. The longest of the words was "beautiful," and he spent all afternoon memorizing it. "B-e-a-u-t-i-f-u-l. B-e-a-u-t-i-f-u-l. B-e-a-u-t-i-f-u-l." It became a song to him, a refrain that wormed itself inextricably into his mind. Proud of himself, he ran up to his mother—the one person he could lovingly describe with this word—to share his accomplishment. After he finished reciting it, she looked at him with confusion. "You only got through the B's?" Paul was crushed, devastated, and yes: deeply hurt by his mother's lack of validation. He ran to his room crying, leaving "beautiful" behind and devoting himself to immediately learning the rest of the words on his list. He never spoke about his academic work with his mother again.

Remembering this experience now, Paul found himself able to find his way into his feeling of hurt toward Sonia for ignoring him and leaving him behind. Shortly thereafter, as he discussed his recent interactions with Sonia in his therapy sessions, Paul noticed that something strange was happening: He was crying. His therapist encouraged him to actively try to *inhabit* the emotion. Paul located the feeling deep in his gut, and he worked to surrender to it, allowing it to wash over him and move through his body and heart. The therapist invited Paul to put words on what was coming up for him, and Paul expressed, "I feel overwhelmed, and sort of confused about what is happening to me and why I am feeling so emotional. I think this might be the hurt feeling—like I am really wanting to feel close and connected to Sonia, but it seems like she is done with me, and she cares more about everyone else than she does about me."

Paul increasingly utilized these strategies to access and experience his emotions in other areas of his life as well, including his feelings of love for his children, anxieties about his work performance, and shame and inadequacy surrounding his difficulties with emotional dysregulation, which made him feel like he was "weak" and unable to function independently in his own life. Interestingly, as Paul developed an increased ability to feel his feelings, he began to feel more grounded and centered in himself: a decreased sense of numbness and emptiness, diminished dissociation, and a reduced experience of feeling "dead inside." "A lot of the emotions I am accessing are actually quite intense and painful. So I am kind of surprised that, as I connect with them more, I feel weirdly better. I'm not feeling good, but at least I am *feeling*, which is much better than always being a thousand miles away from myself."

While Sonia was relieved that Paul's depression was improving, she continued to feel stressed and overwhelmed by having to manage all of the childcare responsibilities on her own. Paul's therapist called attention to Sonia's feedback that Paul was largely absent in the life of their family—a perspective that Paul always defensively dismissed. Sensing some validity in Sonia's feedback, the therapist recommended that Paul employ the Getting Connected to Reality Toolkit. Prompted by the toolkit, Paul intentionally sought out objective information about his parenting that he did *not* want to consider, and which generated pain and distress in him.

Paul could not ignore all of the things that Sonia was doing for their children: making them breakfast, taking them to and from school, cooking dinner, giving them baths, and putting them to bed, after which she proceeded to do the dishes and clean the house. In contrast, Paul was spending most of his time alone in his office—reading philosophy, writing journal articles, posting on Reddit, and watching YouTube videos about puppies and kittens being friends. He realized it had been months since he had taken the kids out for some fun activity outside of the home, or even read them stories before bedtime, which he used to do all of the time.

Looking at these facts in front of him in black-and-white, Paul was overwhelmed by feelings of guilt and shame. He did not *see* himself as an absent parent, but he was starting to wonder if that might be the case. Once these facts were more fully "on his radar," Paul felt remorse whenever he spent extended periods of time alone in his office. Paul began to simply *hang around* the kitchen during meals. Then one day out of the blue, he asked Sonia, "Is there anything I can do to help?" This progressed to Paul volunteering to take the kids to school, helping to cook meals, and doing dishes with Sonia at the end of the night. Since he was around the kids more, he was able to actually engage with them in a direct way. He asked them questions about their days, offered them support when they were struggling, and even resumed reading them stories before bedtime, the way that he used to do. Over time, Paul came to feel more connected with the children, and Sonia expressed feeling grateful and comforted by no longer having to manage all of these tasks completely on her own.

Despite this progress, Paul continued to struggle in his relationship with Sonia. He felt regularly abandoned by her whenever she focused extensively on other things (e.g., the children, her family, her work), and especially when she did not seek him out to pursue physical intimacy and emotional closeness. In these moments, Paul engaged in a form of "retaliatory withdrawal" from Sonia: He would not make eye contact with her, refrain from initiating conversation, give short answers to her questions, and go to bed early without explanation, rather than spending time watching their shows together after putting the kids to bed. Employing MBT's "naming what is absent" technique (Drozek et al., 2023), Paul's therapist gave him direct feedback about these interactions: "You have acknowledged that Sonia probably feels sad when you engage with her in this way, but you don't seem to *care* that you are potentially causing her pain."

Paul responded, "It's true. I think that I just feel so hurt by her that I don't really think about what she is feeling, and if I do, it doesn't really matter to me." Paul utilized the Getting Connected to Other People Toolkit, in order to try to empathize with Sonia more fully. He started by *identifying* with Sonia, focusing on all of the things they had in common: their similar childhoods growing up with emotionally neglectful parents *[history and background]*; their tendencies toward emotional sensitivity and insecurity *[internal states/personality]*; the various activities that they enjoyed doing together (e.g., exercise, classical music, intellectual discourse, spending time in nature) *[behaviors]*; and their shared professional experience of working in demanding jobs in academia *[circumstances]*, which Paul recognized must be contributing to their high levels of stress *[additional internal states]*.

Paul's therapist also encouraged Paul to "import" Sonia's situation into his own life: What would it be like for *him* if Sonia withdrew from him and refused to communicate? Paul acknowledged, "I would *lose my shit*. I would get completely enraged with her *[emotions]*, and I would probably end up criticizing her and trying to hurt her feelings *[desires]*. I also think I would just feel really panicked and desperate *[emotions]*—feeling like I was not good enough, and worthless because she was pulling away from me *[feelings about self]*. I also would definitely believe that it wasn't right for her to be treating me this way: I'm her husband, so she shouldn't be shutting me out and refusing to engage with me *[perspective on situation]*."

As Paul reflected on these matters, he realized that in fact Sonia had *not* responded with aggression and criticism toward him in this whole situation. "It makes me embarrassed to say it, but she has actually been a lot kinder and more supportive to me than I would have been to her, if the roles were reversed." Paul was then able to take the step of directly validating Sonia's feelings of sadness surrounding his manner of treating her. It made sense that she would feel that way, since she was already feeling highly anxious and overwhelmed by working full-time and caring for their children *[other mental states]*, and then she had to deal with him being quite cold and antagonistic toward her *[external factors in the situation]*.

Humbled by these reflections, Paul also applied the "What's my part?" section of the toolkit, in order to examine how he had contributed to the challenges in their relationship. He recognized his desire to hurt and punish Sonia for not being completely responsive to him *[active empathic deficits]*, as well as his tendencies toward withdrawal, criticism, suicidal planning, and relying extensively on Sonia to regulate his emotional states *[problematic actions/interpersonal approaches]*. In all of this, he had not really been thinking about or motivated by what Sonia had been going through, especially her fear of him killing himself, her stress about managing so many tasks, and her future loss, sadness, and devastation if he had moved forward with committing suicide *[passive empathic deficits]*.

Paul shared with his therapist, "I have always seen myself as this depressed, insecure guy who tends to isolate when things get really dark and bleak. But when I talk about all of these things, I realize that I just sound like a real asshole. I am starting to think that I have been *acting* like a real asshole. I have felt so hurt by Sonia, and I wanted her to make it up to me. But I have never really considered how I am actually hurting *her*, and that could be playing a big role in the difficulties in our relationship."

The therapist challenged Paul to consider: What would it look like for him to relate to Sonia in a more empathic manner—to prioritize her feelings and needs in their interactions with each other? Paul contemplated: "I think that I would just be more focused on what *she* is going through when she is not paying attention to me: feeling concerned about the kids, feeling frustrated about her work projects, or wanting to help out her parents. I would think through how it makes her feel when I ignore her, and hopefully consider that before I start pulling away from her *[focus and curiosity]*. I suspect I would also *feel* more worried about her and what she is going through—actually wanting to do what I can to help her feel more stable and secure in the relationship *[internal states]*."

"On the most basic level, I would ask her more about her day: how the kids are doing, what she has been doing at work, and what is going on with her parents, which I don't really care about but I know is important to her. I would also work on NOT ignoring her and withdrawing from her when I am angry at her, and instead try to communicate with her more directly about what I am feeling. I have never really done that before, so I don't really know what it would look like, but I am willing to try *[actions/interpersonal approaches]*."

"I think that this could really make a difference for Sonia. She would probably feel a lot less sad and upset in our interactions, and like we are actually in a mutual relationship together—both of us considering and supporting each other, rather than just her taking care of me like I am another one of the kids. I bet this would make her feel more comfortable with me, more connected with me, and also more grounded in herself, like she has a solid foundation in our relationship. I think that's the way it used to be with us, and I want to get back to that *[impact on the other person]*."

With these ideas in mind, when Paul was feeling hurt and rejected by Sonia focusing on other things, he actively worked to shift the "center of gravity" from himself to Sonia. Looking at Sonia working with their son on his homework, Paul saw how interested she was in helping him learn and grow, as well as how much she cared about him as a little person. Paul worked to simply "take in" Sonia's experience here—to emotionally resonate with these feelings, and to allow them to matter to him. To Paul's surprise, he felt something: not simply his own feelings about Sonia and their son, but *Sonia's* feelings of love and care for their son, almost reverberating inside of him. Sticking with these emotions, Paul attempted to care about Sonia and this aspect of her experience. Paul accessed a strong sense of love for Sonia, along with a range of other feelings: a desire to make her happy, pleasure and joy about her connecting with their son, and delight and appreciation for who Sonia was as a person—an open-hearted, thoughtful, slightly naive presence who brought warmth and kindness to everyone she encountered.

As Paul became more empathically connected to Sonia, he felt less overwhelmed by his anger, spite, and desire to punish her. When he felt rejected by Sonia, he did everything in his power to *not* withdraw from her, and to utilize MBT's strategies for psychic equivalence to address his certainty that Sonia was treating him in some way that was wrong and problematic (Chapter 12). Sometimes he would communicate his emotions of hurt and rejection to Sonia, but much of the time, he worked to address these emotions *internally*, by considering and empathizing with Sonia's valid motives for occupying herself with other things.

Sonia increasingly came to feel safer and more connected to Paul, and more comfortable focusing on her own interests and responsibilities without feeling like she would incur backlash from Paul. They started spending time together again: sharing about their days with each other, watching TV after the kids went to bed, rekindling sexual intimacy, and hiring a babysitter so that they could resume date nights once a week, the way that they did prior to having children. This all helped Paul feel more secure in their relationship, along with an increased sense of trust that Sonia loved and valued him, even while she was invested in other areas of her life and experience. Paul's mood improved, and his suicidal thinking and behavior faded away, never to return.

As the treatment unfolded, Paul began implementing these same strategies in the therapeutic relationship itself. He actively worked to "take in" his therapist's perspective about the topics he was discussing, rather than focusing exclusively on expressing his own ideas and feelings. He seemed less impatient and bored with the therapist, and genuinely interested in what was leading her to ask particular questions and give specific feedback. From the therapist's perspective, the therapy felt less like a monologue and more like a *dialogue* between two equal participants. Paul's therapist felt more present, engaged, and useful in her sessions with Paul—feelings she suspected must mirror how Sonia felt in response to all of Paul's progress.

In reflecting on this important phase of his life and treatment, Paul now shares: "I used to think that I just needed to *get more* from Sonia, in order to feel OK and not feel suicidal all the time. But I learned that it was just a bottomless pit. The more that I tried to get her to take care of me, the less I could function on my own, and I was never really addressing the real problem: I was completely detached from myself and other people. Now that I can actually feel my feelings *and* empathize with others' emotions, I don't want to die all of the time, and I don't need everyone else to regulate me. For the first time in my life, I feel like I am finally standing on solid ground—connected to myself, but also truly caring about the people around me, even when they are not doing what I want them to do."

Chapter Review 14.1
Pretend Mode: Disconnection and Dissociation

Introduction to Pretend Mode

- Pretend mode involves difficulties with disconnection and dissociation: disconnection from your own emotions and desires, and detachment from other people's mental states as well.

  - The tagline for pretend mode is: "Words without feelings."

- The term "pretend mode" does not imply dishonesty or intentional misrepresentation of facts.

  - The "pretend" in pretend mode derives from pretend play in childhood, where the child is absorbed in a world of their own imagination, and is less attentive to their emotions, other people's emotions, and the world around them.

- Pretend mode develops due to deficits in parental mirroring.

  - When caregivers fail to mentalize the child's emotions, the child internalizes images or "representations" of the caregiver, but those representations do not reflect the child's primary feeling states.

  - This leads to a sense of vacancy and emptiness in the self, along with difficulties empathizing and resonating with others' emotions.

- While some people experience "global" problems with pretend mode, you most likely encounter *context-dependent* pretend mode—that is, the tendency to disconnect from yourself and others under certain emotional or interpersonal conditions.

  - For instance, you might dissociate when you are under stress, or you could find it difficult to empathize with others when they are criticizing you.

Disconnection from Yourself

- In borderline personality disorder (BPD), examples of pretend mode with yourself include:

  - Lack of interest in or curiosity about your own mental states

  - Detachment from your own emotions and desires

  - Chronic feelings of emptiness

  - Dissociative symptoms

  - Overreliance on intellectualization, abstractions, and jargon about yourself

  - Disconnection from certain objective facts about your life

---

[continued on next page]

Disconnection from Other People

- In BPD, common forms of pretend mode with other people include:

  - Lack of interest in or curiosity about others' mental states

  - Overreliance on intellectualization, abstractions, and jargon about other individuals

  - Monologues and self-focused communications

  - Disconnection from certain objective facts about others

  - Deficits in empathy for other people, falling under two broad categories:

    - *Passive empathic deficits*: not being fully attentive and responsive to other individuals' emotions and desires, resulting in self-centeredness, entitlement, and "using" others

    - *Active empathic deficits*: experiencing desires and wishes that undermine other people's dignity or well-being, leading to anger, argumentativeness, aggression, or actions intended to cause others emotional or physical pain

  - These problems with empathy take a range of different shapes, summarized in the table on the following page.

[continued on next page]

Examples of Problems in Empathy	
Person-specific Empathic Deficits	Your ability to empathize gets "turned down" or "shut off" with some individuals in your life: your parents, siblings, boss, former friends, etc.
Group-specific Empathic Deficits	You find it difficult to empathize with people who possess certain personal qualities, belong to specific groups, or serve in distinct vocational or cultural roles.
Interaction-specific Empathic Deficits	You experience decreased empathy when you are engaged in particular kinds of interpersonal interchanges with others (e.g., receiving constructive feedback, pursuing sexual attention, confronting injustice).
Constrained or "Biased" Empathy	You feel less interested in and responsive to specific feelings in others (e.g., anger, sadness, insecurity), or certain emotions might even inspire your aggression or ire.
Emotion-dependent Empathic Deficits	Your ability to empathize with other individuals could be significantly dependent on your own emotions—for example, being highly compassionate when you are in a good mood but struggling with anger and irritability when you are dysregulated.
Situational Empathic Deficits	You find it harder to empathize with others when you encounter certain objective circumstances in your life (e.g., involving work, academics, finances, possessions, health and body, living situation, time of day/year, or your immediate environment).
Global Lack of Empathy	You experience more "across the board" problems with empathy—that is, failing to empathize with people under a broad array of conditions, independently of what you are experiencing internally or externally.

Chapter Review 14.2
Mentalizing Practice Points: Getting Connected

In mentalization-based treatment (MBT), the therapeutic approach for addressing pretend mode can be summed up by the maxim: "Get connected."

This involves first stopping the activities that separate you from yourself and others, and then working to get connected to (a) reality, (b) your own emotions and desires, and (c) other people's feeling states.

"Press Pause" on Your Intellect

Do your best to stop or interrupt all forms of intellectualization: analyzing, rationalizing, thinking and communicating in generalities and abstractions, trying to "explain" people's experiences, utilizing psychological jargon, and focusing on "shoulds" and ideals.

- When you are doing these things in an interpersonal interaction, one helpful strategy is to literally *cease talking*, since that will stop the intellectualization dead in its tracks.

Double Down on Stopping Pretend Mode Problem Behaviors

Do everything that you can to not engage in "dissociative behaviors"—that is, actions and interpersonal approaches that separate you from your emotions, or from other people's feeling states.

To address these behaviors, utilize your MBT Crisis Plan developed in Chapter 5, along with all of the mentalizing practice points recommended in this book to help you "reflect rather than reflex."

Get Connected to Reality

When you are in pretend mode, you often minimize and ignore certain objective facts (e.g., behaviors, circumstances, qualities, or characteristics) about yourself or other people. Utilize the Getting Connected to Reality Toolkit on the next page to reckon with facts about yourself or another person, and then to access the emotions that arise for you in relation to those facts.

[continued on next page]

Getting Connected to Reality Toolkit	
Working to Get Connected to Facts about *(circle one)* Yourself OR Another Person:	
	Describe facts/objective factors that • generate distress in you • you want to avoid considering • contradict your (e.g., overly positive or overly negative) beliefs about the person • have not been on your radar
History and Background	
Actions, Interpersonal Approach, or Manner of Communicating	
Objective Characteristics	
External Circumstances	

[continued on next page]

Try to really FOCUS on these objective factors, to "take in" the fact that they are real. When you do this, what do you feel?		
Emotions	Desires	Feelings about Yourself
Work to actually FEEL, access, and inhabit these feeling states—in your body, and deep in your heart.		

Chapter Review 14.3
Mentalizing Practice Points: Getting Connected to Yourself

When you are disconnected from what you are feeling, start by employing mentalization-based treatment's (MBT) techniques for identifying your own internal states, reviewed in Chapter 9. Then utilize the Getting Connected to Yourself Toolkit below, which compiles a handful of strategies to help you access and experience your emotions and desires.

Getting Connected to Yourself Toolkit
Step 1. Identify the feeling state. *(emotion, desire, or feeling about the self)*
Step 2. Assess your level of connectedness. How connected to the feeling state do you feel right now? Draw an arrow on the Connectedness Meter below. 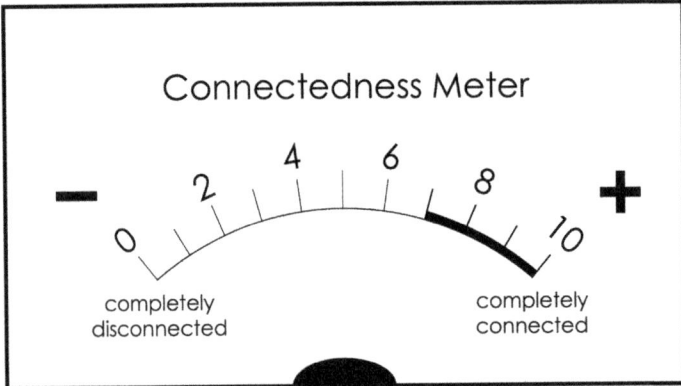 If you feel quite disconnected from the feeling, utilize the strategies below to access it more deeply. As soon as you start accessing the feeling, stop using the toolkit, to avoid becoming too distressed or overwhelmed.

[continued on next page]

Validate the Feeling State.
"It is understandable that I am feeling _____ because of . . ."

My History and Background	My Other Mental States Related to the Emotion	Factors in the External Situation	How Others Feel under Similar Circumstances

Conjure a Validating Companion.

Identify someone who really cares about you. Close your eyes, and picture the person supporting and validating you as you feel the feeling. Who would that individual be? What can you imagine them doing and saying as they empathize with you?

Invoke an Emotional Memory.

Think about a recent experience or situation you associate with the feeling in question. Describe the experience, as well as how it triggered the emotion in you. Try to actually FEEL the feeling, as you remember this.

[continued on next page]

Inhabit the Emotion.

Close your eyes, and actively work to ACCESS, INHABIT, and EXPERIENCE the feeling. Find the feeling in your body, and try to surrender to it, at an emotional level.

Do NOT dismiss or invalidate the emotion. Simply experience it, without taking any action on it.

Chapter Review 14.4
Mentalizing Practice Points: Getting Connected to Other People

When you are struggling to empathize with other people, start by employing mentalization-based treatment's (MBT) techniques for recognizing others' internal states, reviewed in Chapter 9. Then utilize the Getting Connected to Other People Toolkit below, which compiles a range of strategies to help you to emotionally resonate with and care about what others are feeling.

Getting Connected to Other People Toolkit			
Other Person:			
Describe the Other Person's Feeling States. *(emotion, desire, or feeling about the self)*			
Try to Identify with the Other Person. What similarities do you notice between yourself and the other person? These could be present across various domains.			
Internal States/ Personality	Behaviors/ Interpersonal Patterns	Current External Circumstances	History and Background

[continued on next page]

Import the Other Person's Situation.			
What would it be like for you if similar circumstances were happening in your own life?			
Your Emotions	Your Desires	Your Feelings about Yourself	Your Perspective on the Situation

Validate the Other Person's Feeling State.			
"It is understandable that the other person is feeling _____ because of . . ."			
Their History and Background	Their Other Mental States Connected to the Emotion	Factors in the External Situation	How Others Feel under Similar Circumstances

[continued on next page]

"What's my part?"			
Reflect on your own contributions to your challenges with the person, especially how you have engaged with them in maladaptive ways.			
Active Empathic Deficits	Passive Empathic Deficits	Your Problematic Actions/ Interpersonal Approaches	Positive Actions You have NOT Taken
Test-drive a More Empathic Perspective.			
If you were relating to the other person in a more empathic manner, how would your experience with them be different? Consider this question in several domains.			
Your Focus and Curiosity	Your Emotions and Desires	Your Actions/ Interpersonal Approaches	Impact on the Other Person
Try to Care about the Other Person.			
Close your eyes, and actively work to empathize with the other individual. Try to feel what they are feeling—to resonate with them at a deep level. Do NOT dismiss or invalidate what they are going through. Do your best to simply CARE about the person, and to allow their experience to matter to you.			

PART 3

Bringing It All Together

15

Learning How to Trust Other People: The Vantage Points for Mentalizing

At this point in the book, you have learned about all of the core elements in mentalization-based treatment (MBT): strategies for "holding on to your mind" when you encounter your triggers (Chapter 7); techniques for identifying and evolving your attachment style (Chapter 8); how to read emotions in yourself and other people (Chapter 9), and to understand what is leading these feelings to develop (Chapter 10); what to do when you get "stuck" in your mentalizing (Chapter 11); methods for helping you to become more flexible and curious in your thinking (Chapters 12 and 13); and how to get more connected to yourself and other people (Chapter 14).

With all of these elements in place, let's take a moment to consider where you go from here. How do you bring all of these strategies together to move yourself forward in your life—to address your challenges with instability, but perhaps most importantly, to build a life of meaning, purpose, and personal fulfillment? To start tackling these questions, let's return to Katherine, the physician with borderline personality disorder (BPD) we met in Chapter 1, who struggled with a long history of depression, suicidality, and unstable sense of self.

PICKING BACK UP WITH KATHERINE

The last time we heard from Katherine, she had made tremendous progress by the end of her first year in MBT (Chapter 2). She discontinued self-injury, consistently engaged in her work, started online dating, and actively sought to cultivate an identity not strictly organized around her psychiatric symptoms, all the while experiencing decreased feelings of depression and self-hatred.

These improvements opened up space for Katherine to get hired in her first professional job, working as an obstetrics and gynecology (OB/GYN) physician at a prestigious local hospital. She also entered her first romantic relationship, with a man named Matthew—a down-to-earth and kindhearted computer engineer she met on one of the dating apps. After seeing each other for over a year, they moved in together and took the big step of adopting a rescue puppy—a sign to them both that they were committed to moving their relationship forward, over the long term. Katherine shared in her therapy appointments: "I feel like I am coming out of a dark fog, perhaps for the first time in my life. I'm finally starting to do what normal people do: getting a job, having a partner, and even all the mundane stuff like signing up for a Costco membership and going out to brunch with my friends on the weekends."

Despite all of this progress, Katherine continued to struggle with challenges in emotional and interpersonal instability. She felt highly insecure at work, worrying that she would make some mistake that would irrevocably harm her patients. She constantly compared herself to her colleagues, often judging herself as not smart enough, unlikable, and socially awkward. Katherine felt like an imposter in this new world. "Everyone else is so successful and

Mentalization. Robert P. Drozek, Oxford University Press. © Oxford University Press 2025.
DOI: 10.1093/oso/9780198916857.003.0015

accomplished: doing research, publishing papers, serving on hospital committees. I know that I *should* be doing my own research and writing about stuff, but I have no idea what I would even focus on. I feel like I'm a fraud—a psychiatric patient who snuck in through the back door, but I don't really belong here."

Outside of work, Katherine found herself turning these same forms of judgment toward other people. Despite the fact that she called her parents religiously every week, her mother would regularly accuse Katherine of not visiting or checking in on them frequently enough, denouncing her as overly "selfish" and uncaring. Katherine would feel simultaneously guilty and enraged in these moments, responding by defending herself, criticizing her mother as unstable and narcissistic, seeking validation of her views from other people ("Can you believe how crazy she is?"), and ultimately withdrawing from her parents in anger, by ignoring their phone calls and visiting them even less.

In her romantic relationship, while Katherine felt largely loved and supported by Matthew, she remained highly sensitive to any hint of rejection by him. Having spent so many years single and depressed, Katherine would regularly plan activities and trips for them to do together, as a way to finally live her life and feel more engaged in the world. While Matthew was always excited about spending time with Katherine one-on-one, he was far less enthusiastic about attending any activities (e.g., concerts, lectures, dinner with friends) that required more extensive engagement with other people.

Picking up on Matthew's disinterest in these activities, Katherine would respond, "It's fine, it's fine, you don't have to come." She would thus end up going to these events on her own, while Matthew stayed at home playing video games, writing code, and working on electronics projects. Alone at these events, Katherine would feel intensely hurt and rejected by Matthew: "He says that he loves me, but if he really cared about me, he would *want* to do these things that are so important to me." Over time, Katherine increasingly focused on Matthew's perceived deficiencies: He was too shy, he didn't have enough friends or hobbies, he was boring, and he cared more about his machines than he did about interacting with real people.

Katherine would thus experience significant doubts about their relationship, leading her to withdraw from Matthew, or alternatively to criticize him for the issue in question. This led to conflicts, estrangement, and distance in the relationship, which further fueled Katherine's uncertainty and frustration. "I just feel so mad at him, but also mad at myself for getting stuck with him. I mean, I love Matthew, but what does it say about me that I have ended up with someone who is so socially awkward? It's like I am just so ugly and fucked up that this is the best I could do."

Similar processes played out in the therapy as well. When discussing these difficulties in the treatment, in keeping with MBT's therapeutic approach, the therapist would always start by exploring and validating Katherine's emotions and desires surrounding the issue under discussion (Bateman et al., 2023; Drozek et al., 2023). However, whenever the therapist shared his own perspective about the matters at play ("You seem highly attuned to your feelings of anger in the situation, but far less attentive to other emotions that could be coming up for you"), or if he gave Katherine more direct feedback about the scenario ("You seem quite certain that this situation is all Matthew's fault, but you don't appear to be considering your own part in these interactions"), Katherine would become angry and defensive with the therapist: telling him why he was wrong in his views of her, accusing him of criticizing her, and "shutting down" in sessions and refusing to speak.

"I don't WANT to take in your perspective. You are here to validate me—not the other way around. I feel like you're just judging and belittling me all the time, and so I need to fight back against you. If I didn't, I would feel horrible about myself, like I was just letting you walk all over me." The therapist felt stuck in this dynamic, as if he had to choose between two bad options: He could exclusively validate Katherine, in which case he would not be helping her with her core interpersonal challenges, or he could continue calling attention to these challenges, in which case Katherine would not effectively engage in the treatment.

In all of these disruptions, Katherine was struggling with a fundamental challenge facing people with BPD, as they start to get better in treatment: how to trust and connect with other individuals, and to "hold on to" their own perspectives while genuinely taking in and considering others' viewpoints.

THE VANTAGE POINTS FOR MENTALIZING

When you mentalize, you are usually mentalizing ABOUT something. You have a target—a "focal point" for your curiosity and reflection. As we discussed in Chapter 3, this focus can variously be thoughts and feelings in yourself, thoughts and feelings in other people, or more often than not, a little bit of both. Throughout this book, we have been reviewing MBT's strategies for reflecting on these factors, and for what to do when you get "stuck" in your efforts to think about what you and others are feeling.

You might remember Anthony Bateman, the co-developer of MBT introduced in Chapter 5, who was kind enough to write the foreword to this book. In recent years, Anthony has been calling attention to another important facet of mentalizing that had previously not been sufficiently appreciated in the MBT literature: the issue of not simply "what you are looking at" when you are mentalizing, but the position FROM WHICH you are mentalizing. We can refer to this as the *vantage point* for mentalizing—the interpersonal location that you occupy when you are trying to understand yourself and other people.

Broadly speaking, there are four different vantage points for mentalizing:

- *I-mode*, or considering mental states from your own viewpoint;
- *You-mode*, or examining mental states from other people's perspectives;
- *Me-mode*, or contemplating yourself from other people's standpoints;
- *We-mode*, or reflecting on yourself and other people simultaneously, from a shared position of mutuality and connectedness that transcends the outlook of any particular member of the dyad.

See Figure 15.1 for a pictorial representation of these standpoints.

In a series of important writings on these topics, Anthony and his collaborators have suggested that these vantage points are essential to understanding some of the challenges that people experience in BPD, as well as the progress that they make as treatment unfolds (Bateman, Campbell, et al., 2021; Bateman et al., 2023; Drozek et al., 2023).[1] This will thus be the final topic that we cover in the book: understanding the different vantage points for mentalizing, and applying these ideas to help you recover from your symptoms of BPD. So let's review the different vantage points for mentalizing, along with the problems you might encounter when these modes are less developed in your experience.

I-mode. "I-mode" is the experience of considering mental states from your own viewpoint. This includes being in touch with YOUR opinion about things, and what you

[1] Since this topic is perhaps the newest theoretical and clinical development in MBT, we are still working out the most helpful manner of delineating these concepts. For example, Bateman and colleagues (2023) outline the tripartite model of I-mode, me-mode, and we-mode, whereas elsewhere I (along with Brandon Unruh and Anthony Bateman) propose the four-part division of I-mode, me-mode, personalized me-mode, and we-mode (Drozek et al., 2023). Here, I am adding the notion of "you-mode" to refer to the process of considering mental states from other people's perspectives. Anthony Bateman (personal communication) supports this framing, in order to avoid any potential confusion for readers.

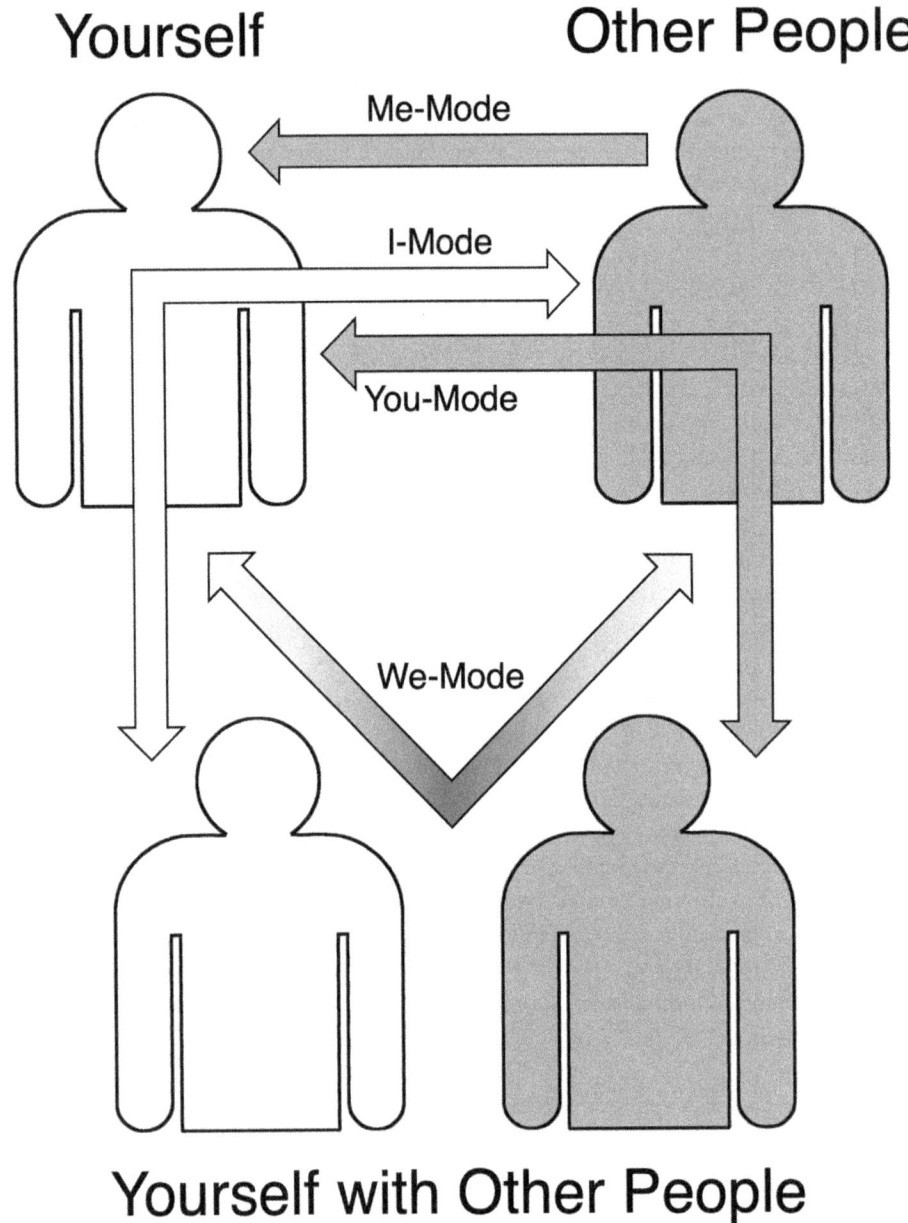

Figure 15.1 The vantage points for mentalizing. I-mode involves considering mental states from your own viewpoint; you-mode entails examining mental states from other people's perspectives; me-mode comprises contemplating yourself from others' standpoints; and we-mode encompasses reflecting on yourself and other people simultaneously, from a shared position of mutuality and connectedness.

actually believe about yourself, other people, and the world around you. I-mode also entails recognizing the *validity* of your perspective—remaining grounded in the fact that your thoughts and feelings have some level of justification, in light of your history, your psychology, and the facts of the situation itself. "It is understandable that I feel this way, given that. . . ." When you are in I-mode, you feel a sense of agency and confidence in your own viewpoint and emotions. *This is my experience. It is mine, and it matters BECAUSE it is mine. No one can take that away from me.* I-mode involves a sense of trust in your own perceptions, along with a connectedness to your own value as a person. You feel emboldened to be yourself, and that you deserve to have your feelings and rights respected in your relationships.

You-mode. "You-mode" is the process of examining mental states from other people's perspectives. This might be seen as a fundamentally impossible endeavor, as you are never truly able to abandon your own standpoint and enter into another person's experience. Instead, you end up utilizing your awareness of your personal mental states (e.g., your thoughts, emotions, desires) in order to understand others' thoughts and feelings. For example, you remember *your* experience of anxiety, which informs what you imagine your partner feels when they talk about "feeling anxious." On this view, you can only really make your way to you-mode through the pathway of I-mode.

When you are in you-mode, you are genuinely *trying* to understand another's mind—not only considering what they are feeling from your own position (the "Other" pole of mentalizing reviewed in Chapter 11), but actively working to inhabit the other individual's internal world, as if from "within their skin." Like I-mode, you-mode involves recognizing the inherent validity of other people's outlooks—the idea that others have *good reason* to feel the way that they do, in light of their history, current circumstances, and personal psychology. "It makes sense that they feel this way, due to the fact that. . . ." Along these lines, you-mode consists of actively empathizing with other people, allowing yourself to be motivated by them, and engaging with them in a manner consistent with their emotions, needs, and rights as human beings.

Me-mode. "Me-mode" is the process of contemplating yourself from other people's perspectives. As with you-mode, this stance might seem practically unattainable. How can you truly "get into" another person's head and understand how they see you? Once again, me-mode simply involves *trying* to enter into the other's experience of you, such that you are able to notice and appreciate their views of you, their feelings about you, and their desires toward you. Like all of the standpoints for mentalizing, me-mode entails recognizing the *validity* of the experience in question, in this case the legitimate, understandable reasons why the person feels this way about you. This involves not simply considering the things about them that lead them to look at you in a certain manner (e.g., their history, personality, current life circumstances), but also acknowledging *your* contributions to how they perceive you: your past actions, broader interpersonal patterns, non-verbal communications, actions you have NOT taken, or even your feelings and motives, which others can often reflexively "read" in their interactions with you.

It is important to note that me-mode is *not* tantamount to worrying and ruminating about what other people think of you. As discussed later, these ruminative tendencies (which are highly common in BPD) are really me-mode "unbuffered" by I-mode and you-mode, such that other individuals' feelings about you end up *determining* your experience of yourself. In contrast, when you are in me-mode, you apprehend others' sense of you, while also reflecting on the role you have played in leading others to see you in this way (Chapter 10). You are thus able to emotionally resonate with others' feelings about you, and to allow these feelings to impact and influence how you engage in your relationships.

We-mode. Finally, "we-mode" is the process of reflecting on yourself and other people simultaneously, from a shared position of mutuality and connectedness. In Chapter 4, we discussed how BPD is often associated with anxiety, fear, and mistrust of others, such that you struggle to feel safe and connected to the people in your life. We-mode is the antidote to these difficulties—on one view, the main psychological and interpersonal experience we have been working to cultivate throughout this book.

We-mode essentially joins together all of the vantage points for mentalization we have reviewed thus far in the chapter. When you are in we-mode, you are simultaneously grounded in yourself *[I-mode]*, engaged with another person's thoughts and feelings *[you-mode]*, and attentive to the other's experience of you *[me-mode]*—all while engaged with another individual who is ALSO connected to themself, you, and your experience of them. In this way, unlike the other vantage points for mentalizing, we-mode is a fundamentally intersubjective process. You cannot achieve we-mode on your own. Rather, you need to be connected to another person who is able to mentalize themself *and* you in real time, such that you are both "reading" and responding to each other in a largely mutual, reciprocal, and personally authentic fashion.

At the same time, we-mode is not simply geared toward two "individuals" interacting with each other. Anthony Bateman explains this further in our recent book, which reviews the different vantage points for mentalization:

> We need to share our inner states and let others know our underlying beliefs, goals, thoughts, and feelings. In so doing, we build a shared mind and generate common goals, from infancy to adulthood through attachment processes that underpin the evolution of mentalization. . . . When we take into account the inferred inner states of others, a shared reality is achieved, building social bonds.
>
> (Drozek et al., 2023)

On this view, when you are connected to another person who is also connected to you, something new is created which transcends either person: a shared experience and reality that encompasses *both* people's perspectives, while also giving rise to joint goals, intentions, and purposes that could never be possible with each individual alone. This is the vantage point of *we-ness*—not simply considering mental states in yourself and others, but doing so from a position of irreducible relatedness and kinship with other individuals.

With these ideas about the vantage points for mentalization in mind, take a moment to complete Worksheet 15.1, which walks you through applying these concepts to your own life.

Worksheet 15.1
Surveying the Vantage Points for Mentalization

I-mode

(1) *I-mode* is the process of considering mental states from your own perspective. This includes remaining connected to your beliefs and opinions, recognizing the validity of your experience, trusting yourself, and acknowledging your value and rights in your relationships. Provide at least three examples where you have been able to inhabit I-mode in your life.

(2) Describe the psychological and interpersonal circumstances in which you experience I-mode. What factors inside of you (e.g., emotions, desires, feelings about yourself) and around you (e.g., events, particular relationships or interactions with others) make it easier for you to enter into and remain in this mode?

You-mode

(3) *You-mode* is the process of examining mental states from other people's position and viewpoint. This involves actively trying to enter into others' perspectives, while also affirming the inherent validity of others' feelings and experience. Provide at least three examples where you where you have been able to occupy you-mode in your life.

[continued on next page]

(4) Describe the psychological and interpersonal circumstances in which you experience you-mode. What factors inside of you (e.g., emotions, desires, feelings about yourself) and around you (e.g., events, particular relationships or interactions with others) make it easier for you to enter into and remain in this mode?

Me-mode

(5) *Me-mode* is the process of contemplating yourself from others' perspectives. This encompasses trying to understand how people are seeing you, recognizing the potential validity of their experience of you, and considering the role you have played in impacting their feelings about you. Provide at least three examples where you have been able to inhabit me-mode in your life.

(6) Describe the psychological and interpersonal circumstances in which you experience me-mode. What factors inside of you (e.g., emotions, desires, feelings about yourself) and around you (e.g., events, particular relationships or interactions with others) make it easier for you to enter into and remain in this mode?

[continued on next page]

We-mode

(7) *We-mode* is the process of reflecting on yourself and other people simultaneously, from a shared position of mutuality and connectedness. This involves remaining grounded in yourself, engaging with another person's thoughts and feelings, and attending to the other's experience of you—all while the other individual also mentalizes themself and you. Provide at least three examples where you have been able to achieve we-mode in your life.

(8) Describe the psychological and interpersonal circumstances in which you experience we-mode. What factors inside of you (e.g., emotions, desires, feelings about yourself) and around you (e.g., events, particular relationships or interactions with others) make it easier for you to enter into and remain in this mode?

DISPARITIES IN THE VANTAGE POINTS FOR MENTALIZING

The aforementioned vantage points for mentalization play an essential role in psychological health and stability. In an MBT framework, health is constituted by the capacity to move flexibly from one vantage point for mentalizing to another, depending on your own internal experience at the time, as well as the events and interactions unfolding in your relationships. At times, you may be more focused on yourself and your perspective *[I-mode]*, but then depending on what is going on around you, you find yourself prioritizing the other person's needs and experiences *[you-mode]*. Perhaps you then notice that they seem to be having a negative response to you *[me-mode]*, which leads you to re-evaluate how you are engaging with them. How can you simultaneously consider *both* your outlook and the other individual's viewpoint, thus working toward a position of mutual consideration and understanding *[we-mode]*?

In these ways, you are able to "meet the demands of the moment" in your relationships—sometimes prioritizing yourself in your mentalizing, sometimes prioritizing others, and sometimes mentalizing from a more communal, collaborative position. This approach leads to increased stability and connectedness in your life, where you are able to care about other people's feelings without sacrificing your own needs and perspective.

In BPD, trouble arises when certain vantage points for mentalizing remain underdeveloped in your experience, such that you end up relying extensively on only certain vantage points in order to navigate your interactions with others. Your life becomes like a three-legged stool: Those legs could be solid on their own, but since the fourth leg is missing, everything gets wobbly and unstable, and the whole structure starts to topple.

See here for the major disparities you may experience surrounding the different vantage points for mentalization:

- *You-mode without I-mode:* You might focus extensively on other people's thoughts and feelings *[you-mode]*, while ignoring and neglecting your own emotions, desires, and needs *[I-mode]*. Your life remains "all about other people," and not about you. This can show itself in people-pleasing, caretaking of others, and self-sacrificing patterns in relationships. You might also end up idealizing other individuals and devaluing yourself, focusing more on what you think you "should" be doing and feeling than on the validity of what you are *actually* experiencing. You criticize yourself, dismiss your own experience, and naturally assume that others' perspectives are somehow more valid than your own. In the worst case scenario, people can mistreat you and take advantage of you without you even knowing it, since you struggle to honor your own needs and rights in your relationships.
- *You-mode without me-mode:* In some cases, you may ground yourself in other people's lives and experiences, for example by focusing on their moods, desires, and life challenges, and perhaps even devoting yourself to helping them and accommodating their needs *[you-mode]*. However, you might be less attuned to how they experience YOU, and what you might be doing to contribute to such perceptions *[me-mode]*. You thus could remain somewhat "clueless" about how you are coming across to others, inadvertently alienating people even as you are trying to prioritize them.
- *I-mode without you-mode:* At times, you could concentrate on the validity of your perspective, but you feel less curious about what *other people* are thinking and feeling, and what is leading them to experience things in this way *[you-mode]*. This can lead to difficulties with arrogance, certainty, stubbornness, dismissiveness, and "digging in your heels" with other people—regularly feeling like you are right and that others are wrong (Chapter 12).
- *I-mode without me-mode:* Similarly, you might get absorbed with how you are seeing things *[I-mode]*, without fully understanding how you are coming across to other people—their beliefs about you, as well as the full range of their emotions,

desires, and intentions toward you *[me-mode]*. This can manifest itself in social awkwardness, self-centeredness, and failing to read social cues in your interactions with other individuals. You also might find yourself "jumping to conclusions" about what others think of you—fixating on certain mental states toward you (e.g., anger, judgment, dislike) but overlooking their other, potentially more positive feelings toward you (e.g., concern, respect, desire to connect with you).

- *Me-mode without I-mode:* At times, you could think a lot about how other people feel about you *[me-mode]*, but you are far less connected to your own beliefs, preferences, and needs *[I-mode]*. This is the identity diffusion associated with BPD, where you get confused about who you are as a person, mold yourself to fit the people around you (i.e., the "chameleon effect" in BPD), and allow other people's views of you to significantly shape how you feel about yourself. *This person is judging me, so I must be bad.* These processes can lead to instability and volatility in your life: You become like a leaf in the breeze, always getting blown around this way and that, completely at the mercy of what is going on around you.

- *Me-mode without you-mode:* You also might be highly vigilant to other people's views of you *[me-mode]*, but you pay less attention to other facets of their internal worlds, including their beliefs, emotions, and desires that have little or nothing to do with you *[you-mode]*. This can cause significant difficulties in your relationships, since others can feel like you are not fully taking them in as people, that you do not fully care about them for their own sake, or that you are somehow only using them meet your own needs. In addition, you can end up "taking things personally" in your interactions with others. For instance, you reflexively assume that a colleague is ignoring your e-mail because they do not respect you *[me-mode]*, whereas they could simply be feeling overwhelmed and stressed by all of their other work responsibilities *[you-mode]*, and so they have not yet had the chance to respond.

- *"Mismatch" between I-mode and me-mode:* At other times, you may be able to understand how other people are seeing you *[me-mode]*, but their views of you do not "match" your own self-experience *[I-mode]*. For example, you feel strongly that you are a highly empathic person, but your friend accuses you of being aggressive and unkind. Or you see yourself as competent and skilled at your job, but your boss keeps passing you over for a promotion. Why would she do that if she really recognized your talents? In BPD, such "mismatches" can be highly destabilizing, leading to difficulties with emotional dysregulation, panic, shame, and rage. In such cases, you might be operating in a highly precarious form of I-mode, ready to topple over into me-mode when confronted with an image of you that contradicts your fragile view of yourself (see Bateman et al., 2023; Drozek et al., 2023).

Mentalizing Warm-up

Now that you have learned about the various disparities in the vantage points for mentalizing, return to Katherine's story on page 411. What specific disparities do you notice Katherine experiencing in her life? How do these challenges impact her mood, self-esteem, relationships, and functionality?

Employing Worksheet 15.2, try relating these ideas to your own experience. How have you struggled to fully occupy the different vantage points for mentalizing in your life and relationships?

Worksheet 15.2
Disparities in the Vantage Points for Mentalizing

Vantage points for mentalizing are the interpersonal locations that you occupy when you are trying to understand yourself and other people. If certain vantage points remain under-developed in your experience, you might experience instability in your mood, self-esteem, relationships, and functionality.

See below for the different disparities that people encounter in the vantage points for mentalization. For each disparity, describe any examples of these difficulties in your life, as well as the factors inside of you (e.g., emotions, desires, feelings about yourself) and around you (e.g., events, particular relationships or interactions with others) that lead you to experience these challenges.

(1) *You-mode without I-mode:* Prioritizing other people's internal states *[you-mode]*, while ignoring and dismissing your own emotions, desires, and needs *[I-mode]*.

(2) *You-mode without me-mode:* Extensively grounding yourself in other people's experiences (e.g., focusing on their moods, desires, and life challenges; trying to continuously help and accommodate them) *[you-mode]*, while being less attuned to how they experience YOU, and what you might be doing to contribute to such perceptions *[me-mode]*.

(3) *I-mode without you-mode:* Focusing on the validity of your perspective *[I-mode]*, but feeling less curious about what other individuals are thinking and feeling, and what is leading them to experience things in this way *[you-mode]*.

[continued on next page]

(4) *I-mode without me-mode:* Concentrating on how you are seeing things *[I-mode]*, without fully understanding how you are coming across to other people—how THEY are experiencing you *[me-mode]*.

(5) *Me-mode without I-mode:* Fixating on what others think of you *[me-mode]*, while feeling less connected to your own beliefs, preferences, and needs *[I-mode]*.

(6) *Me-mode without you-mode:* Thinking excessively about other people's views of you *[me-mode]*, while paying less attention to other facets of their experience, including their beliefs, emotions, and desires that have little or nothing to do with you *[you-mode]*.

(7) *"Mismatch" between I-mode and me-mode:* Experiencing emotional and interpersonal instability when other individuals' views of you *[me-mode]* contradict or undermine how you see yourself *[I-mode]*.

MENTALIZING PRACTICE POINTS: WORKING TOWARD WE-MODE

MBT helps you to address your challenges occupying the different vantage points for mentalization. While this process looks different depending on the person, over the course of an MBT treatment, this often unfolds along a common trajectory: first getting connected to yourself *[I-mode]*, then entering into other people's perspectives *[you-mode]*, next considering yourself from others' standpoint *[me-mode]*, and finally cultivating deeper relationships with other people, such that you are able to consider yourself and others from a shared position of mutual understanding *[we-mode]*.

In these ways, MBT helps you to finally achieve a sense of trust and connectedness with the people around you. You feel safer with others, as if they are seeing you for who you are, and they care about your growth and well-being as a person. At the same time, you feel genuinely invested in them as people: attuned to *their* thoughts and emotions, and motivated to meet their needs and goals. You learn how to be yourself in the interaction, while also accepting other individuals as they are, without feeling like you need to change them in order to get your needs met. You start to feel like you and others are "in this together"—working with each other toward a shared task, whatever your differences and personal vulnerabilities. This all gives rise to a sense of meaning, purpose, and fulfillment in your life, and a sense that you are part of something greater than yourself.

This is what it means to be in a relationship. And this is our main aim in MBT: By helping you to mentalize yourself and other people, you move yourself closer to others, while simultaneously becoming more grounded in your own experience.

So how do you strengthen your capacity to occupy the various vantage points for mentalizing? MBT's therapeutic strategies here follow one broad principle: When you are feeling unsteady in a particular vantage point, work to ground yourself more fully in the outlook in question. You can do this by deploying all of the forms of mentalizing reviewed in this book: first examining mental states in the person *[content-mentalizing]*, then validating the experience *[context-mentalizing]*, next reflecting on your own agency in the vantage point *[context-mentalizing]*, and finally, working to become more emotionally connected to the perspective in question *[process-mentalizing]*.

As always in MBT, these steps involve engaging in certain forms of reflection or "question-asking"—inquiries that you can only really consider by entering into the specific mode of reflection (e.g., I-mode, you-mode, me-mode, we-mode). Over time, you develop an increased ability to move in and out of the different vantage points, including the experience of mutual understanding and "co-mentalizing" with other people.

So now let's review MBT's strategies for strengthening the vantage points for mentalizing.

Strengthen I-mode. If you are struggling to remain grounded in your own experience, utilize MBT's techniques for bolstering I-mode, summarized in the Strengthening I-mode Toolkit below. Start by reflecting on your own mental states, from deep within your own perspective. "Leaving aside what other people think, what do I actually believe about this issue? What is MY opinion here?" Or: "What are my desires and preferences in this situation? What do I really want to happen, in the best case scenario?"

Strengthening I-mode Toolkit
If you are struggling to "hold on to" your own perspective . . .

Content-mentalizing: Reflect on Your Own Mental States	**Thoughts and Beliefs:** • "Leaving aside what other people think, what do **I** actually believe about this issue? What is my opinion here?" • "If no one else were around, what would I be thinking about all of this?" • "If someone else were going through this, what would I think about what is happening? Could any of that apply to me?" **Emotions:** • "What emotions am I experiencing right now?" • "What would I like to do in this scenario? What would I genuinely enjoy?" **Desires:** • "What are my desires and preferences in this situation? What do I really want to happen, in the best case scenario?" • "What do I want for my life in this domain? What circumstance is most consistent with my long-term goals, and who I am as a person?" • "Is there anything about which I am truly curious here? If I had a crystal ball, what would I want to know?" **Values and Ethics:** • "What are my values surrounding this topic? Do I have any strong opinions about how I should behave and relate to other people?" • "What are my rights in this situation? What do I deserve, and how do I deserve other people to be treating me?"
Context-mentalizing: Validate Your Experience	"It is understandable that I feel this way because of _____." Make reference variously to • Your history and background • Your other mental states (e.g., additional thoughts, emotions, desires, or feelings about yourself) related to the experience • Factors in the external situation • How others would feel under similar circumstances

Context-mentalizing: Mentalize Your Agency in I-mode	• "What would it look like for me to approach this situation more authentically—in a manner that reflects my beliefs, emotions, desires, and who I am as a person?" • "How could I express my own emotions to the other person, and give voice to my own desires and preferences?" • "What do I feel like the right thing to do is? What behaviors feel most consistent with my values and ethics?" • "What actions would I take, in order to respect my own dignity, worth, and what I deserve from other people?" • "How would I be acting and relating to others, in order to pursue my long-term goals and interests?" If you identify any potential actions through these questions, before taking them, make sure to "cross-check" them against the other vantage points for mentalizing.
Process-mentalizing: Get Connected to Your Own Perspective	Actively work to • "Own" your beliefs and viewpoints • Access and inhabit your emotions • Experience your wishes and desires • Respect your own dignity, rights, and ethical principles.

Then proceed to *validate* your own experience (Chapter 14), namely by contextualizing it in terms of (a) your history and background, (b) your other mental states (e.g., emotions, desires, values, feelings about yourself) related to the experience, (c) factors in the external situation (e.g., other people's actions, interpersonal interactions between yourself and others, impersonal events), or (d) how others would feel under similar circumstances. "It is understandable that I am feeling angry at my mother, since she spoke to me in a really aggressive manner *[factors in external situation]*. I have a long history of being abused by her *[history and background]*, and I think that a lot of people would feel upset about this *[others' similar experience]*. I don't deserve to be treated that way, especially by someone who is supposed to love and support me *[other mental states: values and ethics]*."

Next try to consider what you would actually *do* in your life, if you were to truly honor and respect your own perspective surrounding the matter at hand. For example, you might ask yourself: "What would it look like for me to approach this situation more authentically—in a manner that reflects my beliefs, emotions, desires, and who I am as a person?" Or you could wonder: "What actions would I take, in order to respect my own dignity, worth, and what I deserve from other people?"

If you end up identifying a specific action you could take along these lines (e.g., sharing your emotions and wishes to a romantic partner, setting a boundary with a family member), make sure to "cross-check" it against the other vantage points for mentalizing, to determine if the action is consistent/inconsistent with those viewpoints. For example, from the perspective of I-mode, you might determine that you want to criticize your best friend for neglecting you since she started a new romantic relationship, but from the perspective of we-mode, you worry that this feedback could endanger your friendship, which you really value. This approach ensures that the new behavior reflects the full range of vantage points available to you, rather than just the one that you happen to be occupying in the moment.

Finally, work to get *emotionally* connected to your own position. This can involve authentically "owning" your beliefs, accessing and fully experiencing your emotions and desires, and honoring your own dignity, rights, and ethical principles. Do your best to pursue these processes at an internal level, not simply at the level of behavior. The goal here is to FEEL a sense of connectedness to your own perspective, such that you attain something of an experiential anchor in the standpoint of I-mode. By engaging in the above forms of reflection, and then by affectively inhabiting your mental states identified in this process, you ground yourself more deeply in your own viewpoint and position.

Strengthen you-mode. If you are finding it challenging to enter into another person's perspective, employ MBT's strategies for moving toward you-mode, outlined in the Strengthening You-mode Toolkit below. Begin by reflecting on the other person's mental states, in general or in the scenario in question. "What emotions could the other individual be feeling right now?" "What really matters to the person? What is important to them, as a person?" To the degree that it is in your power, try to wrestle with these questions *from* the other person's perspective, rather than simply expressing your own view on what is happening for the person. For example, rather than concluding, "My sister just wants to get back at me, because she is jealous of me for being dad's favorite" (a belief likely born out of your own strong opinions about your sister), consider your *sister's* view of her own experience: "She would probably say that she is worried about me, and she is trying to give me feedback so that I can get my life back on track." In this way, you can shift out of a primarily "I-mode interpretation" of others to a predominantly "you-mode" perspective, which is more fully situated in other people's unique personal vantage points.

Strengthening You-mode Toolkit
If you are struggling to enter into another individual's perspective . . .

| Content-mentalizing: Reflect on the Other Person's Mental States | **Thoughts and Beliefs:**
• "What are the other person's thoughts and beliefs about this matter?"
• "What is the person's perspective on this situation? How are they experiencing all of this?"

Emotions:
• "What emotions could the other individual be feeling right now?"
• "How might the person be feeling about themselves? Where is their self-worth and self-esteem?"

Desires:
• "What are the other person's desires and preferences in this situation? What do they really hope will happen, in the best case scenario?"
• "What does the person want for their life more broadly? What are their long-term goals and aspirations?"
• "How do they want other people to see them, and to feel about them?"
• "What are the person's desires for other people? What do they most want for you—in your life and in their relationship with you?" |

	Values and Ethics: • "What really matters to the other individual? What is important to them, as a person?" • "What are their values and ethics? What do they expect of themself and other people?" • "What does this person deserve in this situation? What are their needs and rights?" • "How should other people (including me) be treating them?"
Context-mentalizing: Validate the Other Person's Experience	"It is understandable that the other person feels this way because of _____." Make reference variously to • Their history and background • Their other mental states (e.g., additional thoughts, emotions, desires, or feelings about themself) related to the experience • Factors in the external situation • How others would feel under similar circumstances
Context-mentalizing: Mentalize Your Agency in You-mode	• "What would it look like for me to prioritize the other person in my interactions with them?" • "What actions would I be taking, in order to be more responsive to their emotions, desires, and long-term interests?" • "How could I affirm and validate the person's feelings and perspective?" • "What could I do, in order to better respect the individual's dignity, worth, and rights?" • "How can I genuinely be of service to this person?" If you identify any potential actions through these questions, before taking them, make sure to "cross-check" them against the other vantage points for mentalizing.
Process-mentalizing: Get Connected to the Other Person's Perspective	Actively work to • Value and appreciate the other person's beliefs and viewpoints • Empathize with the person's emotions and feelings about themself • Respect the individual's rights, dignity, and worth • Resonate with the other's wishes and desires • CARE ABOUT the individual as a person

Once you have identified key facets of the other person's experience, work to *validate* the mental states in question. What makes it reasonable and understandable that the other individual sees things in this way, or feels the way that they do? As discussed in

Chapter 14, you can validate another person's feelings by reflecting variously on (a) their history and background, (b) their other mental states (e.g., emotions, desires, values, feelings about themselves) related to the experience, (c) factors in the external situation (e.g., other people's behaviors, interpersonal interactions, impersonal events, actions *you* have taken in your relationship with the individual), or (d) how others would feel under similar circumstances. "It makes sense that my girlfriend has felt depressed lately, since she has been feeling more lonely and disconnected in her friendships *[other mental states]*. She used to receive a ton of support from her friends *[history and background]*, but a lot of them have gotten married and started having kids, so she is spending much more time by herself, without much social interaction *[external factors]*. I think this is a really common experience for people at her age, and in her life stage *[others' similar experience]*."

Next consider what it would look like to *behaviorally* prioritize the other person's feelings and perspective. For example, you might ask yourself, "What actions would I be taking, in order to be more responsive to the other person's emotions, desires, and long-term interests?" Or: "How could I affirm and validate the other person's feelings and perspective?" By reflecting in these ways, you are able to shift your felt sense of agency more fundamentally toward other people's personal viewpoints, such that your naturally arising motives and desires increasingly reflect others' internal worlds.

Finally, attempt to inhabit the other individual's perspective at an *emotional* level. This could variously involve appreciating the person's beliefs and views, empathizing with their emotional states, resonating with their wishes and desires, and striving to experience a feeling of respect for their rights, dignity, and worth. At the same time, endeavor not simply to connect with the other person's mental processes, but to value and care about the other person *as a person*—to feel a sense of warmth, concern, and interest in who they are and what matters to them. As you feel more affectively engaged in the other person's emotional life, you become more fundamentally grounded in what it is like to be them, from their own position and vantage point.

Strengthen me-mode. If you are experiencing difficulties considering how other people view you, try out MBT's techniques for cultivating me-mode, reviewed in the Strengthening Me-mode Toolkit on the next page. To start, itemize relevant "facts" in your relationship with the other person. For example, ask yourself, "What actions has the other individual taken in our interactions? How have they treated me, and how have I responded to that?" Or: "Are there any things I have done, or things that have happened between us, that the person would cite as noteworthy in our relationship?" In BPD, it is all too easy to "hyper-mentalize" other people—that is, to ruminate and worry about what they think of you, in a manner that often departs from the reality of their experience of you. By remaining grounded in the FACTS surrounding your interactions with the other person, you keep your mentalizing accountable to what is *actually happening* between yourself and the person.

	Strengthening Me-mode Toolkit
	If you are struggling to consider yourself from another person's perspective . . .
Content-mentalizing: Reflect on the Other Person's Experience of You	**Relevant Facts about Your Relationship with the Person:** • "What are important events and circumstances in our relationship with each other?" • "What actions have I taken in our interactions? How have I treated the person, and how have they responded to that?" • "What actions has the other individual taken in our interactions? How have they treated me, and how have I responded to that?" • "Are there any things I have done, or things that have happened between us, that the person would cite as noteworthy in our relationship?" **Thoughts and Beliefs:** • "When I did/said _____, what did the other individual think about me?" • "When the person did/said _____, what was their impression of me?" • "What is the person's view of me? How do they see me, and what are their beliefs about me as a person?" **Emotions:** • "When I did/said _____, what emotions was the individual feeling?" • "When the person did/said _____, how were they feeling about me?" • "How does the person seem to feel about me as a person, and in our interactions with each other?" **Desires:** • "When I did/said _____, what was the other person wanting?" • "When the person did/said _____, what desires were they experiencing? What was motivating them?" • "What are the individual's wishes in relation to me? What do they want me to think, fccl, and desire?" **Values and Ethics:** • "What does this person expect of me? What standards do they hold for me—in this situation and in general?" • "How do they think I should be behaving, living my life, and approaching my interactions with them?" • "What do they believe I deserve in my life—in the areas of mood, relationships, external circumstances, and how other people are treating me?"

Context-mentalizing: Validate the Other Person's Feelings about You	"It is understandable that the other person experiences me in this way because of _____." Make reference variously to • Events in your relationship and interactions • Actions you have taken, and ways you have treated the individual • The other individual's history and background • The person's other mental states (e.g., wishes thoughts, emotions, desires, or feelings about themself) concerning themself or their life apart from you • Factors in the external situation • How others would feel under similar circumstances
Context-mentalizing: Mentalize Your Agency in Me-mode	• "What could I do—or stop doing—in order to impact how the other person experiences me?" • "How might I approach the relationship, so that the other person might see me in a more positive light?" • "What would it look like for me to accept and tolerate how the other person is viewing me?" • "When relevant, how could I affirm and validate the other person's beliefs about me?" • "What behaviors could I engage in, in order to be more responsive to the person's feelings about me, desires toward me, and values in our interactions with each other?" If you identify any potential actions through these questions, before taking them, make sure to "cross-check" them against the other vantage points for mentalizing.
Process-mentalizing: Get Connected to the Other Person's Experience of You	Actively work to • Value and appreciate the other person's views of you • Empathize with the person's feelings about you • Resonate with the individual's wishes toward you: what they want you to think, feel, desire, and do • Respect the person's ethics and values for you and your interactions

Now holding these behaviors and interactions in mind, reflect on the other individual's feelings about you. "When I refuse to turn my camera on in the Zoom meeting, what might my colleagues think about me?" Or: "When my husband told me that he wanted me to go inpatient, what emotions and desires was he experiencing?" Still attending to these objective events, you can also ponder the person's mental states about you more broadly in the relationship. "What are the individual's desires in relation to me? What do they want me to think, feel, and desire?"

Once you identify the other person's thoughts and feelings about you, work to contextualize and validate these experiences. Since your current aim is orienting yourself in me-mode, it is usually most helpful to focus primarily on your *own* actions and interpersonal approaches in the dynamic, and how these processes have impacted how the other person experiences you. "It is understandable that my girlfriend doesn't really trust me right now, since I have lied quite a bit about my drinking, and I haven't been following through with all of my responsibilities at work and around the house."

At the same time, feel free to validate the person's feelings about you by invoking other factors in their experience, including their history and background, current external situation, their other mental states about their life apart from you, and how others would feel under similar circumstances. For example, continuing with the example of the mistrustful girlfriend, the person might add, "She has a long history of partners lying to her *[history and background]*, so she always feels worried that people are going to hurt and betray her *[other mental states]*. Her boss has also been really critical and demanding of her recently *[current external situation]*, which would probably make anyone feel more stressed out and paranoid *[others' similar experience]*."

To center yourself more fully in me-mode, you can also reflect on additional behavioral approaches you might take, in light of people's mental states about you. For example, you might wonder, "What could I do—or stop doing—in order to impact how the other person experiences me?" Or you could ask yourself: "What behaviors could I engage in, in order to be more responsive to the person's feelings about me, desires toward me, and values in our interactions with each other?" The goal here is not to reflexively contort yourself to other people's preferences for you, but rather simply to allow others' experience of you to play *some* role in influencing your motives and intentions, and ultimately how you engage in the relationship in question. Sometimes you could decide to do what other people want you to do, but under other circumstances, you might conclude that you need to "hold your ground" and follow your own desires and values—that is, allowing I-mode to trump me-mode. Wherever you end up in these deliberations, by wrestling with these inquiries, you are successfully "expanding your agency" to reflect a broader range of vantage points, including other people's outlook on you.

As a final step, strive to "get connected" to the other person's perceptions of you, at an emotional level rather than a strictly intellectual one. This might sound like a tall order, especially if the person is seeing you in a negative light, and this makes you feel hurt, angry, or upset. That said, a key facet of mentalizing is "delight in different perspectives" (Bateman & Fonagy, 2016), or to use the terms of the present discussion, an embrace of the different vantage points for mentalizing. So regardless of how the other individual experiences you, try to FEEL a sense of compassion for that experience, from their standpoint rather than simply your own. This could show itself in various ways, including appreciating and valuing the other person's views of you, empathizing with their feelings about you, resonating with their wishes for you (e.g., what they want you to think, feel, desire, and do), and respecting their ethics and values for you and your interactions with each other.

In the above ways, you strengthen your ability to enter into others' views of you—allowing these perspectives to enrich how you feel in your relationships, and how you engage with the people around you.

Strengthen we-mode. As we discussed, "we-mode" is the process of reflecting on yourself and other people simultaneously, from a shared position of mutuality, connectedness, and trust. To foster that experience, apply the MBT techniques described in the Strengthening We-mode Toolkit on the following page. The focus of these strategies is the joint experience of you and another person in a particular relationship, so select a relationship in which you would like to develop a greater sense of closeness and collaboration. You can try out these techniques on your own, or if it seems appropriate to the relationship (e.g., with certain family members, romantic partners, or close friends), you are welcome to share the toolkit with the other person, so that you can both work on "strengthening we-mode" together!

Strengthening We-mode Toolkit	
How to cultivate collaboration, trust, and connectedness in a specific relationship	
Content-mentalizing: Reflect on Mental States in the Relationship	**Thoughts and Beliefs:** • "What thoughts and beliefs do we share with one another, in general or about this specific matter?" • "How are we seeing things differently from each other?" • "What have I learned from the other person? What do I think they have learned from me?" **Emotions:** • "How might we be experiencing similar emotions right now? More broadly in our lives, where do I notice parallels in our moods and emotions?" • "At the level of emotions and mood, how are we different from each other?" • "In what ways do we both trust each other? How do we feel 'seen' and understood by the other person as unique individuals?" **Desires:** • "What desires and wishes do we have in common with each other, in this scenario or in general?" • "What are our joint goals, projects, and plans?" • "How are our desires and plans different from each other?" **Values and Ethics:** • "How are our values similar to each other? What is important to us both?" • "What shared expectations do we both have for ourselves, other people, and this relationship?" • "How are our values and expectations different, in this scenario or as people?" • "What rights do we have in common in this situation? How should we both be treating ourselves, and each other?" • "What do we both deserve—in this relationship and more broadly in our lives?"
Context-mentalizing: Validate Your Joint Experience of the Relationship	"It is understandable that we feel this way because of _____." Make reference variously to • Your history together in the relationship, including your interactions with each other • Actions you have taken, actions the other person has taken • Other mental states (e.g., additional thoughts, emotions, desires, or feelings about yourselves) you each have about the relationship • Factors in the external situation that impact both of you • Your respective personal experiences: histories, external situations, and other mental states (e.g., beliefs, emotions, desires, personalities, feelings about yourselves) • How others would feel under similar circumstances

Context-mentalizing: Mentalize Your Agency in We-mode	• "How can I help the other person feel more 'seen' and understood by me, while also giving voice to my own perspective?" • "How can I affirm and validate the other individual's emotions and desires, and at the same time express my own emotions and desires?" • "What could I do to honor and respect the other's expectations and values in our interactions, while simultaneously respecting my own values and needs?" • "How could I pursue our shared goals and values in this relationship?" • "How could I engage with this person in a more mutual, collaborative manner?" • "What would it look like for me to place more trust in the other person? How could I BE more trustworthy in this interaction, and in this relationship?" If you identify any potential actions through these questions, before taking them, make sure to "cross-check" them against the other vantage points for mentalizing.
Process-mentalizing: Get Connected to Your Shared Experience in the Relationship	Actively work to • Value and appreciate the other person's beliefs and viewpoints, while also holding on to your own beliefs and convictions • Empathize with the person's emotions and desires, while authentically accessing your own emotions and desires • Invest emotionally in your common goals and values in this relationship • FEEL a sense of trust in the other person, yourself, and the relationship • Full-throatedly accept yourself exactly as you are, and the other person exactly as they are • Respect the rights, dignity, and worth of yourself and the other person • CARE ABOUT the individual as a unique person, while also embracing and cherishing who you are as a person

Start by examining the various areas of similar mental states in the relationship, for example by asking, "What thoughts and beliefs do we share with one another, in general or about this specific matter?" Or: "What are our joint goals, projects, and plans?" And taking this all further: "In what ways do we both trust each other? How do we feel 'seen' and understood by the other person as unique individuals?" We-mode also entails considering areas of difference or divergence in your experience with others: "How are we seeing things differently from each other?"

Once you have considered your experience with another person, work to *validate* that experience, namely by invoking (a) your history with the other individual; (b) actions you have taken with each other; (c) other mental states (e.g., additional thoughts, emotions, desires, or feelings about yourselves) that you each have about the relationship; (d) factors in the external situation that impact both of you; (e) your personal experiences in your respective lives (e.g., involving your individual histories, life situations, and psychological processes); and (f) how others would feel under similar circumstances.

For example, you could reflect: "It makes sense that my boyfriend and I both want to move in together right now *[shared mental state]*. We've been with each other for like three years *[history in the relationship]*, and things have been going really well with us recently: We're not having as many arguments, he's been saying 'I love you' more, and I basically stay over his place almost every night already *[actions taken with each other]*. We'd also save a lot of money having one place rather than two *[external circumstances]*. Perhaps most importantly, I've been much more stable for a while now *[personal experience]*, and I bet he's finally feeling confident that we actually could make it as a couple *[other mental states about the relationship]*. Looking at the whole picture, I think that a lot of people—including our families—feel like it's time for us to take the next step *[others' similar experience]*."

You can also reflect on your own potential actions and interpersonal approaches, from the perspective of the relationship and your shared experience with the other person. In we-mode, this always entails trying to honor *both* people's preferences and interests, while simultaneously advancing your common goals and intentions in the relationship. For example, you might ask yourself, "How can I help the other person feel more 'seen' and understood by me, while also giving voice to my own perspective?" Or: "What would it look like for me to place more trust in the other person? How could I BE more trustworthy in this interaction, and in this relationship?"

As always, if you feel moved to engage in a certain behavior based on these considerations, make sure to "cross-check" the behavior with the other toolkits in this chapter (e.g., related to I-mode, you-mode, and me-mode), to ensure that the action does not undermine other important perspectives in your and others' experience. For example, you might conclude that you could place more trust in another person by sharing openly about your psychiatric history (a we-mode consideration), but then you recognize that the person in question is actually your *boss*, so this decision would probably not be consistent with your own long-term professional interests and goals (an I-mode concern).

As a final step in advancing we-mode, work to connect more deeply to your areas of joint experience with the other individual. This could involve appreciating the other person's beliefs, while also holding on to your own opinions and convictions; empathizing with the person's emotions and desires, and simultaneously accessing your own feelings and wishes; and investing emotionally in your common goals and values in this relationship. Taking these processes even further, strive to embrace yourself and the other individual *as people*: respecting and valuing each other as distinct but connected individuals; feeling a sense of trust in the other person, yourself, and the relationship; full-throatedly accepting yourself and the person, exactly as you are in the current moment; and endeavoring to actually CARE ABOUT the individual as a unique person, while also embracing and cherishing who you are as a person.

By "getting connected" in these ways, you are not simply considering your own perspective, or the other person's perspective. You are grounding yourself emotionally in a new standpoint that encompasses *both* people's perspectives simultaneously—an experience of trust and mutuality that helps you feel more connected to yourself, other people, and the broader world.

Mentalizing Cool-down

With these strategies in your back pocket, return to Katherine's story on page 411. How might Katherine work to strengthen the different vantage points for mentalizing, in order to address her difficulties with instability arising in her work, personal relationships, and individual therapy?

MOVING FORWARD WITH KATHERINE: THE COAT METAPHOR

To help Katherine work toward greater emotional and interpersonal stability, Katherine's therapist introduced the concept of the vantage points for mentalizing. The therapist and Katherine worked together to catalogue Katherine's challenges occupying these different vantage points, exemplified in the following ways:

- Comparing herself to her colleagues at work: assuming that other people were more successful, healthy, and accomplished than her, and that she was fundamentally inferior to her co-workers *[you-mode without I-mode]*
- Fixating on what she "should" be doing at work (e.g., conducting research, writing, publishing, serving on committees), but feeling less grounded in the validity of her own interests and preferences there *[you-mode without I-mode]*
- Experiencing emotional dysregulation, anger, and behavioral disruptions (e.g., defensiveness, withdrawal, argumentativeness) when other people's views of her contradicted her own self-experience (e.g., her mother seeing her as selfish and uncaring, her therapist giving her feedback about her potential problems in mentalizing) *[mismatch between I-mode and me-mode]*
- Focusing extensively on her views about her mother's problematic qualities and tendencies, while reflecting less on the legitimacy of her mother's feelings and perspective *[I-mode without you-mode]*
- Feeling hurt and rejected by Matthew's aversion to social engagements, without considering other factors in Matthew's experience that could be contributing to this tendency *[me-mode without you-mode]*
- Getting caught-up in her negative judgments of her partner Matthew (e.g., that he was too shy, boring, socially awkward), but feeling less curious about Matthew's own experience and motives in these moments *[I-mode without you-mode]*
- Continuing to struggle with negative judgments of herself for not living up to certain standards (e.g., concerning likability, intelligence, attractiveness, ambition, success, psychiatric stability, and social skills), but feeling less grounded in the emotional validity of her own experience *[you-mode without I-mode]*
- When her therapist provided her with feedback in sessions, feeling convinced that the therapist was judging and criticizing her, but reflecting less on his other feelings about her potentially leading him to make these comments *[I-mode without me-mode]*
- Being highly dismissive and argumentative with her therapist, while experiencing less interest in the therapist's own feelings and perspective *[I-mode without you-mode]*

Katherine and her therapist worked together to begin addressing these different disparities in mentalizing. When Katherine felt drawn to criticize herself and compare herself to others at her job, she utilized the Strengthening I-mode Toolkit to connect with her *own* values and preferences around work and vocation. In these moments, she began asking herself questions like "What are my favorite parts about working here?" and "What do I most want to do right now, on this shift?" On the most basic level, Katherine recognized how much she truly enjoyed spending time with her patients: caring for them throughout their pregnancies, shepherding the miraculous process of delivery and childbirth, and supporting them as they adjusted to the overwhelming but exciting experience of being new mothers. Katherine also especially appreciated teaching medical students and OB/GYN residents. She felt like she was good at it, but she also found this genuinely stimulating and fun—to be helping new doctors get excited about how to best serve their patients.

Sharing these reflections in therapy, the therapist encouraged Katherine to explicitly validate her emotions and preferences along these lines. How was it reasonable and understandable that she was invested in these things? Katherine observed, "It makes sense that I derive so much meaning from helping people. I mean, I spent my whole childhood tending to my mother's emotional needs *[history and background]*, so it feels like second nature to me! Also most of my patients come from poor and disadvantaged backgrounds *[external circumstances]*, so it makes me feel good about myself to be helping them—like I am really making a difference in their lives, and in the lives of their children and families *[other mental states]*. I just find this so much more fulfilling than writing a paper or serving on some stupid committee, which feels more like a chore than a privilege—something I 'should' be doing rather than something I really want to do *[other mental states]*."

Continuing with the Strengthening I-mode Toolkit, Katherine considered what her work life would look like if she truly respected and "owned" these parts of herself. She acknowledged that she would probably spend less time comparing herself to her colleagues, instead trying to throw herself into the parts of her job (e.g., teaching, treating her patients) that she found most personally compelling. As she moved throughout her shifts, Katherine thus tried to get "out of her head and into her heart," working to authentically inhabit the internal processes arising in her as she engaged in her work: anxiety and excitement when responding to challenging clinical situations; a growing confidence in her own knowledge and abilities; and satisfaction and joy when she felt like she was truly able to help someone. Over time, Katherine's feelings of insecurity and inadequacy began to fall away, and she increasingly experienced a sense of connectedness to herself and her own agency in the workplace.

As Katherine's experience at work improved, she turned her attention to addressing challenges in her relationship with Matthew. Noticing her tendency to prioritize her own perspective in their interactions, Katherine employed the Strengthening You-mode Toolkit to ground herself more fully in *Matthew's* emotions and viewpoint. So when Matthew seemed reluctant to attend the social outings she had planned, rather than focusing on her anger and criticisms toward him, she began asking herself, "How is Matthew feeling right now, and what is he wanting?" Katherine knew that Matthew felt quite anxious and uncomfortable in social interactions, like he had to be "on" for other people in a way that he found overwhelming. While Katherine felt enlivened by being around people, this was torture for Matthew—something that had to be endured before he could relax and recharge his emotional battery. In contrast, Matthew felt highly content and invested in working on his computer projects. Not only was he excited about this, but he appeared to feel almost comforted and soothed by taking time by himself to noodle around with his devices.

Katherine shared in therapy: "It really makes sense that he likes spending time in these ways. He grew up as an only child in the Midwest, and computers and video games were a big part of what he did for fun—there wasn't much else to do! *[history and background]* He also works really hard during the day *[external circumstances]*, so I think that writing code is a way for him to emotionally decompress and get grounded in himself again *[other mental states]*. I can relate to that—sort of like when I just want to curl up on the couch and read a book at the end of the day, in order to unwind *[others' similar experience]*."

When discussing these matters, Katherine's therapist called her attention to those moments when she invited Matthew to these social outings, and she withdrew the invitation as soon as she suspected he did not want to attend. However, *Matthew was not actually declining the invitations*. What did Katherine make of that fact? "I mean, I know that he wants to be with me, and to spend time with me. I think he just really doesn't want to go out in the world for these events, but he probably *would* be willing to go, if I told him that it was important to me."

As Katherine increasingly sought to understand and validate Matthew's perspective, she began to take his desire to avoid social outings less personally. Matthew had been this way for his entire adult life, long before they ever met. Appreciating that perhaps these difficulties were not related to how much he cared about her, she felt less hurt, rejected, and angry with Matthew as they navigated these issues together. Over time, Katherine noticed herself softening toward Matthew: feeling compassion for him, craving connection with him even in the midst of these tensions, and experiencing a desire for Matthew to feel more secure and comfortable in their interactions, rather than simply wanting to punish him. Katherine stopped criticizing Matthew for the ways that he liked to spend his time, actively working to remain emotionally connected to him even when he made choices different from her own. Matthew and Katherine's arguments decreased, and they experienced an increased sense of connectedness, stability, and equanimity in the relationship.

Despite Katherine's progress at work and in her romantic relationship, she continued to struggle with defensiveness and dismissiveness with her therapist and parents. Her therapist suggested that Katherine try out the Strengthening Me-mode toolkit, in order to begin considering herself from other people's perspectives. Katherine started by surveying the brute "facts" around these charged interactions with her therapist. Such interchanges would usually start with Katherine sharing her feelings of anger, annoyance, and judgment about some situation that was unfolding in her life. While the therapist would initially respond by exploring and validating Katherine's feelings about the situation, he would often end up highlighting some facet of the scenario where she might be struggling to mentalize. She knew that the therapist's comments were not explicit criticisms of her, but he often looked quite serious when he was saying these things, which made her *feel* like he was judging her. Katherine would usually respond by immediately disagreeing with the feedback, and then doubling down on her view of the issue under discussion. Rarely would she work to "take in" and consider her therapist's perspective, the way that he encouraged her to do.

Continuing with the toolkit, Katherine tried to consider: How was her therapist feeling toward her in these moments? When she was judging and criticizing other people for an extended period of time, Katherine suspected that her therapist was probably becoming a bit anxious and concerned. Maybe this is why he got so serious when he was looking at her: One of her goals in therapy was *treating* her judgments toward others, so he might feel worried that she was not really working on that goal, and thus that she was becoming more agitated and overwhelmed in her life more broadly. Accordingly, when her therapist would give her feedback about her challenges with mentalizing, he probably was wanting to help her somehow—to understand how she was getting "stuck" in her thinking, so that hopefully she could feel better and have stronger relationships. When she responded by refusing to consider his feedback, he possibly felt angry at her for dismissing him, or even hurt by her lack of interest in him and his perspective.

Thinking about her therapist in this way, Katherine thought it was understandable that he would have these various feelings toward her. For one, she could be highly negative and "blamey" of other people in her therapy sessions *[her behaviors/interpersonal approach]*, especially whenever she talked about Matthew or her parents. It made sense that her therapist might feel worried about this, and concerned that she was relating to these relationships in a manner that was harmful to her. And if the therapist's motive genuinely was to help her, then she understood why he would be hurt and angry by her refusal to consider his views. She truly was being aggressive and unkind to her therapist *[her behaviors/interpersonal approach]*, and most people (including her!) would not appreciate being treated in this way *[others' similar experience]*. As Katherine increasingly appreciated the potential validity of her therapist's experience of her, she started feeling a bit embarrassed and sheepish about her manner of approaching their interactions, and a greater sense of empathy for her therapist's various feeling states (e.g., hurt, anger, desires to help her) in their interactions together.

Now feeling more open and receptive to her therapist's experience, Katherine turned her attention to the Strengthening We-mode Toolkit, as an aid to building greater trust and connectedness in their relationship. She started by considering areas of shared experience with her therapist. She suspected that they both were feeling a bit anxious and uncomfortable in their interactions lately, due to this impasse they were facing, and the lack of clarity about how to communicate together more effectively.

Katherine also knew that they were both deeply committed to her therapeutic progress and psychological well-being. They had been through a lot together in the treatment so far. Katherine had started out in therapy basically unable to function (e.g., highly suicidal, missing work, self-injuring, requiring inpatient admission), and her therapist had stuck with her, even when she was not being the most polite and accommodating patient. Especially as she made so much progress, she had come to trust that her therapist knew what he was doing, that he understood her and cared about her as a person, and that he genuinely wanted her to continue moving forward in her life. In this respect, they were definitely on the same page. She had come so far, and she did not want this little hiccup of "how to communicate in therapy" to derail all of her success. At the same time, Katherine and her therapist clearly had different ideas about what steps she needed to take in order to maintain her gains. Her therapist was very focused on Katherine pursuing "mutuality" and "collaboration" in her relationships, but Katherine was often more interested in *receiving* validation from other people, especially her therapist.

Prompted by the Strengthening We-mode Toolkit, Katherine tried to reckon with the question: "How could I help the other person feel more 'seen' and understood by me, while also giving voice to my own perspective?" Katherine communicated in the therapy, "I know how I *should* be answering this question. Just like I would with anybody, I should try to listen to what you are saying, and to consider if there is any value in your perspective. But I just notice such a powerful resistance in me to doing this. Even though I know this isn't true, at an emotional level, it feels like you are criticizing me and trying to control me. I am worried that, if I take in your viewpoint, it is just going to become MY viewpoint, and I am going to lose myself to you."

Katherine's therapist validated these concerns, also affirming the real importance of Katherine not simply "absorbing" his views, but simply *considering* them, while also holding on to her own way of seeing things. The therapist explained: "In MBT, we call this the 'coat metaphor.' If you went to the store to buy a new coat, you wouldn't just buy the first coat that you see. What would you do? *You would try it on for size.* You'd think about what you like about the coat: maybe its color, its shape, its size, or how it feels on your body. But then you'd also assess what you don't like about the coat. Perhaps it feels a bit too tight in the shoulders, or you worry that the hem hangs down too low, given your height. In the end, you might decide that you love the coat and want to purchase it, or you may realize that the coat just isn't right for you. Either way, there would be this moment in the process where you are truly open to buying the coat, and you are just trying to get a sense of whether or not it is right for you."

"Mentalizing is like the process of trying on that new coat. Your only job is to 'try on' and consider this other perspective or viewpoint. First reflect on what *supports* the view. What makes sense about it? What might be helpful about seeing things in this way? But you would not just automatically accept the viewpoint and assume that it is definitely true. Also consider the 'strikes against' the perspective. How might you disagree with the idea? What does not feel right about it to you? In all of this, I don't want you to 'lose yourself' to me, or to anyone else. On the contrary, YOU are the person who is doing the reflecting, and so these are YOUR ideas about whatever perspective you are considering. So by reflecting in these ways, my hope is that you feel even more connected to yourself and your position. It's just that 'your' position comes through engagement and connection with others, rather than something you arrive at all on your own."

The Coat Metaphor in MBT

Mentalizing is like the process of purchasing a new coat at the store. Just as you try on the coat and see how it fits before you buy it, your job is to "try on" and consider the new perspective or viewpoint. What supports the new view? What might be helpful about seeing things in this way?

   At the same time, consider how you might disagree with the idea. What does not feel right about it to you? By reflecting in these ways, you get more connected to your own position, other people's outlooks, and a new vantage point of connectedness and trust in your relationships.

Katherine felt relieved hearing all of this. It opened up the possibility that "taking in" her therapist's beliefs did not mean that she needed to AGREE with them. "I don't really have any experience with this way of approaching things. When I was growing up, my mother's perspective was the only allowable perspective in our family. The only way that I could feel separate from her was to get angry at her and focus on her defects, which allowed me to 'keep her mind away from mine.' And that is basically what I have continued to do, whenever I feel like I am on a different page from other people. But if I can remember that you are just asking me to CONSIDER your viewpoint, and at the end of the day, I get to decide what I want to believe, that feels much less threatening to me. I still don't know how to stop feeling like you are criticizing me, but I guess I can continue to work on that."

"Is there anything that *I* could be doing differently, to make this all easier for you?", the therapist asked.

Katherine wondered aloud if, whenever her therapist was about to give her feedback about some area where she was struggling, perhaps he could explicitly "warn" her that the feedback was coming, or even remind her that he was not intending to disparage her by sharing his observations. The therapist was grateful for these suggestions: "I can't really stop sharing my ideas here, but if approaching things this way would make this all feel less horrible to you, I really want to do that."

Thus commenced a period in the therapy where Katherine and her therapist worked in earnest to engage with each other in a more mutual, collaborative manner. The therapist continued to actively explore and validate Katherine's emotions, but when he reached a point in their sessions when he felt compelled to give Katherine feedback about her potential problems in mentalizing (e.g., intellectualization, empathic deficits, certainty or rigidity in her thinking), he started to "forecast" his comments in advance, and to attain Katherine's consent prior to moving forward in these communications. "The more that we talk about this argument with your mother, something is coming across to me about how you've been thinking about all of this. It doesn't *feel* like a criticism to me, but I can't be sure how it will land with you. Are you up for discussing this a bit?" Aided by these prefaces, Katherine felt less blindsided and overwhelmed by her therapist's observations. She also experienced an increased sense of autonomy in these conversations, as if she was *choosing* to take in these observations, rather than having them forced onto her in an aggressive way.

In turn, Katherine actively worked to "take in" and consider her therapist's feedback about the challenges she was experiencing in her life. For example, when Katherine was discussing her anger at her mother for insisting that they plan a family get-together for the holidays, the therapist shared his view that Katherine appeared to be feeling quite certain that her mother was doing something wrong in the scenario *[I-mode]*, and she seemed far less interested in considering the potential validity of her mother's motives and desires in the scenario *[you-mode]*. Katherine reflected on these ideas in their therapy appointment: "I hear what you are saying. Given how crazy and problematic my mother has been my whole life, I just assume that she is *always* being crazy and problematic. But I guess it is a pretty common thing for parents to try to get everyone together around the holidays, and I haven't really been thinking about that. That said, my mother has still been kind of intrusive in the party-planning: texting me all of the time, and trying to get me to stay longer than I agreed to. So even though it is understandable that she is planning this event, she still seems to be going about it in a controlling manner."

In this way, Katherine increasingly sought to consider other people's views and positions, without sacrificing her own agency in the process. She became far less defensive and argumentative in her interactions with her therapist, and more able to reflect on the feedback that he was offering to her, in a balanced manner that increasingly affirmed the experiences of the various people in her life: herself, her colleagues, her friends, her partner, her therapist, and yes, even her parents.

Utilizing the approach that Katherine developed with her therapist, when her mother got angry at Katherine for not communicating with them frequently enough, Katherine attempted to refrain from criticizing and attacking her mother in return. Instead, Katherine worked to accept and tolerate her mother's disapproval of her *[me-mode]*, and to remain simultaneously grounded in the validity of her own needs and preferences in their relationship *[I-mode]*. She was an adult woman who was in a serious relationship with a full-time, demanding job. Talking to her parents once a week was completely reasonable—perhaps even more frequent than many people her age spoke with their parents. Katherine attempted to explicitly validate and empathize with her mother's feelings around these issues, while also acknowledging her own boundaries and preferences: "I can see how hurtful and upsetting this is for you, especially since it feels like me not calling you every day means that I do not care about you. While I understand this is your perspective, for me, it doesn't feel like this says anything about how I feel about you. I love you, and I want to be connected to you. It's just that, given the nature of my life and responsibilities, this is what works for me right now. I know that it's not perfect, but I hope that we can find a way to stay in touch with each other that we can both live with."

While Katherine's mother was unsurprisingly disappointed by Katherine's position on these matters, she felt far more "seen" and understood by Katherine's efforts to engage with her in a more supportive, collaborative fashion. They experienced less strife and conflict in their relationship, and Katherine stopped withdrawing from her parents in a retaliatory fashion. Over time, as Katherine gained practice non-defensively "owning" her needs and preferences in her interactions with her mother, Katherine's mother became far less critical of her, seemingly developing a reluctant acceptance of Katherine's preferred manner of engaging with them.

This sort of progress has proliferated across Katherine's life and experience. Katherine has close friends whom she sees regularly, and with whom she maintains genuinely open, affectionate, and mutual relationships. She feels both fulfilled and confident in her role as an OB/GYN, even receiving a formal promotion to medical school faculty so that she is able to integrate her passion for teaching with her deep commitment to women's reproductive health. Even as Katherine became more accepting of Matthew's social preferences, when important events came up that she really wanted them to attend as a couple (e.g., weddings, concerts, dinner with friends), she would express these wishes to Matthew, in an open and non-demanding manner. Since he loved her and wanted to meet her needs, he would happily agree to go with her. As a couple, they were thus able to achieve a balance between both people's perspectives and preferences, in a way that felt workable and satisfying to them both.

After several years of being together, Matthew and Katherine got married, bought a house, and started the process of building a family of their own. Katherine became an important support and advocate for her parents as they grew older—a role that was practically impossible for her when she was struggling with her previous difficulties with defensiveness and reactivity. Now three years after starting in MBT, Katherine no longer experiences suicidal thinking, depression, or impulses to harm herself—her longest period of remission from these symptoms in her adult life.

Katherine shares about her experience in the therapy: "It's hard to fathom how much my life has changed in just a few years. Before I started in treatment, I used to think that my problems were inherent to me—who I was as a person. I was depressed, worthless, ugly, and fundamentally *bad*, and no one was ever going to want to be with me. Little did I know that I had a highly treatable disorder, and I had simply never received evidence-based treatment for it. In this case, it turns out that the treatment was really just reflection: getting connected to what I was feeling, trying to understand and empathize with other people's feelings, and becoming curious enough to start to question all of those things that I had always just assumed were true about me. And for the first time that I can remember, I can say that I am glad to be alive. I feel good about myself, like I have a reason for being here. But I guess the most important thing is that I don't feel so alone anymore. I finally feel connected to other people—that I can trust them, they can trust me, and I am actually contributing to the world around me."

Chapter Review 15.1
The Vantage Points for Mentalizing

Take-aways on the Vantage Points for Mentalizing

- A *vantage point* for mentalizing is the interpersonal location that you occupy when you are trying to understand yourself and other people.

  - It is not "what you are looking at" when you mentalize, but the position FROM WHICH you are mentalizing.

- There are four different vantage points for mentalizing.

  - **I-mode:** considering mental states from your own viewpoint

    - I-mode involves being in touch with your own opinions and beliefs, the validity of your experiences, your own sense of agency, and your rights as a person.

  - **You-mode:** examining mental states from other people's perspectives

    - Even though you can only ever understand another person by making reference to your own mental states ("If that were happening to me, I would feel sad . . . "), you-mode entails actively TRYING to put yourself in the other individual's shoes, recognizing the legitimacy of their viewpoint, and empathizing with them.

  - **Me-mode:** contemplating yourself from other people's standpoints

    - Me-mode is NOT tantamount to worrying and ruminating about how people see you.

    - Rather, me-mode encompasses seeking to understand other people's experience of you (e.g., their beliefs, feelings, and desires related to you), the validity of the experience in question, and the role you have played in leading others to see you in this way.

  - **We-mode:** reflecting on yourself and other people simultaneously, from a shared position of mutuality and kinship that transcends the outlook of any particular member of the dyad.

    - We-mode encompasses all of the other vantage points of mentalization: remaining grounded in your own perspective *[I-mode]*, appreciating other people's viewpoints *[you-mode]*, attending to others' experience of you *[me-mode]*, and operating from a standpoint of trust and connectedness with other individuals *[we-mode]*.

The Coat Metaphor in MBT

Mentalizing is like the process of purchasing a new coat at the store. Just as you try on the coat and see how it fits before you buy it, your job is to "try on" and consider the new perspective or viewpoint. What supports the new view? What might be helpful about seeing things in this way?

At the same time, consider how you might disagree with the idea. What does not feel right about it to you? By reflecting in these ways, you get more connected to your own position, other people's outlooks, and a new vantage point of connectedness and trust in your relationships.

[continued on next page]

An Illustration of the Vantage Points for Mentalizing

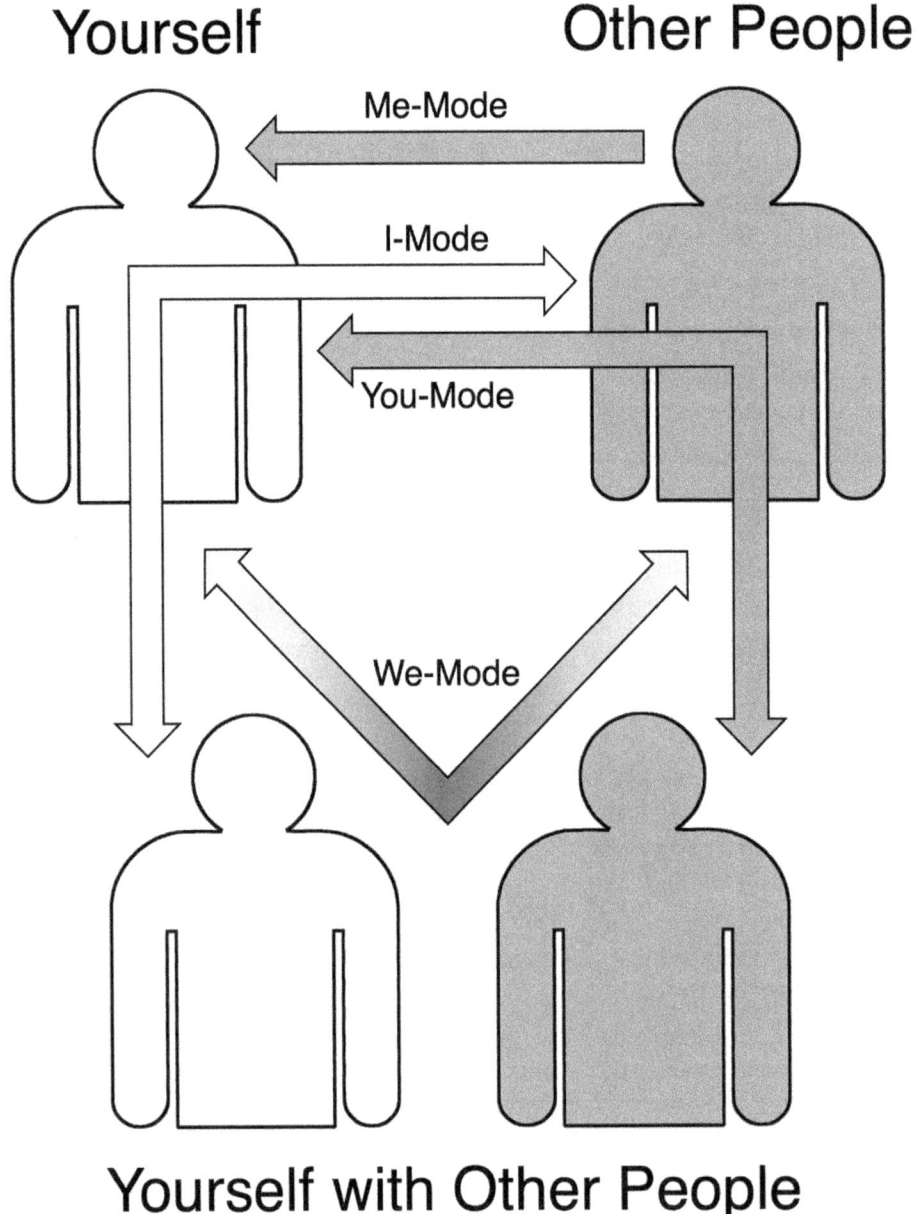

Chapter Review 15.2
Disparities in the Vantage Points for Mentalizing

- According to mentalization-based treatment (MBT), health is constituted by the capacity to move flexibly from one vantage point for mentalizing to another, depending on your own internal experience at the time, as well as the events unfolding in your relationships.

- In borderline personality disorder (BPD), certain vantage points for mentalizing remain underdeveloped in your experience, such that you end up relying extensively on only certain vantage points in order to navigate your interactions with others.

- Common disparities in the vantage points for mentalization include:

  - **You-mode without I-mode:** Prioritizing other people's internal states *[you-mode]*, while ignoring and dismissing your own emotions, desires, and needs *[I-mode]*.

  - **You-mode without me-mode:** Extensively grounding yourself in other people's experiences *[you-mode]*, while being less attuned to how they experience YOU, and what you might be doing to contribute to such perceptions *[me-mode]*.

  - **I-mode without you-mode:** Focusing on the validity of your perspective *[I-mode]*, but feeling less curious about what other individuals are thinking and feeling, and what is leading them to experience things in this way *[you-mode]*.

  - **I-mode without me-mode:** Concentrating on how you are seeing things *[I-mode]*, without fully understanding how you are coming across to other people— how THEY are experiencing you *[me-mode]*.

  - **Me-mode without I-mode:** Fixating on what others think of you *[me-mode]*, while feeling far less connected to your own beliefs, preferences, and needs *[I-mode]*.

  - **Me-mode without you-mode:** Thinking excessively about other people's views of you *[me-mode]*, while paying less attention to their beliefs, emotions, and desires that have little or nothing to do with you *[you-mode]*.

  - **"Mismatch" between I-mode and me-mode:** Experiencing emotional and interpersonal instability when other individuals' views of you *[me-mode]* contradict how you see yourself *[I-mode]*.

Chapter Review 15.3
Mentalizing Practice Points: Grounding Yourself in Your Own Perspective

When you are feeling unsteady in a particular vantage point for mentalizing, work to ground yourself more fully in the outlook in question.

You can do this by deploying all of the forms of mentalizing reviewed in this book: first examining mental states in the person *[content-mentalizing]*, then validating the experience *[context-mentalizing]*, next reflecting on your own agency in the vantage point *[context-mentalizing]*, and finally, working to become more emotionally connected to the perspective in question *[process-mentalizing]*.

Strengthening I-mode Toolkit
If you are struggling to "hold on to" your own perspective . . .

Content-mentalizing: Reflect on Your Own Mental States	**Thoughts and Beliefs:** • "Leaving aside what other people think, what do **I** actually believe about this issue? What is my opinion here?" • "If no one else were around, what would I be thinking about all of this?" • "If someone else were going through this, what would I think about what is happening? Could any of that apply to me?" **Emotions:** • "What emotions am I experiencing right now?" • "What would I like to do in this scenario? What would I genuinely enjoy?" **Desires:** • "What are my desires and preferences in this situation? What do I really want to happen, in the best case scenario?" • "What do I want for my life in this domain? What circumstance is most consistent with my long-term goals, and who I am as a person?" • "Is there anything about which I am truly curious here? If I had a crystal ball, what would I want to know?" **Values and Ethics:** • "What are my values surrounding this topic? Do I have any strong opinions about how I should behave and relate to other people?" • "What are my rights in this situation? What do I deserve, and how do I deserve other people to be treating me?"

[continued on next page]

Context-mentalizing: Validate Your Experience	"It is understandable that I feel this way because of _____." Make reference variously to • Your history and background • Your other mental states (e.g., additional thoughts, emotions, desires, or feelings about yourself) related to the experience • Factors in the external situation • How others would feel under similar circumstances
Context-mentalizing: Mentalize Your Agency in I-mode	• "What would it look like for me to approach this situation more authentically—in a manner that reflects my beliefs, emotions, desires, and who I am as a person?" • "How could I express my own emotions to the other person, and give voice to my own desires and preferences?" • "What do I feel like the right thing to do is? What behaviors feel most consistent with my values and ethics?" • "What actions would I take, in order to respect my own dignity, worth, and what I deserve from other people?" • "How would I be acting and relating to others, in order to pursue my long-term goals and interests?" If you identify any potential actions through these questions, before taking them, make sure to "cross-check" them against the other vantage points for mentalizing.
Process-mentalizing: Get Connected to Your Own Perspective	Actively work to • "Own" your beliefs and viewpoints • Access and inhabit your emotions • Experience your wishes and desires • Respect your own dignity, rights, and ethical principles.

Chapter Review 15.4
Mentalizing Practice Points:
Appreciating Other People's Perspectives

Strengthening You-mode Toolkit
If you are struggling to enter into another individual's perspective . . .

	Thoughts and Beliefs: • "What are the other person's thoughts and beliefs about this matter?" • "What is the person's perspective on this situation? How are they experiencing all of this?" **Emotions:** • "What emotions could the other individual be feeling right now?" • "How might the person be feeling about themself? Where is their self-worth and self-esteem?" **Desires:** • "What are the other person's desires and preferences in this situation? What do they really hope will happen, in the best case scenario?" • "What does the person want for their life more broadly? What are their long-term goals and aspirations?" • "How do they want other people to see them, and to feel about them?" • "What are the person's desires for other people? What do they most want for you—in your life and in their relationship with you?" **Values and Ethics:** • "What really matters to the other individual? What is important to them, as a person?" • "What are their values and ethics? What do they expect of themself and other people?" • "What does this person deserve in this situation? What are their needs and rights?" • "How should other people (including me) be treating them?"
Content-mentalizing: Reflect on the Other Person's Mental States	

[continued on next page]

Context-mentalizing: Validate the Other Person's Experience	"It is understandable that the other person feels this way because of _____." Make reference variously to • Their history and background • Their other mental states (e.g., additional thoughts, emotions, desires, or feelings about themself) related to the experience • Factors in the external situation • How others would feel under similar circumstances
Context-mentalizing: Mentalize Your Agency in You-mode	• "What would it look like for me to prioritize the other person in my interactions with them?" • "What actions would I be taking, in order to be more responsive to their emotions, desires, and long-term interests?" • "How could I affirm and validate the person's feelings and perspective?" • "What could I do, in order to better respect the individual's dignity, worth, and rights?" • "How can I genuinely be of service to this person?" If you identify any potential actions through these questions, before taking them, make sure to "cross-check" them against the other vantage points for mentalizing.
Process-mentalizing: Get Connected to the Other Person's Perspective	Actively work to • Value and appreciate the other person's beliefs and viewpoints • Empathize with the person's emotions and feelings about themself • Respect the individual's rights, dignity, and worth • Resonate with the other's wishes and desires • CARE ABOUT the individual as a person

Chapter Review 15.5
Mentalizing Practice Points: Understanding Other
People's Views of You

Strengthening Me-mode Toolkit	
If you are struggling to consider yourself from another person's perspective . . .	
Content-mentalizing: Reflect on the Other Person's Experience of You	**Relevant Facts about Your Relationship with the Person:** • "What are important events and circumstances in our relationship with each other?" • "What actions have I taken in our interactions? How have I treated the person, and how have they responded to that?" • "What actions has the other individual taken in our interactions? How have they treated me, and how have I responded to that?" • "Are there any things I have done, or things that have happened between us, that the person would cite as noteworthy in our relationship?" **Thoughts and Beliefs:** • "When I did/said _____, what did the other individual think about me?" • "When the person did/said _____, what was their impression of me?" • "What is the person's view of me? How do they see me, and what are their beliefs about me as a person?" **Emotions:** • "When I did/said _____, what emotions was the individual feeling?" • "When the person did/said _____, how were they feeling about me?" • "How does the person seem to feel about me as a person, and in our interactions with each other?" **Desires:** • "When I did/said _____, what was the other person wanting?" • "When the person did/said _____, what desires were they experiencing? What was motivating them?" • "What are the individual's wishes in relation to me? What do they want me to think, feel, and desire?" **Values and Ethics:** • "What does this person expect of me? What standards do they hold for me—in this situation and in general?"

[continued on next page]

	• "How do they think I should be behaving, living my life, and approaching my interactions with them?" • "What do they believe I deserve in my life—in the areas of mood, relationships, external circumstances, and how other people are treating me?"
Context-mentalizing: Validate the Other Person's Feelings about You	"It is understandable that the other person experiences me in this way because of _____." Make reference variously to • Events in your relationship and interactions • Actions you have taken, and ways you have treated the individual • The other individual's history and background • The person's other mental states (e.g., additional thoughts, emotions, desires, or feelings about themself) concerning themself or their life apart from you • Factors in the external situation • How others would feel under similar circumstances
Context-mentalizing: Mentalize Your Agency in Me-mode	• "What could I do—or stop doing—in order to impact how the other person experiences me?" • "How might I approach the relationship, so that the other person might see me in a more positive light?" • "What would it look like for me to accept and tolerate how the other person is viewing me?" • "When relevant, how could I affirm and validate the other person's beliefs about me?" • "What behaviors could I engage in, in order to be more responsive to the person's feelings about me, desires toward me, and values in our interactions with each other?" If you identify any potential actions through these questions, before taking them, make sure to "cross-check" them against the other vantage points for mentalizing.
Process-mentalizing: Get Connected to the Other Person's Experience of You	Actively work to • Value and appreciate the other person's views of you • Empathize with the person's feelings about you • Resonate with the individual's wishes toward you: what they want you to think, feel, desire, and do • Respect the person's ethics and values for you and your interactions

Chapter Review 15.6
Mentalizing Practice Points: Developing Trust and
Connectedness with Other People

Strengthening We-mode Toolkit
How to cultivate collaboration, trust, and connectedness in a specific relationship

Content-mentalizing: Reflect on Mental States in the Relationship	**Thoughts and Beliefs:** • "What thoughts and beliefs do we share with one another, in general or about this specific matter?" • "How are we seeing things differently from each other?" • "What have I learned from the other person? What do I think they have learned from me?" **Emotions:** • "How might we be experiencing similar emotions right now? More broadly in our lives, where do I notice parallels in our moods and emotions?" • "At the level of emotions and mood, how are we different from each other?" • "In what ways do we both trust each other? How do we feel 'seen' and understood by the other person as unique individuals?" **Desires:** • "What desires and wishes do we have in common with each other, in this scenario or in general?" • "What are our joint goals, projects, and plans?" • "How are our desires and plans different from each other?" **Values and Ethics:** • "How are our values similar to each other? What is important to us both?" • "What shared expectations do we both have for ourselves, other people, and this relationship?" • "How are our values and expectations different, in this scenario or as people?" • "What rights do we have in common in this situation? How should we both be treating ourselves, and each other?" • "What do we both deserve—in this relationship and more broadly in our lives?"

[continued on next page]

Context-mentalizing: Validate Your Joint Experience of the Relationship	"It is understandable that we feel this way because of _____." Make reference variously to • Your history together in the relationship, including your interactions with each other • Actions you have taken, actions the other person has taken • Other mental states (e.g., additional thoughts, emotions, desires, or feelings about yourselves) you each have about the relationship • Factors in the external situation that impact both of you • Your respective personal experiences: histories, external situations, and other mental states (e.g., beliefs, emotions, desires, personalities, feelings about yourselves) • How others would feel under similar circumstances
Context-mentalizing: Mentalize Your Agency in We-mode	• "How can I help the other person feel more 'seen' and understood by me, while also giving voice to my own perspective?" • "How can I affirm and validate the other individual's emotions and desires, and at the same time express my own emotions and desires?" • "What could I do to honor and respect the other's expectations and values in our interactions, while simultaneously respecting my own values and needs?" • "How could I pursue our shared goals and values in this relationship?" • "How could I engage with this person in a more mutual, collaborative manner?" • "What would it look like for me to place more trust in the other person? How could I BE more trustworthy in this interaction, and in this relationship?" If you identify any potential actions through these questions, before taking them, make sure to "cross-check" them against the other vantage points for mentalizing.

[continued on next page]

	Actively work to
Process-mentalizing: Get Connected to Your Shared Experience in the Relationship	• Value and appreciate the other person's beliefs and viewpoints, while also holding on to your own beliefs and convictions • Empathize with the person's emotions and desires, while authentically accessing your own emotions and desires • Invest emotionally in your common goals and values in this relationship • FEEL a sense of trust in the other person, yourself, and the relationship • Full-throatedly accept yourself exactly as you are, and the other person exactly as they are • Respect the rights, dignity, and worth of yourself and the other person • CARE ABOUT the individual as a unique person, while also embracing and cherishing who you are as a person

Akbari, M., Seydavi, M., Hosseini, Z. S., Krafft, J., & Levin, M. E. (2022). Experiential avoidance in depression, anxiety, obsessive-compulsive related, and posttraumatic stress disorders: A comprehensive systematic review and meta-analysis. *Journal of Contextual Behavioral Science, 24*, 65–78.

Al-Shamali, H. F., Winkler, O., Talarico, F., Greenshaw, A. J., Forner, C., Zhang, Y., . . . & Burback, L. (2022). A systematic scoping review of dissociation in borderline personality disorder and implications for research and clinical practice: Exploring the fog. *Australian & New Zealand Journal of Psychiatry, 56*(10), 1252–1264.

Álvarez-Tomás, I., Ruiz, J., Guilera, G., & Bados, A. (2019). Long-term clinical and functional course of borderline personality disorder: A meta-analysis of prospective studies. *European Psychiatry, 56*(1), 75–83.

American Psychiatric Association. (2022). *Diagnostic and statistical manual of mental disorders* (5th ed., text rev.). American Psychiatric Association Publishing.

Arioli, M., Cattaneo, Z., Ricciardi, E., & Canessa, N. (2021). Overlapping and specific neural correlates for empathizing, affective mentalizing, and cognitive mentalizing: A coordinate-based meta-analytic study. *Human Brain Mapping, 42*(14), 4777–4804.

Ballespí, S., Vives, J., Sharp, C., Chanes, L., & Barrantes-Vidal, N. (2021). Self and other mentalizing polarities and dimensions of mental health: Association with types of symptoms, functioning and well-being. *Frontiers in Psychology, 12*, 1–13.

Barazandeh, H., Kissane, D. W., Saeedi, N., & Gordon, M. (2016). A systematic review of the relationship between early maladaptive schemas and borderline personality disorder/traits. *Personality and Individual Differences, 94*, 130–139.

Baron-Cohen, S. (1990). Autism: A specific cognitive disorder of "mind-blindness". *International Review of Psychiatry, 2*(1), 81–90.

Bartholomew, K. (1990). Avoidance of intimacy: An attachment perspective. *Journal of Social and Personal Relationships, 7*(2), 147–178.

Bartholomew, K., & Horowitz, L. M. (1991). Attachment styles among young adults: A test of a four-category model. *Journal of Personality and Social Psychology, 61*(2), 226–244.

Bateman, A. (2020). *The MBT Adherence and Competence Scale manual.* Unpublished manuscript.

Bateman, A., Campbell, C., & Fonagy, P. (2021). Rupture and repair in mentalization-based group psychotherapy. *International Journal of Group Psychotherapy, 71*(2), 371–392.

Bateman, A., Constantinou, M. P., Fonagy, P., & Holzer, S. (2021). Eight-year prospective follow-up of mentalization-based treatment versus structured clinical management for people with borderline personality disorder. *Personality Disorders: Theory, Research, and Treatment, 12*(4), 291–299.

Bateman, A., & Fonagy, P. (1999). Effectiveness of partial hospitalization in the treatment of borderline personality disorder: A randomized controlled trial. *American Journal of Psychiatry, 156*(10), 1563–1569.

Bateman, A., & Fonagy, P. (2001). Treatment of borderline personality disorder with psychoanalytically oriented partial hospitalization: An 18-month follow-up. *American Journal of Psychiatry*, *158*(1), 36–42.

Bateman, A., & Fonagy, P. (2004). *Psychotherapy for borderline personality disorder: Mentalization-based treatment*. Oxford University Press.

Bateman, A., & Fonagy, P. (2006). *Mentalization based treatment for borderline personality disorder: A practical guide*. Oxford University Press.

Bateman, A., & Fonagy, P. (2008). 8-year follow-up of patients treated for borderline personality disorder: Mentalization-based treatment versus treatment as usual. *American Journal of Psychiatry*, *165*(5), 631–638.

Bateman, A., & Fonagy, P. (2009). Randomized controlled trial of outpatient mentalization-based treatment versus structured clinical management for borderline personality disorder. *American Journal of Psychiatry*, *166*(12), 1355–1364.

Bateman, A., & Fonagy, P. (2016). *Mentalization-based treatment for personality disorders: A practical guide*. Oxford University Press.

Bateman, A., & Fonagy, P. (Eds.). (2019a). *Handbook of mentalizing in mental health practice* (2nd ed.). American Psychiatric Publishing.

Bateman, A., & Fonagy, P. (2019b). A randomized controlled trial of a mentalization-based intervention (MBT-FACTS) for families of people with borderline personality disorder. *Personality Disorders: Theory, Research, and Treatment*, *10*(1), 70–79.

Bateman, A., Fonagy, P., Campbell, C., Luyten, P., & Debbané, M. (2023). *Cambridge guide to mentalization-based treatment (MBT)*. Cambridge University Press.

Bateman, A., O'Connell, J., Lorenzini, N., Gardner, T., & Fonagy, P. (2016). A randomised controlled trial of mentalization-based treatment versus structured clinical management for patients with comorbid borderline personality disorder and antisocial personality disorder. *BMC Psychiatry*, *16*(1), 1–11.

Beck, J. S. (2020). *Cognitive behavior therapy: Basics and beyond* (3rd ed.). Guilford Publications.

Belsky, D. W., Caspi, A., Arseneault, L., Bleidorn, W., Fonagy, P., Goodman, M., . . . & Moffitt, T. E. (2012). Etiological features of borderline personality related characteristics in a birth cohort of 12-year-old children. *Development and Psychopathology*, *24*(1), 251–265.

Boon, S., Steele, K., & van der Hart, O. (2011). *Coping with trauma-related dissociation: Skills training for patients and therapists*. W. W. Norton & Company.

Bora, E. (2021). A meta-analysis of theory of mind and "mentalization" in borderline personality disorder: A true neuro-social-cognitive or meta-social-cognitive impairment? *Psychological Medicine*, *51*(15), 2541–2551.

Brennan, K. A., Clark, C. L., & Shaver, P. R. (1998). Self-report measurement of adult romantic attachment: An integrative overview. In J. A. Simpson & W. S. Rholes (Eds.), *Attachment theory and close relationships* (pp. 46–76). Guilford Press.

Buchman-Wildbaum, T., Unoka, Z., Dudas, R., Vizin, G., Demetrovics, Z., & Richman, M. J. (2021). Shame in borderline personality disorder: Meta-analysis. *Journal of Personality Disorders*, *35*(Supplement A), 149–161.

Bud, S., Nechita, D., & Szentagotai Tatar, A. (2023). Emotion regulation strategies in borderline personality disorder: A meta-analysis. *Clinical Psychologist*, *27*(1), 1–18.

Burghart, M., & Mier, D. (2022). No feelings for me, no feelings for you: A meta-analysis on alexithymia and empathy in psychopathy. *Personality and Individual Differences*, *194*, 111658.

Bylsma, L. M., Morris, B. H., & Rottenberg, J. (2008). A meta-analysis of emotional reactivity in major depressive disorder. *Clinical Psychology Review*, *28*(4), 676–691.

Cackowski, S., Reitz, A. C., Ende, G., Kleindienst, N., Bohus, M., Schmahl, C., & Krause-Utz, A. (2014). Impact of stress on different components of impulsivity in borderline personality disorder. *Psychological Medicine*, *44*(15), 3329–3340.

Camoirano, A. (2017). Mentalizing makes parenting work: A review about parental reflective functioning and clinical interventions to improve it. *Frontiers in Psychology*, *8*, 1–12.

Carey, B. (2019, February 8). Dr. John Gunderson, 76, dies; Defined borderline personality disorder. *The New York Times*.

Cassidy, J., & Shaver, P. R. (Eds.). (2016). *Handbook of attachment: Theory, research, and clinical applications* (3rd ed.). Guilford Press.

Cattane, N., Rossi, R., Lanfredi, M., & Cattaneo, A. (2017). Borderline personality disorder and childhood trauma: Exploring the affected biological systems and mechanisms. *BMC Psychiatry*, *17*, 1–14.

Chervonsky, E., & Hunt, C. (2017). Suppression and expression of emotion in social and interpersonal outcomes: A meta-analysis. *Emotion*, *17*(4), 669–683.

Choi-Kain, L. W., Reich, D. B., Masland, S. R., Iliakis, E. A., & Ilagan, G. S. (2020). Longitudinal course of borderline personality disorder: What every clinician needs to know. *Current Treatment Options in Psychiatry*, *7*(3), 429–445.

Coles, N. A., March, D. S., Marmolejo-Ramos, F., Larsen, J. T., Arinze, N. C., Ndukaihe, I. L., . . . & Liuzza, M. T. (2022). A multi-lab test of the facial feedback hypothesis by the Many Smiles Collaboration. *Nature Human Behaviour*, *6*(12), 1731–1742.

Cristea, I. A., Gentili, C., Cotet, C. D., Palomba, D., Barbui, C., & Cuijpers, P. (2017). Efficacy of psychotherapies for borderline personality disorder: A systematic review and meta-analysis. *JAMA Psychiatry*, *74*(4), 319–328.

Crowell, J. A., Fraley, R. C., & Roisman, G. I. (2016). Measurement of individual differences in adult attachment. In J. Cassidy & P. R. Shaver (Eds.), *Handbook of attachment: Theory, research, and clinical applications* (3rd ed., pp. 598–635). Guilford Press.

Crowell, S. E., Beauchaine, T. P., & Linehan, M. M. (2009). A biosocial developmental model of borderline personality: Elaborating and extending Linehan's theory. *Psychological Bulletin*, *135*(3), 495–510.

D'Aurizio, G., Di Stefano, R., Socci, V., Rossi, A., Barlattani, T., Pacitti, F., & Rossi, R. (2023). The role of emotional instability in borderline personality disorder: A systematic review. *Annals of General Psychiatry*, *22*(1), 1–8.

Davies, H., Wolz, I., Leppanen, J., Fernandez-Aranda, F., Schmidt, U., & Tchanturia, K. (2016). Facial expression to emotional stimuli in non-psychotic disorders: A systematic review and meta-analysis. *Neuroscience & Biobehavioral Reviews*, *64*, 252–271.

Decety, J., & Meyer, M. (2008). From emotion resonance to empathic understanding: A social developmental neuroscience account. *Development and Psychopathology*, *20*(4), 1053–1080.

Dennett, D. C. (1971). Intentional systems. *The Journal of Philosophy*, *68*(4), 87–106.

Derks, Y. P., Westerhof, G. J., & Bohlmeijer, E. T. (2017). A meta-analysis on the association between emotional awareness and borderline personality pathology. *Journal of Personality Disorders*, *31*(3), 362–384.

Doward, J., & Hall, S. (2019, April 27). Therapy saved a refugee child. Fifty years on, he's leading a mental health revolution. *The Guardian*.

Drozek, R. P. (2018). Stimulating reflection and curiosity. In B. Palmer & B. Unruh (Eds.), *Borderline personality disorder: A case-based approach* (pp. 11–23). Springer.

Drozek, R. P. (2019). *Psychoanalysis as an ethical process*. Routledge.

Drozek, R. P. (2022). The patient as an ethical subject: Technical implications of the patient's irreducible responsibility. *Contemporary Psychoanalysis*, *58*(1), 77–101.

Drozek, R. P., Bateman, A. W., Henry, J. T., Connery, H. S., Smith, G. W., & Tester, R. D. (2021). Single-session mentalization-based treatment group for law enforcement officers. *International Journal of Group Psychotherapy*, *71*(3), 441–470.

Drozek, R. P., & Henry, J. (2021). Mentalization-based treatment. In R. E. Feinstein (Ed.), *Personality disorders* (pp. 237–258). Oxford University Press.

Drozek, R. P., & Unruh, B. T. (2020). Mentalization-based treatment for pathological narcissism. *Journal of Personality Disorders*, *34*, 177–203.

Drozek, R. P., & Unruh, B. T. (2022). Mentalization-based treatment for a physician with borderline personality disorder. *American Journal of Psychotherapy*, *75*(1), 51–54.

Drozek, R. P., Unruh, B. T., & Bateman, A. W. (2023). *Mentalization-based treatment for pathological narcissism: A handbook*. Oxford University Press.

Duschinsky, R., & Foster, S. (2021). *Mentalizing and epistemic trust: The work of Peter Fonagy and colleagues at the Anna Freud Centre*. Oxford University Press.

Edwards, E. R., Rose, N. L., Gromatsky, M., Feinberg, A., Kimhy, D., Doucette, J. T., . . . & Hazlett, E. A. (2021). Alexithymia, affective lability, impulsivity, and childhood adversity in borderline personality disorder. *Journal of Personality Disorders, 35* (Supplement A), 114–131.

Ellison, W. D., Rosenstein, L. K., Morgan, T. A., & Zimmerman, M. (2018). Community and clinical epidemiology of borderline personality disorder. *Psychiatric Clinics, 41*(4), 561–573.

Ensink, K., Alandin, L., Target, M., Fonagy, P., Sabourin, S., & Berthelot, N. (2015). Mentalization in children and mothers in the context of trauma: An initial study of the validity of the Child Reflective Functioning Scale. *British Journal of Developmental Psychology, 33*(2), 203–217.

Fearon, R. M. P., & Belsky, J. (2016). Precursors of attachment security. In J. Cassidy & P. R. Shaver (Eds.), *Handbook of attachment: Theory, research, and clinical applications* (3rd ed., pp. 291–313). Guilford Press.

Fitzpatrick, S., Ip, J., Krantz, L., Zeifman, R., & Kuo, J. R. (2019). Use your words: The role of emotion labeling in regulating emotion in borderline personality disorder. *Behaviour Research and Therapy, 120*, 1–13.

Fonagy, P. (1989). On tolerating mental states: Theory of mind in borderline personality. *Bulletin of the Anna Freud Centre, 12*(2), 91–115.

Fonagy, P., & Bateman, A. (2008). The development of borderline personality disorder: A mentalizing model. *Journal of Personality Disorders, 22*(1), 4–21.

Fonagy, P., Gergely, G., Jurist, E. L., & Target, M. (2002). *Affect regulation, mentalization, and the development of the self.* Other Press.

Fonagy, P., Luyten, P., & Allison, E. (2015). Epistemic petrification and the restoration of epistemic trust: A new conceptualization of borderline personality disorder and its psychosocial treatment. *Journal of Personality Disorders, 29*(5), 575–609.

Fonagy, P., Luyten, P., Allison, E., & Campbell, C. (2017). What we have changed our minds about: Part 2. Borderline personality disorder, epistemic trust and the developmental significance of social communication. *Borderline Personality Disorder and Emotion Dysregulation, 4*(1), 1–12.

Fonagy, P., Luyten, P., Moulton-Perkins, A., Lee, Y. W., Warren, F., Howard, S., . . . & Lowyck, B. (2016). Development and validation of a self-report measure of mentalizing: The Reflective Functioning Questionnaire. *PLOS One, 11*(7), 1–28.

Fonagy, P., Simes, E., Yirmiya, K., Wason, J., Barrett, B., Frater, A., . . . & Bateman, A. (2025). Mentalisation-based treatment for antisocial personality disorder in males convicted of an offence on community probation in England and Wales (Mentalization for Offending Adult Males, MOAM): A multicentre, assessor-blinded, randomised controlled trial. *The Lancet Psychiatry, 12*(3), 208–219.

Fraley, R. C., Hudson, N. W., Heffernan, M. E., & Segal, N. (2015). Are adult attachment styles categorical or dimensional? A taxometric analysis of general and relationship-specific attachment orientations. *Journal of Personality and Social Psychology, 109*(2), 354–368.

Frías, Á., & Palma, C. (2015). Comorbidity between post-traumatic stress disorder and borderline personality disorder: A review. *Psychopathology, 48*(1), 1–10.

Gagliardini, G., Gatti, L., & Colli, A. (2020). Further data on the reliability of the Mentalization Imbalances Scale and of the Modes of Mentalization Scale. *Research in Psychotherapy: Psychopathology, Process, and Outcome, 23*(1), 88–98.

Gagliardini, G., Gullo, S., Caverzasi, E., Boldrini, A., Blasi, S., & Colli, A. (2018). Assessing mentalization in psychotherapy: First validation of the Mentalization Imbalances Scale. *Research in Psychotherapy: Psychopathology, Process, and Outcome, 21*(3), 164–177.

Gagliardini, G., Gullo, S., Teti, A., & Colli, A. (2023). Personality and mentalization: A latent profile analysis of mentalizing problematics in adult patients. *Journal of Clinical Psychology, 79*(2), 514–530.

Gagliardini, G., Gullo, S., Tinozzi, V., Baiano, M., Balestrieri, M., Todisco, P., . . . & Colli, A. (2020). Mentalizing subtypes in eating disorders: A latent profile analysis. *Frontiers in Psychology, 11*(564291), 1–13.

Goodman, M., Tomas, I. A., Temes, C. M., Fitzmaurice, G. M., Aguirre, B. A., & Zanarini, M. C. (2017). Suicide attempts and self-injurious behaviours in adolescent and adult patients with borderline personality disorder. *Personality and Mental Health*, *11*(3), 157–163.

Gori, A., Arcioni, A., Topino, E., Craparo, G., & Lauro Grotto, R. (2021). Development of a new measure for assessing mentalizing: The Multidimensional Mentalizing Questionnaire (MMQ). *Journal of Personalized Medicine*, *11*(4), 1–16.

Gori, A., & Topino, E. (2023). Exploring and deepening the facets of mentalizing: The integration of network and factorial analysis approaches to verify the psychometric properties of the Multidimensional Mentalizing Questionnaire (MMQ). *International Journal of Environmental Research and Public Health*, *20*(6), 1–16.

Grant, B. F., Chou, S. P., Goldstein, R. B., Huang, B., Stinson, F. S., Saha, T. D., . . . & Ruan, W. J. (2008). Prevalence, correlates, disability, and comorbidity of DSM-IV borderline personality disorder: Results from the Wave 2 National Epidemiologic Survey on Alcohol and Related Conditions. *Journal of Clinical Psychiatry*, *69*(4), 533–545.

Greenberg, D. M., Kolasi, J., Hegsted, C. P., Berkowitz, Y., & Jurist, E. L. (2017). Mentalized affectivity: A new model and assessment of emotion regulation. *PLOS One*, *12*(10), 1–27.

Greenberger, D., & Padesky, C. A. (2016). *Mind over mood: Change how you feel by changing the way you think* (2nd ed.). Guilford Publications.

Griffin, D. W., & Bartholomew, K. (1994). The metaphysics of measurement: The case of adult attachment. In K. Bartholomew & D. Perlman (Eds.), *Advances in personal relationships: Attachment processes in adulthood* (Vol. 5, pp. 17–52). Jessica Kingsley.

Grilo, C. M., & Udo, T. (2021). Association of borderline personality disorder criteria with suicide attempts among US adults. *JAMA Network Open*, *4*(5), 1–13.

Gunderson, J. G. (1996). The borderline patient's intolerance of aloneness: Insecure attachments and therapist availability. *The American Journal of Psychiatry*, *153*(6), 752–758.

Gunderson, J. G., & Lyons-Ruth, K. (2008). BPD's interpersonal hypersensitivity phenotype: A gene–environment–developmental model. *Journal of Personality Disorders*, *22*(1), 22–41.

Hallquist, M. N., & Pilkonis, P. A. (2012). Refining the phenotype of borderline personality disorder: Diagnostic criteria and beyond. *Personality Disorders: Theory, Research, and Treatment*, *3*(3), 228–246.

Harris, R. (2009). *ACT made simple: An easy-to-read primer on acceptance and commitment therapy*. New Harbinger.

Harris, R. (2022). *The happiness trap: How to stop struggling and start living* (2nd ed.). Shambhala.

Hayes, S. C. (2020). *A liberated mind: How to pivot toward what matters*. Penguin.

Herman, J. L., Perry, J. C., & van der Kolk, B. A. (1989). Childhood trauma in borderline personality disorder. *The American Journal of Psychiatry*, *146*(4), 490–495.

Herstell, S., Betz, L. T., Penzel, N., Chechelnizki, R., Filihagh, L., Antonucci, L., & Kambeitz, J. (2021). Insecure attachment as a transdiagnostic risk factor for major psychiatric conditions: A meta-analysis in bipolar disorder, depression and schizophrenia spectrum disorder. *Journal of Psychiatric Research*, *144*, 190–201.

Hertzmann, L., Target, M., Hewison, D., Casey, P., Fearon, P., & Lassri, D. (2016). Mentalization-based therapy for parents in entrenched conflict: A random allocation feasibility study. *Psychotherapy*, *53*(4), 388–401.

Hollander, M. (2017). *Helping teens who cut: Using DBT skills to end self-injury* (2nd ed.). Guilford Press.

Imperatori, C., Corazza, O., Panno, A., Rinaldi, R., Pasquini, M., Farina, B., . . . & Bersani, F. S. (2020). Mentalization impairment is associated with problematic alcohol use in a sample of young adults: A cross-sectional study. *International Journal of Environmental Research and Public Health*, *17*(22), 1–9.

Javaras, K. N., Zanarini, M. C., Hudson, J. I., Greenfield, S. F., & Gunderson, J. G. (2017). Functional outcomes in community-based adults with borderline personality disorder. *Journal of Psychiatric Research*, *89*, 105–114.

Johnson, B. N., Kivity, Y., Rosenstein, L. K., LeBreton, J. M., & Levy, K. N. (2022). The association between mentalizing and psychopathology: A meta-analysis of the reading the mind in the eyes task across psychiatric disorders. *Clinical Psychology: Science and Practice*, *29*(4), 423–439.

Jones, A. P., Happé, F. G., Gilbert, F., Burnett, S., & Viding, E. (2010). Feeling, caring, knowing: Different types of empathy deficit in boys with psychopathic tendencies and autism spectrum disorder. *Journal of Child Psychology and Psychiatry*, *51*(11), 1188–1197.

Jurist, E. (2018). *Minding emotions: Cultivating mentalization in psychotherapy*. Guilford Press.

Juul, S., Lunn, S., Poulsen, S., Sørensen, P., Salimi, M., Jakobsen, J. C., . . . & Simonsen, S. (2019). Short-term versus long-term mentalization-based therapy for outpatients with subthreshold or diagnosed borderline personality disorder: A protocol for a randomized clinical trial. *Trials*, *20*, 1–10.

Juurlink, T. T., ten Have, M., Lamers, F., van Marle, H. J., Anema, J. R., de Graaf, R., & Beekman, A. T. (2018). Borderline personality symptoms and work performance: A population-based survey. *BMC Psychiatry*, *18*, 1–9.

Kaiser, D., Jacob, G. A., Domes, G., & Arntz, A. (2016). Attentional bias for emotional stimuli in borderline personality disorder: A meta-analysis. *Psychopathology*, *49*(6), 383–396.

Kaufman, E. A., & Meddaoui, B. (2021). Identity pathology and borderline personality disorder: An empirical overview. *Current Opinion in Psychology*, *37*, 82–88.

Kernberg, O. (1975). *Borderline conditions and pathological narcissism*. Jason Aronson.

Kim, S. H., Baek, M., & Park, S. (2021). Association of parent–child experiences with insecure attachment in adulthood: A systematic review and meta-analysis. *Journal of Family Theory & Review*, *13*(1), 58–76.

King-Casas, B., Sharp, C., Lomax-Bream, L., Lohrenz, T., Fonagy, P., & Montague, P. R. (2008). The rupture and repair of cooperation in borderline personality disorder. *Science*, *321*(5890), 806–810.

Koenigsberg, H. W. (2010). Affective instability: Toward an integration of neuroscience and psychological perspectives. *Journal of Personality Disorders*, *24*(1), 60–82.

Kohut, H. (1984). *How does analysis cure?* University of Chicago Press.

Kraft, T. L., & Pressman, S. D. (2012). Grin and bear it: The influence of manipulated facial expression on the stress response. *Psychological Science*, *23*(11), 1372–1378.

Krause-Utz, A., Niedtfeld, I., Knauber, J., & Schmahl, C. (2017). Neurobiology of borderline personality disorder. In B. Stanley & A. S. New (Eds.), *Borderline personality disorder* (pp. 83–109). Oxford University Press.

Kreisman, J. J., & Straus, H. (2021). *I hate you—don't leave me: Understanding the borderline personality* (3rd ed.). Penguin.

Kring, A. M., & Moran, E. K. (2008). Emotional response deficits in schizophrenia: Insights from affective science. *Schizophrenia Bulletin*, *34*(5), 819–834.

Liebke, L., Koppe, G., Bungert, M., Thome, J., Hauschild, S., Defiebre, N., . . . & Lis, S. (2018). Difficulties with being socially accepted: An experimental study in borderline personality disorder. *Journal of Abnormal Psychology*, *127*(7), 670–682.

Linehan, M. M. (1993). *Skills training manual for treating borderline personality disorder*. Guilford Press.

Linehan, M. M. (2015a). *DBT skills training handouts and worksheets* (2nd ed.). Guilford Press.

Linehan, M. M. (2015b). *DBT skills training manual* (2nd ed.). Guilford Press.

Linehan, M. M., Armstrong, H. E., Suarez, A., Allmon, D., & Heard, H. L. (1991). Cognitive-behavioral treatment of chronically parasuicidal borderline patients. *Archives of General Psychiatry*, *48*(12), 1060–1064.

Lo, C. K., Chan, K. L., & Ip, P. (2019). Insecure adult attachment and child maltreatment: A meta-analysis. *Trauma, Violence, & Abuse*, *20*(5), 706–719.

Luyten, P., Campbell, C., Allison, E., & Fonagy, P. (2020). The mentalizing approach to psychopathology: State of the art and future directions. *Annual Review of Clinical Psychology*, *16*, 297–325.

Luyten, P., & Fonagy, P. (2015). The neurobiology of mentalizing. *Personality Disorders: Theory, Research, and Treatment*, *6*(4), 366–379.

Luyten, P., & Fonagy, P. (2018). The neurobiology of attachment and mentalizing: A neurodevelopmental perspective. In C. Schmahl, K. L. Phan, & R. O. Friedel (Eds.), *Neurobiology of personality disorders* (pp. 111–138). Oxford University Press.

Lyons-Ruth, K., Bureau, J. F., Holmes, B., Easterbrooks, A., & Brooks, N. H. (2013). Borderline symptoms and suicidality/self-injury in late adolescence: Prospectively observed relationship correlates in infancy and childhood. *Psychiatry Research*, *206*(2–3), 273–281.

Lysaker, P. H., Cheli, S., Dimaggio, G., Buck, B., Bonfils, K. A., Huling, K., . . . & Lysaker, J. T. (2021). Metacognition, social cognition, and mentalizing in psychosis: Are these distinct constructs when it comes to subjective experience or are we just splitting hairs? *BMC Psychiatry*, *21*(1), 1–14.

Magid, M., Finzi, E., Kruger, T. H. C., Robertson, H. T., Keeling, B. H., Jung, S., . . . & Wollmer, M. A. (2015). Treating depression with botulinum toxin: A pooled analysis of randomized controlled trials. *Pharmacopsychiatry*, *25*(6), 205–210.

Mancke, F., Herpertz, S. C., & Bertsch, K. (2015). Aggression in borderline personality disorder: A multidimensional model. *Personality Disorders: Theory, Research, and Treatment*, *6*(3), 278–291.

Manning, S. Y. (2011). *Loving someone with borderline personality disorder: How to keep out-of-control emotions from destroying your relationship*. Guilford Press.

Marich, J. (2023). *Dissociation made simple: A stigma-free guide to embracing your dissociative mind and navigating daily life*. North Atlantic Books.

Martinussen, M., Friborg, O., Schmierer, P., Kaiser, S., Øvergård, K. T., Neunhoeffer, A. L., . . . & Rosenvinge, J. H. (2017). The comorbidity of personality disorders in eating disorders: A meta-analysis. *Eating and Weight Disorders: Studies on Anorexia, Bulimia and Obesity*, *22*, 201–209.

Mason, P. T., & Kreger, R. (2020). *Stop walking on eggshells: Taking your life back when someone you care about has borderline personality disorder* (3rd ed.). New Harbinger Publications.

Meehan, K. B., De Panfilis, C., Cain, N. M., Antonucci, C., Soliani, A., Clarkin, J. F., & Sambataro, F. (2017). Facial emotion recognition and borderline personality pathology. *Psychiatry Research*, *255*, 347–354.

Midgley, N., Besser, S. J., Dye, H., Fearon, P., Gale, T., Jefferies-Sewell, K., . . . & Wood, S. (2017). The Herts and minds study: Evaluating the effectiveness of mentalization-based treatment (MBT) as an intervention for children in foster care with emotional and/or behavioural problems: A phase II, feasibility, randomised controlled trial. *Pilot and Feasibility Studies*, *3*(1), 1–12.

Mikulincer, M., & Shaver, P. R. (2012). An attachment perspective on psychopathology. *World Psychiatry*, *11*(1), 11–15.

Mikulincer, M., & Shaver, P. R. (2016). *Attachment in adulthood: Structure, dynamics, and change* (2nd ed.). Guilford Press.

Miller, C. E., Townsend, M. L., Day, N. J., & Grenyer, B. F. (2020). Measuring the shadows: A systematic review of chronic emptiness in borderline personality disorder. *PLOS One*, *15*(7), 1–49.

Miller, C. E., Townsend, M. L., & Grenyer, B. F. (2021). Understanding chronic feelings of emptiness in borderline personality disorder: A qualitative study. *Borderline Personality Disorder and Emotion Dysregulation*, *8*, 1–9.

Mitchell, A. E., Dickens, G. L., & Picchioni, M. M. (2014). Facial emotion processing in borderline personality disorder: A systematic review and meta-analysis. *Neuropsychology Review*, *24*(2), 166–184.

Mitchell, S. A. (1993). *Hope and dread in psychoanalysis*. Basic Books.

Németh, N., Mátrai, P., Hegyi, P., Czéh, B., Czopf, L., Hussain, A., . . . & Simon, M. (2018). Theory of mind disturbances in borderline personality disorder: A meta-analysis. *Psychiatry Research*, *270*, 143–153.

Newbury-Helps, J., Feigenbaum, J., & Fonagy, P. (2017). Offenders with antisocial personality disorder display more impairments in mentalizing. *Journal of Personality Disorders*, *31*(2), 232–255.

Ohse, L., Zimmermann, J., Kerber, A., Kampe, L., Mohr, J., Schierz, R., . . . & Hörz-Sagstetter, S. (2024). Impairments in cognitive and emotional empathy as markers of general versus specific personality pathology. *Psychopathology*, *57*(2), 136–148.

Oladottir, K., Wolf-Arehult, M., Ramklint, M., & Isaksson, M. (2022). Cluster analysis of personality traits in psychiatric patients with borderline personality disorder. *Borderline Personality Disorder and Emotion Dysregulation*, *9*(1), 1–11.

Olié, E., Doell, K. C., Corradi-Dell'Acqua, C., Courtet, P., Perroud, N., & Schwartz, S. (2018). Physical pain recruits the nucleus accumbens during social distress in borderline personality disorder. *Social Cognitive and Affective Neuroscience*, *13*(10), 1071–1080.

Oud, M., Arntz, A., Hermens, M. L., Verhoef, R., & Kendall, T. (2018). Specialized psychotherapies for adults with borderline personality disorder: A systematic review and meta-analysis. *Australian & New Zealand Journal of Psychiatry*, *52*(10), 949–961.

Porter, C., Palmier-Claus, J., Branitsky, A., Mansell, W., Warwick, H., & Varese, F. (2020). Childhood adversity and borderline personality disorder: A meta-analysis. *Acta Psychiatrica Scandinavica*, *141*(1), 6–20.

Reitz, S., Kluetsch, R., Niedtfeld, I., Knorz, T., Lis, S., Paret, C., . . . & Schmahl, C. (2015). Incision and stress regulation in borderline personality disorder: Neurobiological mechanisms of self-injurious behaviour. *The British Journal of Psychiatry*, *207*(2), 165–172.

Reutter, K. (2019). *The dialectical behavior therapy skills workbook for PTSD: Practical exercises for overcoming trauma and post-traumatic stress disorder*. New Harbinger Publications.

Rhee, S. H., Friedman, N. P., Boeldt, D. L., Corley, R. P., Hewitt, J. K., Knafo, A., . . . & Zahn-Waxler, C. (2013). Early concern and disregard for others as predictors of antisocial behavior. *Journal of Child Psychology and Psychiatry*, *54*(2), 157–166.

Rhee, S. H., Friedman, N. P., Corley, R. P., Hewitt, J. K., Hink, L. K., Johnson, D. P., . . . & Zahn-Waxler, C. (2016). An examination of the developmental propensity model of conduct problems. *Journal of Abnormal Psychology*, *125*(4), 550–564.

Rhee, S. H., Woodward, K., Corley, R. P., du Pont, A., Friedman, N. P., Hewitt, J. K., . . . & Zahn-Waxler, C. (2021). The association between toddlerhood empathy deficits and antisocial personality disorder symptoms and psychopathy in adulthood. *Development and Psychopathology*, *33*(1), 173–183.

Richetin, J., Preti, E., Costantini, G., & De Panfilis, C. (2017). The centrality of affective instability and identity in borderline personality disorder: Evidence from network analysis. *PLOS One*, *12*(10), 1–14.

Rifkin-Zybutz, R. P., Moran, P., Nolte, T., Feigenbaum, J., King-Casas, B., Fonagy, P., & Montague, R. P. (2021). Impaired mentalizing in depression and the effects of borderline personality disorder on this relationship. *Borderline Personality Disorder and Emotion Dysregulation*, *8*(1), 1–6.

Ring, D., & Lawn, S. (2019). Stigma perpetuation at the interface of mental health care: A review to compare patient and clinician perspectives of stigma and borderline personality disorder. *Journal of Mental Health*, *2019*(March), 1–21.

Rosso, A. M., & Airaldi, C. (2016). Intergenerational transmission of reflective functioning. *Frontiers in Psychology*, *7*(1903), 1–11.

Rossouw, T. I., & Fonagy, P. (2012). Mentalization-based treatment for self-harm in adolescents: A randomized controlled trial. *Journal of the American Academy of Child & Adolescent Psychiatry*, *51*(12), 1304–1313.

Salgado, R. M., Pedrosa, R., & Bastos-Leite, A. J. (2020). Dysfunction of empathy and related processes in borderline personality disorder: A systematic review. *Harvard Review of Psychiatry*, *28*(4), 238–254.

Salzer, S., Streeck, U., Jaeger, U., Masuhr, O., Warwas, J., Leichsenring, F., & Leibing, E. (2013). Patterns of interpersonal problems in borderline personality disorder. *The Journal of Nervous and Mental Disease*, *201*(2), 94–98.

Scalabrini, A., Cavicchioli, M., Fossati, A., & Maffei, C. (2017). The extent of dissociation in borderline personality disorder: A meta-analytic review. *Journal of Trauma & Dissociation, 18*(4), 522–543.

Schielke, H., Brand, B. L., & Lanius, R. A. (2022). *The Finding Solid Ground program workbook: Overcoming obstacles in trauma recovery*. Oxford University Press.

Schulze, J., Neumann, I., Magid, M., Finzi, E., Sinke, C., Wollmer, M. A., & Krüger, T. H. (2021). Botulinum toxin for the management of depression: An updated review of the evidence and meta-analysis. *Journal of Psychiatric Research, 135*, 332–340.

Scott, L. N., Wright, A. G., Beeney, J. E., Lazarus, S. A., Pilkonis, P. A., & Stepp, S. D. (2017). Borderline personality disorder symptoms and aggression: A within-person process model. *Journal of Abnormal Psychology, 126*(4), 429–440.

Sebastian, A., Jacob, G., Lieb, K., & Tüscher, O. (2013). Impulsivity in borderline personality disorder: A matter of disturbed impulse control or a facet of emotional dysregulation? *Current Psychiatry Reports, 15*, 1–8.

Shah, R., & Zanarini, M. C. (2018). Comorbidity of borderline personality disorder: Current status and future directions. *Psychiatric Clinics, 41*(4), 583–593.

Sharp, C., Fonagy, P., & Goodyer, I. M. (2006). Imagining your child's mind: Psychosocial adjustment and mothers' ability to predict their children's attributional response styles. *British Journal of Developmental Psychology, 24*, 197–214.

Skoglund, C., Tiger, A., Rück, C., Petrovic, P., Asherson, P., Hellner, C., . . . & Kuja-Halkola, R. (2021). Familial risk and heritability of diagnosed borderline personality disorder: A register study of the Swedish population. *Molecular Psychiatry, 26*(3), 999–1008.

Sleuwaegen, E., Houben, M., Claes, L., Berens, A., & Sabbe, B. (2017). The relationship between non-suicidal self-injury and alexithymia in borderline personality disorder: "Actions instead of words". *Comprehensive Psychiatry, 77*, 80–88.

Sloover, M., van Est, L. A., Janssen, P. G., Hilbink, M., & van Ee, E. (2022). A meta-analysis of mentalizing in anxiety disorders, obsessive-compulsive and related disorders, and trauma and stressor related disorders. *Journal of Anxiety Disorders, 92*, 1–19.

Slotema, C. W., Wilhelmus, B., Arends, L. R., & Franken, I. H. (2020). Psychotherapy for posttraumatic stress disorder in patients with borderline personality disorder: A systematic review and meta-analysis of its efficacy and safety. *European Journal of Psychotraumatology, 11*(1), 1–15.

Smith, M., & South, S. (2020). Romantic attachment style and borderline personality pathology: A meta-analysis. *Clinical Psychology Review, 75*, 1–15.

Smits, M. L., Feenstra, D. J., Bales, D. L., de Vos, J., Lucas, Z., Verheul, R., & Luyten, P. (2017). Subtypes of borderline personality disorder patients: A cluster-analytic approach. *Borderline Personality Disorder and Emotion Dysregulation, 4*, 1–15.

Smits, M. L., Luyten, P., Feenstra, D. J., Bales, D. L., Kamphuis, J. H., Dekker, J. J., . . . & Busschbach, J. J. (2022). Trauma and outcomes of mentalization-based therapy for individuals with borderline personality disorder. *American Journal of Psychotherapy, 75*(1), 12–20.

Snir, A., Rafaeli, E., Gadassi, R., Berenson, K., & Downey, G. (2015). Explicit and inferred motives for nonsuicidal self-injurious acts and urges in borderline and avoidant personality disorders. *Personality Disorders: Theory, Research, and Treatment, 6*(3), 267–277.

Sosic-Vasic, Z., Eberhardt, J., Bosch, J. E., Dommes, L., Labek, K., Buchheim, A., & Viviani, R. (2019). Mirror neuron activations in encoding of psychic pain in borderline personality disorder. *NeuroImage: Clinical, 22*, 1–8.

Stanley, B., & Brown, G. K. (2008). *The safety plan treatment manual to reduce suicide risk: Veteran version*. United States Department of Veterans Affairs.

Stevens, J. S., & Jovanovic, T. (2019). Role of social cognition in post-traumatic stress disorder: A review and meta-analysis. *Genes, Brain and Behavior, 18*(1), 1–10.

Stoffers-Winterling, J. M., Storebø, O. J., Kongerslev, M. T., Faltinsen, E., Todorovac, A., Jørgensen, M. S., . . . & Simonsen, E. (2022). Psychotherapies for borderline personality disorder: A focused systematic review and meta-analysis. *The British Journal of Psychiatry*, *221*(3), 538–552.

Storebø, O. J., Stoffers-Winterling, J. M., Völlm, B. A., Kongerslev, M. T., Mattivi, J. T., Jørgensen, M. S., . . . & Simonsen, E. (2020). Psychological therapies for people with borderline personality disorder. *Cochrane Database of Systematic Reviews*, *2020*(5), 1–512.

Strawson, P. F. (2008). *Freedom and resentment and other essays*. Routledge.

Temes, C. M., Frankenburg, F. R., Fitzmaurice, G. M., & Zanarini, M. C. (2019). Deaths by suicide and other causes among patients with borderline personality disorder and personality-disordered comparison subjects over 24 years of prospective follow-up. *The Journal of Clinical Psychiatry*, *80*(1), 4039.

Temes, C. M., & Zanarini, M. C. (2018). The longitudinal course of borderline personality disorder. *Psychiatric Clinics*, *41*(4), 685–694.

Tomko, R. L., Trull, T. J., Wood, P. K., & Sher, K. J. (2014). Characteristics of borderline personality disorder in a community sample: Comorbidity, treatment utilization, and general functioning. *Journal of Personality Disorders*, *28*(5), 734–750.

Twemlow, S. W., Fonagy, P., & Sacco, F. C. (2005). A developmental approach to mentalizing communities: II. The Peaceful Schools experiment. *Bulletin of the Menninger Clinic*, *69*(4), 282–304.

Urbonaviciute, G., & Hepper, E. G. (2020). When is narcissism associated with low empathy? A meta-analytic review. *Journal of Research in Personality*, *89*, 104036.

Ventura Wurman, T., Lee, T., Bateman, A., Fonagy, P., & Nolte, T. (2021). Clinical management of common presentations of patients diagnosed with BPD during the COVID-19 pandemic: The contribution of the MBT framework. *Counselling Psychology Quarterly*, *34*(3–4), 744–770.

Wagner-Skacel, J., Riedl, D., Kampling, H., & Lampe, A. (2022). Mentalization and dissociation after adverse childhood experiences. *Scientific Reports*, *12*(1), 1–7.

Wimmer, H., & Perner, J. (1983). Beliefs about beliefs: Representation and constraining function of wrong beliefs in young children's understanding of deception. *Cognition*, *13*(1), 103–128.

Witt, K. G., Hetrick, S. E., Rajaram, G., Hazell, P., Salisbury, T. L. T., Townsend, E., & Hawton, K. (2021). Psychosocial interventions for self-harm in adults. *Cochrane Database of Systematic Reviews*, *2021*(4), 1–234.

Wrege, J. S., Ruocco, A. C., Carcone, D., Lang, U. E., Lee, A. C., & Walter, M. (2021). Facial emotion perception in borderline personality disorder: Differential neural activation to ambiguous and threatening expressions and links to impairments in self and interpersonal functioning. *Journal of Affective Disorders*, *284*, 126–135.

Zanarini, M. C., Conkey, L. C., Temes, C. M., & Fitzmaurice, G. M. (2018). Randomized, controlled trial of web-based psychoeducation for women with borderline personality disorder. *The Journal of Clinical Psychiatry*, *79*(3), 16m11153.

Zanarini, M. C., & Frankenburg, F. R. (2008). A preliminary, randomized trial of psychoeducation for women with borderline personality disorder. *Journal of Personality Disorders*, *22*(3), 284–290.

Zanarini, M. C., Frankenburg, F. R., Hennen, J., Reich, D. B., & Silk, K. R. (2005). The McLean Study of Adult Development (MSAD): Overview and implications of the first six years of prospective follow-up. *Journal of Personality Disorders*, *19*(5), 505–523.

Zanarini, M. C., Frankenburg, F. R., Reich, D. B., & Fitzmaurice, G. (2010). Time to attainment of recovery from borderline personality disorder and stability of recovery: A 10-year prospective follow-up study. *American Journal of Psychiatry*, *167*(6), 663–667.

Zanarini, M. C., Frankenburg, F. R., Reich, D. B., & Fitzmaurice, G. (2012). Attainment and stability of sustained symptomatic remission and recovery among borderline patients and axis II comparison subjects: A 16-year prospective follow-up study. *The American Journal of Psychiatry*, *169*(5), 476–483.

Zanarini, M. C., Frankenburg, F. R., Wedig, M. M., & Fitzmaurice, G. M. (2013). Cognitive experiences reported by borderline patients and axis II comparison subjects: A 16-year prospective follow-up study. *The American Journal of Psychiatry*, *170*(6), 671–679.

Zanarini, M. C., Laudate, C. S., Frankenburg, F. R., Wedig, M. M., & Fitzmaurice, G. (2013). Reasons for self-mutilation reported by borderline patients over 16 years of prospective follow-up. *Journal of Personality Disorders*, *27*(6), 783–794.

Zeegers, M. A., Colonnesi, C., Stams, G. J. J., & Meins, E. (2017). Mind matters: A meta- analysis on parental mentalization and sensitivity as predictors of infant–parent attachment. *Psychological Bulletin*, *143*(12), 1245–1272.

Zhang, X., Li, J., Xie, F., Chen, X., Xu, W., & Hudson, N. W. (2022). The relationship between adult attachment and mental health: A meta-analysis. *Journal of Personality and Social Psychology*, *123*(5), 1089–1137.

For the benefit of digital users, indexed terms that span two pages (e.g., 52–53) may, on occasion, appear on only one of those pages.

Tables, boxes, and figures are indicated by *t*, *b*, and *f* following the page number.